Avian Medicine
and Surgery in
Practice
Companion and aviary birds

BOB DONELEY

BVSc, FACVSc (Avian Medicine), CMAVA
Registered Specialist in Bird Medicine
Head of Service, Small Animal Hospital
School of Veterinary Science
University of Queensland, Australia

MANSON PUBLISHING/THE VETERINARY PRESS

Second impression 2011

Copyright © 2011 Manson Publishing Ltd

ISBN: 978-1-84076-112-2

A CIP catalogue record for this book is available from the British Library.

For full details of all Manson Publishing Ltd titles please write to:
Manson Publishing Ltd, 73 Corringham Road, London NW11 7DL, UK
Tel: +44(0)20 8905 5150
Fax: +44(0)20 8201 9233
Website: www.mansonpublishing.com

Commissioning editor: Jill Northcott
Project manager: Jane Fricker
Copy-editors: Joanna Brocklesby and Peter Beynon
Designer: Cathy Martin, Presspack Computing Ltd
Layout: DiacriTech, India
Colour reproduction: Tenon & Polert Colour Scanning Ltd, Hong Kong
Printed by: Grafos SA, Barcelona, Spain

CONTENTS

INTRODUCTION

I graduated from the University of Queensland in 1982. Bird medicine in those days rated two lectures from the small animal lecturer, Charlie Prescott. It was actually just one lecture, but Charlie gave it twice. Those of us who remember Charlie as a lecturer will understand how that came about! In my first year in practice I was asked to give a talk to the local budgie club. With only those two lectures behind me I needed to get some information to do this. The only reference book I had access to was the Proceedings of a bird medicine conference hosted by the University of Sydney Post Graduate Foundation in 1981. This book contained some ground-breaking work, including Ross Perry's description of a feather disorder in cockatoos he described as 'Psittacine Beak and Feather Dystrophy Syndrome', a disease he thought could be viral. It was all new to me and sparked my interest in bird medicine, an interest that has not left me in over 25 years.

In that quarter of a century bird medicine has evolved tremendously. Not only was Ross Perry proved to be right about PBFD, but we now know it affects other parrots. We have sophisticated diagnostic testing for PBFD; and we are investigating the means to protect against PBFD and even treat the disorder. This growth in our knowledge has been due to the hard work of both academics and clinicians, all of whom have contributed, in ways both great and small, to the current state of avian medicine. None can be said to have made an insignificant contribution.

This book is my attempt to summarize much of that knowledge. It is not complete; no book can hope to achieve that. But it is my hope that busy clinicians will be able to use it as a quick reference guide and that students, both undergraduate and postgraduate, can use it as a study guide. I apologize for any errors and omissions (and I am sure there are more than a few); those mistakes are mine, and mine alone. I can only promise to do better next time!

Of course, no one person can produce a book by him- or herself. I owe a vote of thanks to many people: Jill Northcott, Jane Fricker, Peter Beynon and the staff of Manson Publishing who cajoled me into starting (and then finishing) this book, and then produced the finished article; Brian Speer, who provided me with his study notes, which formed the basis of my own study notes and finally this book; John Chitty and Scott Ford, who reviewed the manuscript and made many valuable suggestions; Scott Echols, Bob Schmidt and Shane Raidal, who provided the cytology images used in this book; Larry Nemetz, Angela Lennox, David Phalen and Brian Speer who provided other images; and, of course, the many veterinarians all over the world who have taught me what I know about avian medicine.

There are two other votes of thanks I owe. Firstly, to my staff at the West Toowoomba Veterinary Surgery, who have worked so hard to keep me sane (especially you, Julie). And lastly, and most importantly, to my wife Maree and my children, Liz and Patrick, who have tolerated me, encouraged me and made sacrifices for me throughout my career. Without them I could not have achieved what I have, and without them, it would not have been worth it.

Bob Doneley
Toowoomba

ABBREVIATIONS

ACE	angiotensin converting enzyme
ACH	acetylcholine
ACTH	adrenocorticotrophic hormone
ADH	antidiuretic hormone
ALD	angular limb deformity
ALP	alkaline phosphatase
ALT	alanine aminotransferase
APP	avian pancreatic polypeptide
AST	aspartate aminotransferase
ATP	adenosine triphosphate
AV	atrioventricular
AVT	arginine vasotocin
BELISA	blocking enzyme-linked immunosorbent assay
bpm	beats per minute
BUN	blood urea nitrogen
CAM	chorioallantoic membrane
CBC	complete blood count
CDC	Centre for Disease Control
CF	complement fixation
CK	creatine kinase
CNS	central nervous system
COX	cyclo-oxygenase
CRF	corticotropin-releasing factor
CT	computed tomography
DIC	disseminated intravascular coagulation
DMSO	dimethyl sulfoxide
ECG	electrocardiogram
ECL	electrochemiluminescent
ELISA	enzyme-linked immunosorbent assay
ESF	external skeletal fixation
FA	fluorescent antibody
FSH	follicle stimulating hormone
GABA	gamma-amino butyric acid
GFR	glomerular filtration rate
GGT	gamma glutamyl transferase
GLDH	glutamate dehydrogenase
GnRH	gonadotrophin-releasing hormone
HCG	human chorionic gonadotropin
IFA	immunofluorescent antibody
IPD	internal papilloma disease
IPPV	intermittent positive pressure ventilation
LDH	lactate dehydrogenase
LH	luteinizing hormone
LHRH	luteinizing hormone releasing hormone
LPS	lipopolysaccharide
MCH	mean corpuscular haemoglobin
MCHC	mean corpuscular haemoglobin count
MCV	mean cell volume
MRI	magnetic resonance imaging
MSH	melanotropic hormone
NSAID	nonsteroidal anti-inflammatory drug
PAS	periodic acid–Schiff
PBFD	psittacine beak and feather disease
PCR	polymerase chain reaction
PCV	packed cell volume
PDD	proventricular dilatation disease
PET	positron emission tomography
PG	prostaglandin
PMV	paramyxovirus
PP	pancreatic polypeptide
PsHV	psittacid herpesvirus
PT	prothrombin time
PTFE	polytetrafluoroethylene
PTH	parathyroid hormone
RBC	red blood cell
SGOT	serum glutamate oxaloacetate transaminase
SGPT	serum glutamate pyruvate transaminase
SPF	specific pathogen-free
STC	spontaneous turkey cardiomyopathy
STH	somatotropic hormone
TG	thyroglobulin
TIF	tie-in fixator
TRH	thyrotropin releasing hormone
TSH	thyroid-stimulating hormone
UDCA	ursodeoxycholic acid
USG	urine specific gravity
VPC	ventricular premature contraction
WBC	white blood cell

US AND INTERNATIONAL UNIT (BLOOD VALUES) CONVERSION

	Conventional (US) unit	Conversion factor	SI unit
Haematology			
Red blood cell count	$10^6/\mu l$	1	$10^{12}/l$
Haemoglobin	g/dl	0.1	g/l
MCH	pg/cell	1	pg/cell
MCHC	g/dl	0.1	g/l
MCV	μm^3	1	fl
Platelet count	$10^3/\mu l$	1	$10^9/l$
White blood cell count	$10^3/\mu l$	1	$10^9/l$
Plasma chemistry			
Alkaline phosphatase	u/l	1	IU/l
ALT (SGPT)	u/l	1	IU/l
Albumin	g/dl	10	g/l
Ammonia (NH_4)	µg/dl	0.5871	µmol/l
Amylase	u/l	1	IU/l
AST (SGOT)	u/l	1	IU/l
Bilirubin	mg/dl	17.1	µmol/l
Calcium	mg/dl	0.2495	mmol/l
Carbon dioxide	mEq/l	1	mmol/l
Chloride	mEq/l	1	mmol/l
Cholesterol	mg/dl	0.02586	mmol/l
Cortisol	µg/dl	27.59	nmol/l
Creatine kinase	u/l	1	IU/l
Creatinine	mg/dl	88.4	µmol/l
Fibrinogen	mg/dl	0.01	g/l
Glucose	mg/dl	0.05551	mmol/l
Iron	µg/dl	0.1791	µmol/l
Lipase			
Sigma Tietz	u/dl	280	IU/l
Cherry Crandall	u/l	1	IU/l
Lipid, total	mg/dl	0.01	g/l
Osmolality	mOsm/kg	1	mmol/kg
Phosphate (as inorganic P)	mg/dl	0.3229	mmol/l
Potassium	mEq/l	1	mmol/l
Protein, total	g/dl	10	g/l
Sodium	mEq/l	1	mmol/l
Thyroxine (T_4)	µg/dl	12.87	nmol/l
Urea nitrogen	mg/dl	0.357	mmol/l*
Uric acid	mg/dl	59.48	µmol/l

Modified from: *The Merck Veterinary Manual* (1998) 8th edn. Merck and Co., Whitehouse Station, NJ as adapted from *The SI Manual in Health Care* (1981) Metric Commission, Canada.
*Urea.
SI-International System of Units; MCH-mean corpuscular haemoglobin; MCHC-mean corpuscular haemoglobin count; MCV-mean cell volume; ALT-alanine aminotransferase; SGPT-serum glutamate pyruvate transaminase; AST-aspartate aminotransferase; SGOT-serum glutamate oxaloacetate transaminase.

CHAPTER 1
CLINICAL ANATOMY AND PHYSIOLOGY

INTRODUCTION

Although veterinarians are taught avian anatomy in veterinary school, if one is unfamiliar with its clinical relevance it is always worth refreshing one's memory. This chapter will highlight those features of avian anatomy and physiology that are relevant to the clinician. It will not seek to be a comprehensive review of the subject. The focus in this chapter is on companion birds and, as such, anatomical structures such as the phallus will not be discussed. Without a basic understanding of anatomy and physiology, it becomes difficult to understand the pathophysiology of disease and how treatment will affect the patient as a whole.

THE SKIN, FEATHERS, NAILS AND BEAK

Avian skin is attached to both the underlying muscles and to the skeleton. It consists of the thin epidermis (only 10 cell layers deep) and the thicker underlying dermis. Feather follicles originate from the dermis. True glands are absent from much of the skin, although epidermal cells may secrete a lipoid sebaceous material. The external ear has glands that secrete a waxy material, but the only other gland found on the skin is the uropygial gland. This gland, absent in ratites, many pigeons, woodpeckers and some parrots (*Amazona*, *Anodorhynchus* and *Cyanospitta*), is a bilobed gland on the dorsum of the tail. It secretes a lipoid sebaceous material, spread over feathers during grooming, which may assist in waterproofing, cleaning and reducing skin infections. It is thought it may also have a role in sex identification; uropygial secretions may play a role in ultraviolet reflectivity, which in turn may be used by birds for sex differentiation.

Scales, raised areas of highly keratinized epidermis separated by folds of less keratinized skin, cover the nonfeathered part of the leg, known as the podotheca. The claws, which enclose the terminal phalanx of each digit, are made up of two plates: the strongly keratinized dorsal plate enclosing dorsal and lateral aspects of the phalanx, and the softer ventral plate forming the sole of the claw. The dorsal plate grows faster than the ventral plate, therefore the nails curve downwards.

The bones of the upper and lower jaw are covered in horny keratin, called rhamphotheca (**1**); the mandibular rhamphotheca is known as the gnathotheca and the maxillary rhamphotheca is called the rhinotheca. The dorsal midline of the rhinotheca is the culmen and the ventral midline of the gnathoceca is the gonys. The cutting edge of both the upper and lower beak is the tomia, while the soft tissue between the mandibular rami is

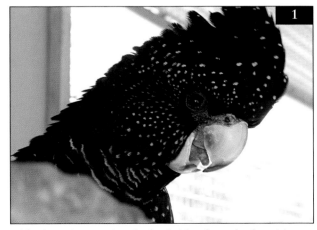

1 The keratin covering the beak (the rhamphotheca) is histologically similar to skin.

the inter-ramular region (**2**). Histologically the rhamphotheca resembles skin, with the dermis attached to the periosteum of the underlying bone. The epidermis is modified, in that the stratum corneum is thickened and hardened, as the cells contain free calcium phosphate and crystals of hydroxyapatite. The neurological innervation of the upper beak is the ophthalmic and maxillary divisions of the trigeminal nerve, while the mandibular division of the trigeminal nerve innervates the lower beak. The cere, the fleshy area around the nares, is found only in owls, parrots and pigeons.

The unique structure of avian skin is the feathers. These arise from feather follicles, arranged in tracts around the body known as pterylae. The featherless skin between these tracts is called apterylae. Each follicle is a cylindrical pit in the skin, lined with epidermis and dermis. At the base of the follicle is the dermal papilla, a small mound of dermis that enters the proximal shaft of the feather (the calamus) through a small hole known as the inferior umbilicus. The epidermis covering the dermal papilla is continuous with the calamus and with a thin layer of epidermis covering the dermal papilla (**3**).

Each feather shaft consists of the calamus, embedded in follicle, and the rachis, the main shaft beyond the calamus. They are distinguished by the distal (superior) umbilicus, a small opening into the shaft found at the junction of the rachis and calamus. Occasionally there is an after feather (the hypopenna), a small extra feather on the rim of the distal umbilicus (**4**, **5**).

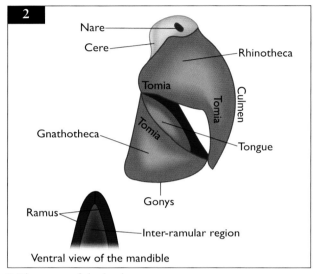

2 The parts of the beak.

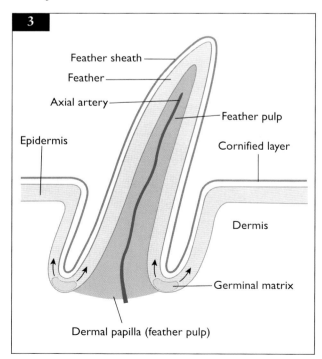

3 The feather follicle.

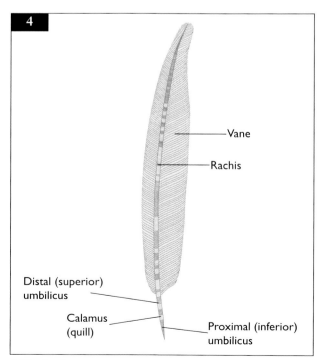

4 The feather.

Coming off the rachis are the barbs and coming off the barbs are the barbules, filaments that interlock to form the vane (6). This is the pennaceous region. The vanes are asymmetrical, with the external vane narrower than the internal vane. On the dorsal wing the external vane of one feather overlaps the internal vane of the next. Just below the vane is the plumaceous region, where a few downy barbs fail to interlock.

Within the calamus of an immature feather is the pulp, a loose reticulum of mesoderm with an axial artery and vein. This pulp retracts as the feather matures, leaving pulp caps (empty chambers within the calamus).

There are seven types of feathers (7): contour, semiplume, down, powder down, hypopenna, filoplume and bristle.

5 Closer view of the calamus and rachis of the feather.

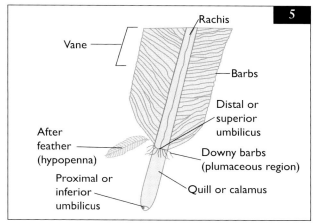

6 Closer view of the pennaceous portion of the feather.

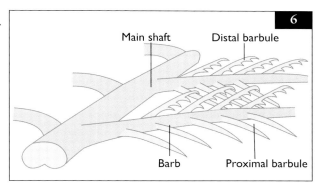

7 Types of feathers.

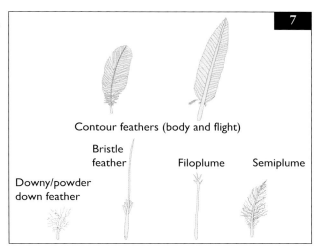

- Contour feathers include the flight feathers and the body feathers. The flight feathers on the tail are called the retrices. The flight feathers on the wings are known as the remiges: the primaries (9–11) arise from the periosteum of the metacarpus; the secondaries (6–32) arise from the periosteum of the ulna; and the tertiaries arise from the humeral area. Overlying them are the coverts (**8**).
- Semiplume feathers have a wholly fluffy vane, with the rachis longer than barb. They lie along pterylae margins, acting as insulation.
- Down feathers are also wholly fluffy, but the rachis is either absent or shorter than the longest barb. Distribution varies between species.
- Powder down feathers are structured like down feathers, although some are semiplumes or contour feathers. They shed a fine waxy powder, which is actually keratin flakes. This powder forms a waterproofing coat over the contour feathers and may play a role in keeping the bird clean. Powder down feathers are usually grouped in patches (e.g. on the thigh), although some species have them widely distributed. They are found in herons, parrots, toucans, pigeons and bowerbirds.
- Hypopennae (1–5) are small feathers projecting from the distal umbilicus of pennaceous and plumaceous feathers (after feathers). They are usually not associated with retrices or longer remiges.
- Filoplumes have a long fine shaft with a tuft of short barbs/barbules at the end. They possibly have a sensory/proprioceptive role and are found close to the follicles of contour feathers.

- Bristles have a stiff rachis, with either a few barbs at the proximal end or no barbs at all. They are found around the mouth, nares and eyes, and possibly have a tactile function.

The colour of feathers is the result of the combination of pigments and feather structure. Carotenoids or psittacins (yellow pigments absorbed from the diet, including reds, oranges and pinks) create the foreground colour. Melanins are the grey pigments (including black, grey and brown) that create the background and also the foreground colour. Each feather barb has a cortex (an outer layer) containing either carotenoid pigments (psittacins) or melanin pigments. If melanin is in the cortex, it is known as foreground colour and produces black, greys, dark browns and chestnut reds. This is the marking seen in many birds. The barb also has a medulla, which only ever contains melanin (background melanin). All of these pigments are distributed in different layers and, when combined with special features of barb structure that affect the passage of light, produce the spectrum of colours seen.

Moulting, the shedding of old, worn feathers and the renewal of plumage, is a regular event. It is controlled by a wide range of factors including thyroid activity, reproductive hormones, photoperiod, body condition, age and diet. After a series of juvenile moults to attain adult plumage, most birds go on to moult one to two times annually. These moults, often referred to as the prenuptial and postnuptial moults, occur in spring and autumn respectively. The pattern of moulting is orderly and in the following progression (with some overlap): the inner primaries;

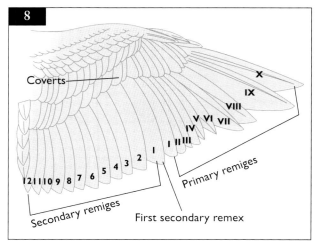

8

Coverts

X
IX
VIII
V VI VII
IV
I II III
1 2 3 4 5 6 7 8 9 10 11 12

Primary remiges

Secondary remiges

First secondary remex

8 The feathers of the wing of a parrot.

the outer primaries; the secondaries and tail feathers; and finally the body contour feathers. It is usually bilaterally symmetrical and is paced so as to avoid loss of flight capacity at any time.

When it is time to moult an old feather, a proliferation of epidermal cells at the base of the follicle (the epidermal collar) separates the old feather from the dermal papilla and allows it to shed. These epidermal cells then start to group themselves into two series of spiral barb ridges. The tips of these ridges end along a longitudinal line on the ventral aspect of the feather (the seam). On the dorsal side of feather the epidermis thickens to form the rachis. Within this structure is the dermal core, consisting of the axial blood vessels, with mesoderm around them. As it grows the feather emerges from the follicle as a pointed projection with a dermal core and an epidermal cover (sheath). This sheath then progressively ruptures, freeing the barbs that have separated along the seam and allowing the feather to open. Much of the increased grooming activity seen in birds at this time is to remove this sheath.

Because birds lack sweat glands, they rely on evaporative heat loss from the respiratory tract and heat transfer through apterylae (the featherless tracts of skin) to cool their bodies. To do this, many birds hold their feathers close to the body and may extend their wings, exposing the apterylae. Conversely, to retain body heat when ill or cold, they fluff their feathers up to trap body heat against the skin. (Ostriches do the reverse, i.e. they raise their feathers to promote heat loss and hold them close to conserve body heat.)

THE SKELETON
GENERAL
Bones serve two major functions: they provide structural support for the muscular system and they act as a reservoir for calcium and phosphorus (9). Although the structural make-up of bone is similar across all animal species, there are some specific differences between mammalian and avian bones. The requirement for flight means that birds have evolved with bones that are lightweight, but aerodynamically strong. They have thin brittle cortices and wide medullas that may, in some species and some bones, be

9 The skeleton of a bird.

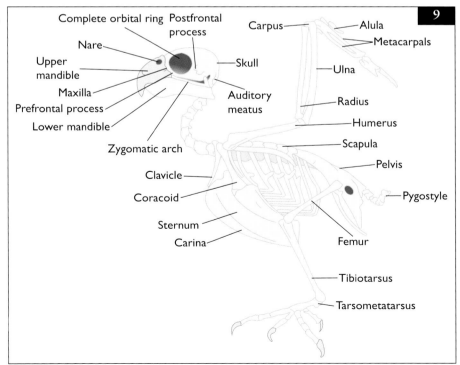

pneumatic. Under the influence of oestrogen during the breeding season, many hens will lay down medullary bone (extra bone in the medullary cavities of the long bones) to form a calcium reservoir for egg production.

The blood supply to bones arises from periosteal, medullary, metaphyseal and epiphyseal vessels. The periosteal blood supply is the predominant source of blood to the bone and its disruption, either by trauma or surgical repair of a fracture, may result in delayed healing or even complete failure to heal (a nonunion).

Healing of avian bones can be achieved through:
- Primary healing. Bone to bone healing through the Haversian system, with minimal callus formation. This is only achieved with rigid fixation with perfect bone apposition.
- Endosteal callus formation. Occurs rapidly where bones are well aligned. This is the most important part of bone healing.
- Periosteal callus formation. Occurs when fractures are not aligned and there is movement at the fracture site.

The rate of healing of a fractured bone is therefore dependent on:
- Displacement of bone fragments. Segmental fractures will heal well, so long as periosteal blood supply is intact. If devitalized, the fragment can be incorporated into the fracture site as a cortical bone graft. Healing is slower, as cancellous bone first bridges the gap, then the segment is demineralized and becomes cancellous itself. This form of healing may take 9–18 weeks.
- Damage to blood supply. Periosteal blood supply is very important in callus formation, and its importance exceeds that of the medullary blood supply.
- Presence of infection. Sequestra can actually add to the stability of a fracture and should not be removed until a bony callus has formed.
- Movement at the fracture site creates a large haematoma requiring a large cartilaginous bridge.

Stable, well aligned fractures will heal faster in birds than in mammals. Clinical stability of a fracture may be achieved at 2–3 weeks and may precede radiographic evidence of healing, usually visible at 3–6 weeks. Complete bony union will usually take eight weeks.

SKULL

The upper jaw of companion birds consists of three bones: the premaxilla, the nasal bone and the maxilla (**10**). Together they form a rigid block hinged to the braincase by the prokinetic craniofacial joint (**11**). The elastic zone of this joint allows movement of the upper jaw. The palate, made up of the palatal processes of the premaxillary and maxillary bones, the palatine bones, the vomers, jugal arches, pterygoids and the quadrate bones, is not a complete shelf between the oral and the nasal cavities. The left and right quadrate bones articulate between the mandible, the braincase,

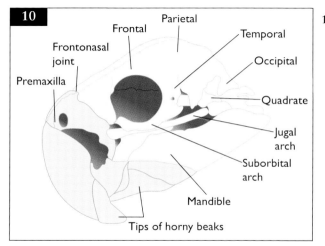

10 Psittacine skull.

the jugal arches and the pterygoid bones. Rostral rotation pushes the jaw open and *vice versa*. The eye orbit is complete only in psittacines. There is a very thin interorbital septum with the orbital nerves running through the caudal edge of this septum. The lower jaw consists of two mandibular rami fused at a symphysis.

VERTEBRAE

The requirements of flight have limited the flexibility of the avian spinal column. The most mobile part is the cervical spine, made up of 11–12 vertebrae in psittacines. They provide sufficient flexibility for a parrot to reach its tail and uropygial gland. The thoracic vertebrae, carrying the ribs, are somewhat flexible in psittacines, but are fused in many other species to form the notarium. Caudal to the thoracic vertebrae/notarium are a few mobile vertebrae, the last of which articulates with the synsacrum. The synsacrum consists of 10–23 fused thoracic, lumbar, sacral and caudal vertebrae. It is followed by five to eight free caudal vertebrae and then the pygostyle (four to ten fused caudal vertebrae), which supports the tail retrices.

RIBS

There are three to nine pairs of ribs, each with a dorsal vertebral component (made of bone) and a ventral sternal component (made of ossified cartilage). There is an uncinate process (caudodorsal process) on vertebral ribs.

STERNUM

The size of the sternum increases with increasing flight or swimming abilities, as it serves as the attachment of the pectoral muscles needed for flight. There is a prominent ventral medial keel (the carina) in many species.

THORACIC GIRDLE

The thoracic girdle is made up of the scapulae, the coracoids and the clavicles. The scapula is strongly attached to the ribs and, in some species, reaches to the ilium. The coracoid is massive in most birds, functioning to hold the wing away from the sternum during flight. The clavicles fuse ventrally to form the furcula. In many parrots they are united only by cartilage or fibrous tissue. The ventral part of the furcula is attached to the apex of the sternal keel by ligaments. The clavicles serve as a transverse spacer, bracing the wings apart, and for attachment of muscles that produce the downstroke of the wings. These three bones come together at the canalis triosseus (foramen triosseum, triosseal canal), through which the tendon of the supracoracoid muscle passes. This muscle lifts the humerus for the upstroke of the wing. The glenoid cavity, formed by the scapula and coracoid, is directed laterally and allows abduction and adduction of the wing.

WINGS

The humerus, in most pet species, is a pneumatic bone; the lateral diverticulum of the clavicular air sac enters through the pneumatic foramen on the medial side of the greater tuberosity. In flight the dorsal edge of the humerus becomes the trailing edge of the wing, demonstrating the range of movement that the humerus is capable of, a range of movement that includes elevation, depression, protraction, retraction and dorsal and ventral rotation. The ulna is larger

11 Prokinesis.

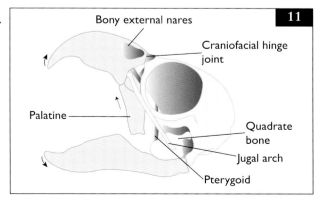

than the radius. The secondary flight feathers are anchored to the ulna by ligaments. The 'wrist' joint is formed by the radial carpal bone (cranial) and the ulnar carpal bone (caudal) articulating with the carpometacarpus. This consists of the metacarpal bones and the digits. The major and minor metacarpals are fused proximally and distally with an interosseus space. There are three digits: the alular digit with one phalanx; the minor digit, also with one phalanx; and the major digit with two phalanges. See **12**.

PELVIC GIRDLE

The pelvic girdle contains the ilium, ischium and pubis, all partially fused with each other and the synsacrum. The girdle is incomplete ventrally for passage of large fragile eggs (the pelvic symphysis is present only in ostriches and rheas).

LEGS

The femur is a stout and relatively short bone that slopes cranially to bring the legs forward towards the centre of gravity. A patella is present in most birds. The tibiotarsus is formed by the fusion of the tibia and the proximal row of tarsal bones; the hock joint, therefore, is actually an intertarsal joint. The fibula extends two-thirds of the way down the tibiotarsus, to which it is fused. The reduction in its size limits rotation of the leg. The tarsometatarsus, formed by the fusion of the distal row of tarsal bones to the three main metatarsal bones of digits II, III and IV, is usually shorter than the tibiotarsus except in long-legged birds. There are four digits in parrots: I has two phalanges and is usually directed backwards; II has three phalanges; III has four phalanges; and IV has five phalanges. The fourth digit is directed caudally in parrots. See **13** and **14**.

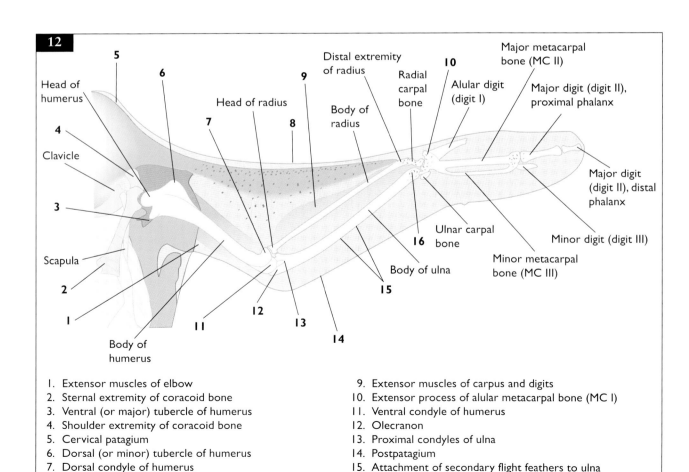

1. Extensor muscles of elbow
2. Sternal extremity of coracoid bone
3. Ventral (or major) tubercle of humerus
4. Shoulder extremity of coracoid bone
5. Cervical patagium
6. Dorsal (or minor) tubercle of humerus
7. Dorsal condyle of humerus
8. Propatagium
9. Extensor muscles of carpus and digits
10. Extensor process of alular metacarpal bone (MC I)
11. Ventral condyle of humerus
12. Olecranon
13. Proximal condyles of ulna
14. Postpatagium
15. Attachment of secondary flight feathers to ulna
16. Distal condyles of ulna

12 The bones of the wing.

13 Lateral view of the leg.

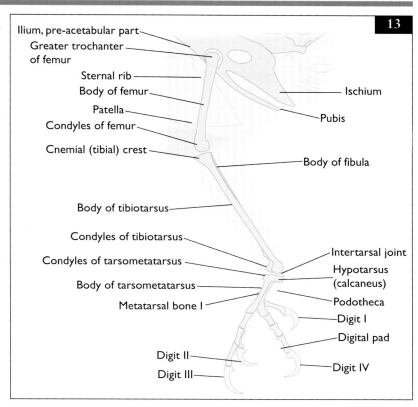

Ilium, pre-acetabular part
Greater trochanter of femur
Sternal rib
Body of femur
Patella
Condyles of femur
Cnemial (tibial) crest
Body of tibiotarsus
Condyles of tibiotarsus
Condyles of tarsometatarsus
Body of tarsometatarsus
Metatarsal bone I
Digit II
Digit III
Ischium
Pubis
Body of fibula
Intertarsal joint
Hypotarsus (calcaneus)
Podotheca
Digit I
Digital pad
Digit IV

14 Craniocaudal view of the leg.

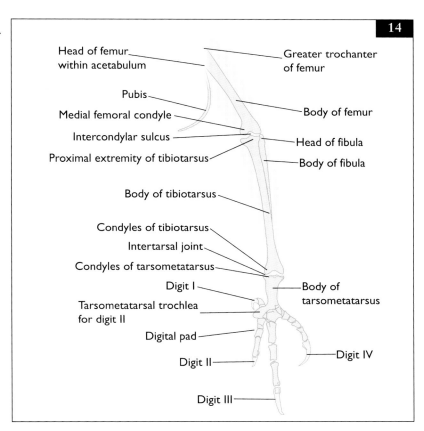

Head of femur within acetabulum
Pubis
Medial femoral condyle
Intercondylar sulcus
Proximal extremity of tibiotarsus
Body of tibiotarsus
Condyles of tibiotarsus
Intertarsal joint
Condyles of tarsometatarsus
Digit I
Tarsometatarsal trochlea for digit II
Digital pad
Digit II
Digit III
Greater trochanter of femur
Body of femur
Head of fibula
Body of fibula
Body of tarsometatarsus
Digit IV

THE DIGESTIVE TRACT

OROPHARYNX

The choana is a median fissure in the palate connecting the oropharynx to the nasal cavity. The palate is usually ridged laterally and rostrally to the choana, and is associated with the dehusking of seed and other foods. Caudal to the choana and palate is the infundibular cleft, a slit-like opening in the midline that is common to the right and left pharyngotympanic (Eustachian) tubes. This cleft cannot be closed by atmospheric pressure, making changes in altitude while flying possible. There is also lymphatic tissue (the pharyngeal tonsil) abundant in wall of the cleft.

The tongue is supported by the hypobranchial (hyoid) apparatus. It has many adaptations for collecting and manipulating food and for swallowing. Only parrots have intrinsic muscles within the tongue. Just caudal to the tongue is the laryngeal mound, which carries the glottis. It has several rows of backward-pointing papillae to aid in swallowing.

The salivary glands are found in: the roof of the oropharynx (maxillary, palatine and sphenopterygoid glands); the angle of the mouth and cheeks; and the floor of the oropharynx (mandibular, lingual, and cricoarytenoid glands). They are best developed in birds that evolved on a dry diet.

OESOPHAGUS AND CROP

The oesophagus is thin-walled and distensible, with a relatively greater diameter than that found in mammals (**15, 16**). Longitudinal folds on the internal surface allow for this distension; the size and degree of these folds is proportional to the size of the food particles swallowed. The oesophagus is lined with incompletely keratinized squamous epithelial cells and mucus glands (especially in the thoracic oesophagus).

The crop is an enlargement of the oesophagus found in many (but not all) birds (e.g. it is very prominent in psittacines, but very small in most passerines). Its lining is similar to that of the oesophagus, except that it has no mucus glands. It serves as a food storage area for birds that eat rapidly and then move to a safer area to give the food time to pass further down the digestive tract. The exit from the crop into the thoracic oesophagus is at the level of the thoracic inlet, on the right side of the midline of the neck. A fold of crop tissue lies over the exit, which then makes an S-shaped turn into the thoracic oesophagus.

PROVENTRICULUS AND VENTRICULUS

There is no obvious boundary between the thoracic oesophagus and the proventriculus, other than a lack of internal folds. The proventriculus is lined with mucus-secreting columnar epithelial cells. Within the laminar propria are the gastric glands, multi- or unilobular glands lined with tall columnar mucus cells. They discharge into an alveolus, which then drains into the central cavity of the lobule. Secondary ducts collect from different glands, which then empty into a primary duct and this empties into the proventricular lumen. These glands may be present throughout the proventriculus or contained in defined tracts or areas. They produce hydrochloric acid and pepsin.

Between the proventriculus and the gizzard is the intermediate zone, a variably developed region with a microscopic structure somewhere between the two. It may narrow to form an isthmus between the proventriculus and gizzard.

The gizzard (or ventriculus) varies in size and shape between species. Those species that eat soft food (e.g. lorikeets) have smaller, rounder gizzards, which can be difficult to distinguish from the proventriculus. Other species have a thickened, biconvex gizzard, with a wall consisting of smooth muscle bands, rich in myoglobin. Asymmetrical arrangement of these muscle bands results in both rotatory and crushing movements when the gizzard contracts. The gizzard is lined with simple columnar epithelium, with crypts containing exits for tubular glands in the lamina propria. These tubular glands secrete hard vertical rods that interconnect laterally for greater strength. Between them is a softer horizontal matrix of carbohydrate–protein complex secreted by the cells of the epithelium and crypts. This matrix hardens with the effect of hydrochloric acid. The vertical rods project slightly out from the horizontal matrix. This layer of rods and matrix is known as the cuticle or koilin layer. When combined with the asymmetrical rotatary grinding of the ventricular muscles, these rods and the matrix are very effective at crushing and grinding food into a soft pulp.

There is also a pyloric region connecting the gizzard to the duodenum. Its lining is microscopically intermediate between gizzard and duodenum. Its function is unclear.

INTESTINAL TRACT

The duodenum forms a narrow U-shape on the right side of the gizzard, with the descending duodenum proximal to the ascending duodenum. It is lined with mucus-secreting goblet cells. The bile and pancreatic ducts often open near to each other in the distal end of the ascending duodenum. There may be two bile ducts (the common hepatoenteric duct and the cystoenteric duct) and two to three pancreatic ducts.

The jejunum and ileum are usually arranged in a number of narrow U-shaped loops at the edge of the dorsal mesentery on the right side of the abdominal cavity. The vitelline (Meckel's) diverticulum is the short blind remnant of the yolk sac; it can be used to differentiate jejunum from ileum.

The large intestine is very short, separated from the ileum by the ileorectal sphincter. In some species, caeca arise from the rectum at the junction of the rectum with the ileum. Their form and size vary, and they are reduced or absent in parrots, swifts and pigeons. See **15** and **16**.

PANCREAS

The avian pancreas consists of three lobes. The dorsal and ventral lobes are supported and separated by the pancreatic artery within the duodenal loop, and the splenic lobe runs more laterally up to the spleen, as an extension of the ventral lobe. See **15** and **16**. The pancreas has both endocrine and exocrine functions.

15 Ventral view of the gastrointestinal tract.

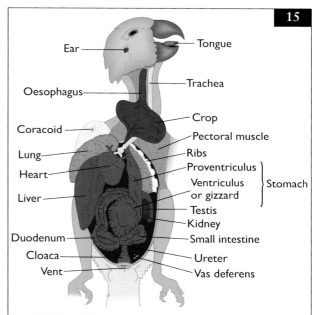

16 Lateral view of the gastrointestinal tract.

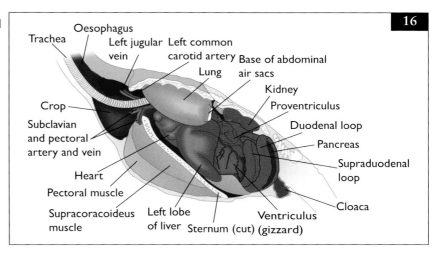

While the amount of endocrine tissue is proportionally greater than that of mammals, over 99% of the pancreatic mass has an exocrine function. The exocrine pancreas consists of compound tubuloacinar glands divided into lobules. These glands secrete amylase, lipase, proteolytic enzymes and sodium bicarbonate into the ascending duodenum via pancreatic ducts. Pancreatic secretion, which is at a higher rate than that of mammals, is controlled by both neural and hormonal mechanisms. Immediately a bird starts eating, pancreatic secretion begins, apparently via a vagal reflex. Distension of the proventriculus stimulates a hormonal response involving a vasoactive intestinal polypeptide; this results in pancreatic secretion. Diet can also affect the rate of secretion, with diets high in fat and carbohydrates increasing the activity of amylase and lipase.

LIVER

The avian liver consists of the right and left lobes joined cranially in the midline. The right lobe is larger than the left, with each lobe having several small processes. The liver is enclosed in a thin and slightly elastic capsule of connective tissue, allowing its expansion. Blood is supplied to the liver by the right and left hepatic arteries and hepatic portal veins. The hepatic arteries arise from the coeliac artery, while the portal veins drain blood from the proventriculus, ventriculus, duodenum, pancreas, intestines and cloaca. Two hepatic veins join the caudal vena cava cranial to the liver, draining blood away from the liver.

Terminal portal venules and arterioles empty into sinusoids between plates of hepatocytes. The low pressure in these sinusoids allows the hepatocytes to absorb molecules from the blood. Phagocytic Kupffer cells are also present in the sinusoids, collecting particulate matter and microorganisms. The now 'filtered' blood drains into the hepatic veins and on to the heart. The oxygenated arterial blood maintains the viability of the hepatocytes. Bile canaliculi form between three to five hepatocytes and drain into a bile ductule.

A portal triad of arteriole, portal venule and bile ductule, along with associated hepatocytes, bile canaliculi and sinusoids, forms the basic functional unit of the liver: the hepatic acinus. Hepatocytes close to these portal triads are said to be 'periportal'. Those further away, near the hepatic venules, are called 'periacinar'. The intermediate area is termed the 'midzone'. The hepatocytes in these different areas, although morphologically the same, are biochemically different and react differently to incoming chemicals and metabolites.

Bile is produced by hepatocytes and enters the bile canaliculi and then the ductules in the portal triad, which then empty into the interlobular ducts. These in turn form the right and left hepatic ducts, which join to become the common hepatoenteric duct emptying into the duodenum. A branch of the right hepatic duct either forms the right hepatoenteric duct (emptying into the duodenum) or, in those birds with a gall bladder, the hepatocystic duct entering the gall bladder. (Pigeons, most psittacines and ostriches do not have gall bladders.) From there the cystoenteric duct runs to the duodenum. Birds thus have two bile ducts emptying into the duodenum.

The liver has several functions in the body:

- Digestion. Bile contains bile acids, synthesized in the liver from cholesterol. (In birds the primary bile acid is chenodeoxycholic acid.) In the distal duodenum these bile acids emulsify fat, facilitating its digestion. Bile acids are then resorbed in the jejunum and ileum and recirculated through the liver. Bile also plays a role in the digestion of carbohydrates and protein. It contains amylase and helps to activate pancreatic amylase and lipase in the duodenum. Because of the lack of biliverdin reductase and glucuronyl transferase in birds, the primary bile pigment is biliverdin, giving avian bile its characteristic green colour.

- Carbohydrate metabolism. The portal blood supply, carrying nutrient-rich blood from the gastrointestinal tract, supplies the liver with these nutrients before any other major organs. Hepatic enzymes carry out glycogenesis, protein synthesis and lipogenesis in the well-fed bird. The glycogen, protein and triglycerides produced in the liver enter the circulation and are used (or stored) throughout the body. If a bird is fasted (for any reason), the resultant hypoglycaemia stimulates glucagon production, which in turn activates liver enzymatic pathways to produce glucose through glycogeolysis, gluconeogenesis and lipolysis. The liver therefore plays a major role in carbohydrate metabolism.

- Metabolism of metabolites, drugs and chemicals. The liver, through its microsomal drug-metabolizing enzyme system in the periacinar hepatocytes, processes both endogenous metabolites and exogenous chemicals. Hydrophobic, lipid-soluble molecules (which are difficult to eliminate) are converted by the liver to hydrophilic, water-soluble molecules and excreted in bile and urine. This is done in two phases; in the first, enzymes modify the molecules by oxidation or reduction; in the second they are enzymatically conjugated with other molecules to become sufficiently water soluble. The best example of this is the synthesis of urea and uric acid from protein in the liver.

- Protein synthesis. The liver is the primary site of synthesis of a range of essential proteins:
  - Albumin.
  - Fibrinogen, prothrombin and clotting factors I, II, V, VII, VII, IX and XII.
  - Molecules involved in the transport of metals, hormones, and lipids (e.g. ceruloplasmin and macroglobulins).
- Antimicrobial effect. The Kupffer cells in the sinusoids are important in the clearance of microorganisms entering the portal circulation in cases of intestinal infections or surgery. They also play a role in the detoxification of bacterial endotoxins.

CLOACA

The cloaca is the common exit for the gastrointestinal, urinary and reproductive tracts. As a point of terminology, the cloaca is the chamber; its opening to the skin is the vent. The cloaca is divided internally by two mucosal folds into three compartments: the coprodeum, the urodeum and the proctodeum (**17**). This structure is similar in all birds; the main variation is the presence or absence of the phallic structures of the proctodeum.

The coprodeum is the most cranial, and largest, compartment. There is no distinction between rectum and coprodeum (except in the ostrich, which has a rectocoprodeal fold, and Anatidae, where there is an abrupt change in gross appearance of the mucosa). Some species have villi and folds on the mucosa; others have none.

The urodeum is the middle and smallest compartment, separated from the other two compartments by two circular mucosal folds. The coprourodeal fold is a cranial annular fold that stretches to become a thin diaphragm if the coprodeum is full of faeces; it may close during egg laying to prevent defecation while the bird is laying an egg. The uroproctodeal fold is a caudal, semicircular dorsolateral fold that fades out ventrally. The urogenital ducts open into the urodeum on the dorsolateral mucosa (the ureters dorsally, the genital ducts laterally). The ureter opens via a simple opening; the ductus deferens opens via a conical papilla. In immature hens a homologue of the ductus deferens papilla may be present, but it disappears with maturity. In the mature hen the left oviduct opens ventrally and laterally relative to the left ureter. There may be a small mound at its opening. In immature birds it is covered with a membrane that disappears at maturity.

The proctodeum is the short caudal compartment between the lips of the vent and the uroproctodeal fold. In immature birds an opening in the dorsal wall leads into the cloacal bursa.

The vent is a transverse slit guarded by dorsal and ventral lips. This horizontal arrangement is the reason why purse-string sutures are unsuitable to close the vent in birds.

17 The cloaca.

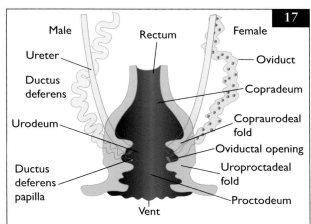

THE URINARY SYSTEM

The kidneys lie in the renal fossae of the synsacrum, each divided into three divisions: the caudal, middle and cranial divisions (**18**). (Note: these are not lobes.) The distinctions between these divisions are not always clear. The spinal nerves and sacral plexus pass through the kidneys between the middle and caudal divisions. The surface of the kidney is covered in rounded projections, the renal lobules.

Each renal lobule is a pear-shaped elongated piece of tissue wedged between the interlobular veins and enclosed by its perilobular collecting tubules. At the tapering end of the lobule the collecting tubules converge to form the medullary collecting tubules (medullary region or cone of the lobule); this tapering end also contains the nephronal loops (loops of Henle) of the medullary nephrons. The wide part of the lobule is the cortical region; it contains nephrons of both cortical and medullary nephrons (but not the medullary nephronal loops).

Several lobular medullary regions converge into a single cone-shaped assembly of collecting tubules in a connective tissue sheath (known as the medullary region of a renal lobe) draining into a single collecting duct. Several of these ducts combine to form a secondary branch of the ureter.

Although there is a lobular cortex and medulla, there are no distinct renal cortical and medullary regions because both lobes and lobules are embedded in tissue at differing depths in the kidney. There is a higher number of medullary regions in birds that conserve water and, therefore, a smaller volume of cortical regions. This implies a higher proportion of mammalian-type nephrons and, therefore, a better counter-current concentration.

There are two types of nephron: cortical (or reptilian) nephrons with no nephronal loop; and medullary (or mammalian) nephrons with a nephronal loop penetrating the medullary region. Both types start with a renal corpuscle: a glomerular capsule (Bowman's) enclosing the glomerulus (tuft of capillaries). Collecting tubules lie both superficially on the surface of the cortical region (perilobular) and within the medullary region (medullary). Several form a collecting duct, which then forms a secondary branch of the ureter.

The arterial blood supply to the kidneys comes from the cranial, middle and caudal renal arteries. The kidney also receives a venous supply via the cranial and caudal renal portal veins, which form a venous ring encompassing both kidneys. Blood enters this ring from the external iliac vein, the ischiadic veins, the internal iliac veins and the caudal mesenteric veins. Afferent renal veins come off the ring and enter the renal parenchyma to become the interlobular veins. The renal portal valve is located in the common iliac vein; when it is open (adrenergic stimulation), blood is diverted into the caudal vena cava and away from the kidney.

The ureter starts within the depth of the cranial division and continues caudally in a groove on the ventral surface of the middle and caudal divisions. It receives primary branches, which in turn receive secondary branches from the collecting ducts draining several renal lobes. The ureter opens into the urodeum.

The urine:plasma osmolar ratio in most birds can only reach 2.0–2.5, compared with 25–30 in mammals. Birds will excrete 1% of filtered water, compared with mammals who excrete less than 0.1%. The concentration ability of the avian kidney lies with the mammalian nephrons; because most birds have more reptilian nephrons than mammalian nephrons, they do not produce concentrated urine. This is believed to be, in part, due to the need for water to transport the more viscous uric acid through renal tubules. Uric acid, the end product of protein metabolism in birds, is produced in the liver and removed from the blood by a combination of filtration in the glomerulus (10%)

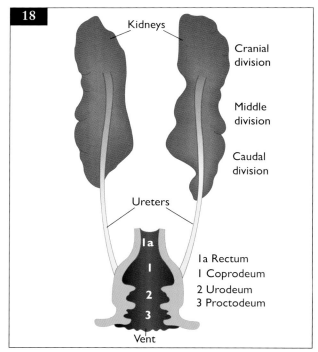

18

Kidneys

Cranial division

Middle division

Caudal division

Ureters

1a Rectum
1 Coprodeum
2 Urodeum
3 Proctodeum

Vent

18 The urinary system.

and tubular secretion in the proximal part of the nephron (90%).

Urine production is controlled by arginine vasotocin (AVT), the avian equivalent of antidiuretic hormone (ADH). Increased plasma osmolality stimulates the hypothalamus to produce AVT. This in turn constricts afferent arterioles of the reptilian nephrons (reducing the glomerular filtration rate [GFR]) and increases the permeability of the collecting ducts of the mammalian nephrons. The end result is decreased urine production and therefore decreased plasma osmolarity.

Water resorption also occurs in the rectum during retrograde flushing from the cloaca. Up to 15% of urine water can be resorbed in this manner, but this is reduced by polyuria and stress-induced defecation. If the urine is too concentrated, a concentration gradient across the rectal mucosa cannot be achieved and so resorption would be limited. But, as urine osmolality increases, birds are able gradually to increase plasma osmolality, thus preserving the urine:plasma osmolar ratio and allowing water resorption. Birds with functional salt glands can decrease plasma osmolality by excreting salt, but this is not applicable to psittacines.

Effective osmoregulation therefore requires:
- Normal plasma osmolalarity.
- Sufficient functional nephrons.
- Normal production of, and response to, AVT.
- Efficient cloacal water resorption.

THE RESPIRATORY TRACT
UPPER RESPIRATORY TRACT
The size and shape of the nares (nostrils) is variable between species. They are located at the top of the beak (except in the kiwi, where they are located at the tip of the beak). In parrots and pigeons (and owls) they are located within the fleshy cere. Just inside the nares is the operculum, a cornified flap of tissue.

The nasal septum is partly bony and partly cartilaginous. It is complete in parrots and many other species, and separates the nasal cavity to the level of the choana. Within the nasal cavity are the nasal conchae (turbinates), usually divided into three parts: the scroll-like highly vascular rostral turbinates with their stratified squamous epithelial lining; the middle turbinates, also scroll-like but with a mucociliary lining; and the caudal turbinates with an olfactory epithelial lining innervated by the olfactory nerve. The vascularity of the turbinates assists in the control the rate of water and heat loss from the body. The infraorbital sinus network is connected to the nasal cavity in the middle and caudal regions of the nasal cavity. However, the connections between

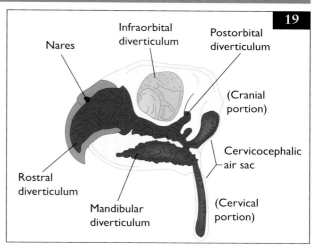

19 The sinus network within the skull.

the nasal cavity and the sinuses are such that it is difficult to sample the sinuses by a nasal flush.

The infraorbital sinuses are located around the eye, the upper beak, the mandible and the pneumatized sections of skull (**19**). They are classified as rostral (in the maxillary rostrum or bill), periorbital/ preorbital (rostral to the orbit), infraorbital (medial to the eye), mandibular (mandibular rostrum) and postorbital (surrounding the opening of the ear). The right and left sides communicate and have diverticula in Anseriformes, Psittaciformes and insectivorous Passeriformes. They do not communicate in noninsectivorous Passeriformes.

Each infraorbital sinus has five diverticula and two chambers:
- Rostral diverticulum. Within the beak, surrounded by premaxillary bone.
- Maxillary chamber. Underneath the nares, lateral to the rostral diverticulum, extending back to the preorbital diverticulum.
- Preorbital diverticulum. In the space between the nares and the rostral aspect of the orbit. It is bordered medially by the nasal cavity and dorsolaterally by the nasal and frontal bones. It connects to the suborbital chamber.
- Suborbital chamber. Beneath the bony orbit. It is bordered medially by the caudal extent of the nasal cavity and laterally by the jugal and prefrontal bones.
- Infraorbital diverticulum. Above the suborbital chamber, extending behind the suborbital arch and medial to the eye. It is the largest diverticulum.

- Postorbital diverticulum. This has two parts: the caudal portion is the preauditory diverticulum, extending caudally to the bony orbit and bound by the temporal and quadrate bones laterally; and the cranial portion is immediately caudal to the orbit.
- Mandibular diverticulum. Communicating with the maxillary portion near the postorbital diverticulum. Occupies the mandibular bone.

In addition the cervicocephalic air sac communicates with the most caudal aspect of the infraorbital sinus. This air sac does not play a role in gas exchange, nor does it communicate with the lower respiratory tract. It has two divisions: the cranial cephalic (from occipital region to just behind the cere), which is not found in many species, including the macaw; and the cervical (from the tympanic area and extending in two columns bilaterally down the neck). It is thought to play several roles: insulation for heat retention, control of buoyancy, reducing the force of impact with water in fish-eating birds, and support of the head during sleep or flight. Jugular venepuncture may result in blood entering this air sac and appearing as epistaxis.

The upper respiratory tract serves several functions: it provides a sense of smell; it filters airborne debris; it plays a role in thermoregulation; and it plays a role in water conservation.

LOWER RESPIRATORY TRACT

Birds do not have a true larynx as such, but rather have a glottis. This has no role in voice production; its main role is preventing food passing into the trachea. There are four cartilage structures in the glottis: the cricoid, a scoop-shaped cartilage with left and right lateral wings; the procricoid, a small cartilage that articulates with the cricoid wings on the dorsal midline; and the two arytenoids that form the margins of the glottis. The glottis is located in the laryngeal mound behind the tongue. During inspiration the glottis is raised to the choana and opened, allowing air to be inspired without opening the mouth.

Unlike mammals, the avian trachea is composed of complete cartilaginous rings, each shaped like a signet ring, with the broad part forming the left and right walls, alternately. These rings therefore partially overlap each other. They may be ossified in passerines and some larger species. The tracheal lumen diameter progressively reduces caudally, but is still larger than that of a comparative mammal: the typical avian trachea is 2.7 times longer and 1.29 times wider than that of comparably sized mammals. This means that the avian tracheal dead space is 4.5 times greater than that of comparably sized mammals. Birds compensate for this with a low respiratory frequency (one-third of that of mammals) and an increased tidal volume (four times that of mammals). It is important to understand this anatomy when intubating birds. Noncuffed tubes are preferable, but if cuffed tubes are used they should not be inflated, and smaller tubes than at first appreciated are necessary to prevent iatrogenic trauma to the tracheal lining caudal to the glottis.

Most companion birds will have a tracheobronchial syrinx: the last of the tracheal rings fuse into a syringeal box, which joins to the first of the bronchial rings. (There are also tracheal and bronchial syrinxes in other species, e.g. storks and owls.) The syrinx consists of a number of variably ossified cartilages and vibrating soft structures.

The syringeal cartilages consist of:
- The tympanum. A direct continuation of the trachea, formed by the fusion of several tracheal rings. It is commonly ossified.
- The tracheal syringeal cartilages. C-shaped flattened cartilages, attached to the pessulus at one end and free at the other.
- The pessulus. A wedge-shaped cartilage with the blade lying dorsoventrally, dividing the airway vertically.
- The bronchial syringeal cartilages. Three to five paired C-shaped rings forming the divided part of the syrinx.

The vibrating structures of syrinx include:
- The paired medial tympaniform membranes that form the medial surface of the divided part of syrinx, held between free ends of bronchial syringeal cartilages.
- The paired lateral tympaniform membranes that form the membranous areas between the cartilages on the lateral aspect of the syrinx.
- The lateral labium. A pad of elastic tissue projecting into the lumen of the syrinx from the cartilage of the lateral wall.
- The medial labium projecting into the lumen from the pessulus.

The syrinx is controlled by both intrinsic and extrinsic muscles. The number of intrinsic muscles varies between species: songbirds have five pairs; parrots have only two pairs; and some ratites and Galliformes have none at all. There are three sets of extrinsic muscles: one pair of cleidohyoid muscles, from the clavicle to the glottis, which pulls the trachea caudally and relaxes the muscles around the syrinx; the tracheolateral muscle, from the caudal trachea to the syrinx, enclosing the trachea ventrally and laterally, which tenses the syrinx; and the sternotracheal muscle, from the craniolateral sternum to the trachea, just cranial to the syrinx, which fuses with the tracheolateral muscle.

There are two theories on how birds vocalize. The first holds that vibration of the tympaniform membranes produces sound; the second that compression of the bronchial elements against the median parts of syrinx forms narrow slots through which air is forced during expiration, causing whistling sounds.

Avian lungs are not lobed as are mammalian lungs. Approximately one-quarter of the lung volume is enclosed between ribs; avian lungs weigh about the same as those of mammals (on a weight basis), but are more compact and take up 50% as much space as in mammals. They extend from the first to the seventh rib in Psittaciformes, but may extend to the ilia in some species (**20, 21**).

Each lung receives one of the two primary bronchi, formed by the bifurcation of the trachea at the syrinx.

20 Schematic drawing of the avian lower respiratory tract.

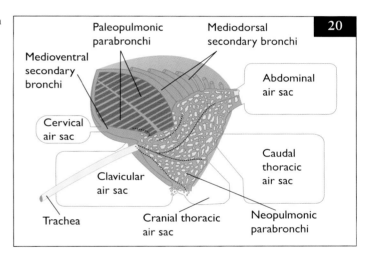

21 Ventral view of the avian lower respiratory tract.

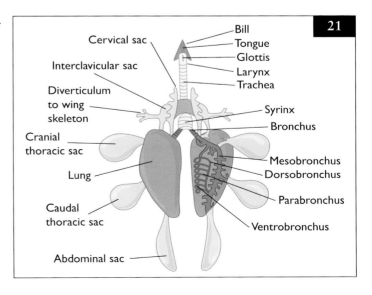

The bronchus enters the lung ventrally and obliquely at the junction of the cranial and middle third of the lung and then passes dorsolaterally to the lung surface and turns caudally to its opening into the abdominal air sac. The bronchi have a well developed internal, circular, smooth muscle layer and longitudinally orientated smooth muscles. Acetylcholine, pilocarpine and histamine induce contraction and atropine blocks these effects. Each primary bronchus gives off four groups of secondary bronchi:

- Mediodorsal (seven to ten). Originate from the dorsal wall of the primary bronchus and are located over the costal surface of the lung.
- Lateroventral (eight). Arise from ventral wall of the primary bronchus and are located in the ventral part of the costal surface of the lung; they enter the abdominal and caudal thoracic air sac.
- Laterodorsal (variable number). Arise from the lateral wall of the primary bronchus and extend laterally towards the costal surface.
- Medioventral (four to six). Arise from the dorsomedial wall of the cranial third of the primary bronchus and run medially on the ventral (septal) surface of the lung, servicing three-quarters of the septal surface of the lung. They are the largest of the secondary bronchi.

The secondary bronchi give rise to the parabronchi (tertiary bronchi), which anastomose with other parabronchi. They are divided into two groups: the paleopulmonic and the neopulmonic parabronchi. The paleopulmonic parabronchi come off the mediodorsal and medioventral secondary bronchi. They form the medioventral–mediodorsal system in the cranial and dorsal region of the lung, making up about two-thirds of the lung. Air flows unidirectionally, caudal to cranial, in this region of the lung, which is the major site of gas exchange and is more efficient than the neopulmonic lung. The remainder of the lung (ventrolateral) is the neopulmonic region. It is most advanced in chickens, pigeons and passerines; absent in emus and penguins; and minimal in storks, cormorants, cranes, ducks, gull, owls and buzzards. Air in this region changes direction with each phase of breathing (i.e. it is bidirectional).

The parabronchi are uniform in diameter throughout the lung and lined with simple squamous epithelium. The inner lining of these parabronchi is pierced by numerous openings into individual chambers, called atria. Atria are pocket-like polygonal cavities, lined with flat or cuboidal epithelium and coated in surfactant. The openings into the atria are surrounded by smooth muscle with parasympathetic and sympathetic innervation. At the bottom of each atrium are infundibula: openings that lead to air capillaries. These air capillaries branch and freely anastomose with each other; their small diameter means that the pressure gradient for oxygen diffusion is greater than in mammals. They are intimately entwined with a network of blood capillaries, making them the site of gaseous exchange.

Extending from the lungs are the air sacs. Embryos have six pairs, two of which fuse in most birds at, or soon after, hatching to form the clavicular air sac. Adult birds, therefore, have nine air sacs: the unpaired clavicular and the paired cervical, anterior thoracic, posterior thoracic and abdominal air sacs. (Chickens and some other species fuse their cervical air sacs, leaving them with eight air sacs.)

The clavicular air sac is a large unpaired and complicated sac occupying the thoracic inlet and extending into the extrathoracic diverticula (the humerus, coracoid, scapula and clavicle) and the intrathoracic diverticula (around the heart and along the sternum). The first, second and third medioventral bronchi form the main connections to the clavicular air sac.

The cervical air sacs arise from the first medioventral bronchus. They form two median chambers lying between lungs and dorsal to the oesophagus, leading into a pair of vertebral diverticula on each side of the vertebral column, one inside the neural canal and one outside. They also invade the vertebrae.

The cranial thoracic air sacs arise from medioventral secondary bronchi and lie dorsolaterally in the coelom. The caudal thoracic air sacs are found caudal to the cranial thoracic air sacs and arise from lateroventral secondary bronchi and primary bronchi.

The abdominal air sacs arise from lateroventral secondary bronchi and primary bronchi and lie between the caudal thoracic air sacs. They are the most variable in size, but are often the largest air sacs. They carry air to leg and pelvic bones through perirenal and femoral diverticula.

Although the mesenteric oblique septum separates the thoracic and abdominal cavities, there is no muscular diaphragm to aid in respiration. Instead, birds rely on the movement of the ribs and sternum to move air through the respiratory tract. During inspiration the external intercostal muscles pull the ribs cranially, laterally and ventrally. At the same time the sternum, coracoids and furcula move ventrally and cranially, pivoting at the shoulder joint. Combined, these movements have the effect of increasing the coelomic volume. Expiration is simply a reversal of these movements, using the internal intercostal muscles and the abdominal muscles.

The air moves through the airways on a two-breath cycle (**22**):
- First inspiration. Air moves through the trachea into the primary bronchus and neopulmonic region, and then into the caudal air sacs. Some air may enter the paleopulmonic region and start gaseous exchange.
- First expiration. Air moves from the caudal air sacs into the paleopulmonic region; a small volume of air (12%) escapes from the caudal air sacs through the bidirectional neopulmonic region to escape through the trachea.
- Second inspiration. Air moves from the paleopulmonic region into the cranial air sacs.
- Second expiration. Air moves from the cranial air sacs out through the bronchi and trachea; a small volume of air (12%) escapes from the caudal air sacs through the bidirectional neopulmonic region to escape through the trachea.

As mentioned earlier, gaseous exchange occurs in the air capillaries. The cross-current arrangement between parabronchial air flow and parabronchial blood capillaries in the paleopulmonic region provides a highly efficient system of gaseous exchange, so efficient that birds need less ventilation to achieve a higher level of oxygenation of blood than mammals.

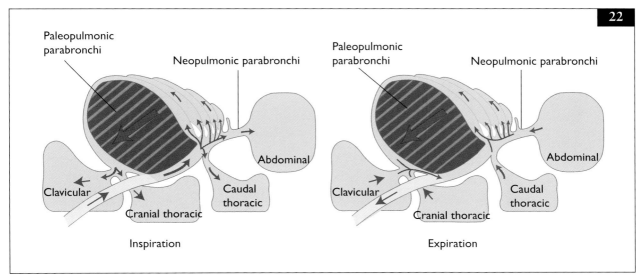

22 Air flow through the respiratory tract.

THE REPRODUCTIVE TRACT
FEMALE REPRODUCTIVE TRACT

The avian embryo has two ovaries and two oviducts. During incubation the left gonadal region receives more germ cells than the right, leading to asymmetrical development. The right ovary and oviduct usually regress, so most birds have only a left ovary and oviduct (with the exception of the kiwi and some raptors) (**23**).

The ovary is located beside the cranial division of the left kidney, adjacent to the adrenal gland. The ovarian blood supply enters the ovarian hilus where it is in close contact with the dorsal coelomic wall. The arterial supply comes from the ovario-oviductal branch of the left cranial renal artery, while venous drainage is via two ovarian veins directly into the caudal vena cava. This vascular anatomy makes ovariectomy a difficult and dangerous procedure to undertake, requiring optical magnification and specialized ligating instruments.

In seasonal laying birds (e.g. psittacines) three phases of ovarian growth can be recognized:
- Prenuptial acceleration. At the beginning of the breeding season the ovary begins to enlarge.

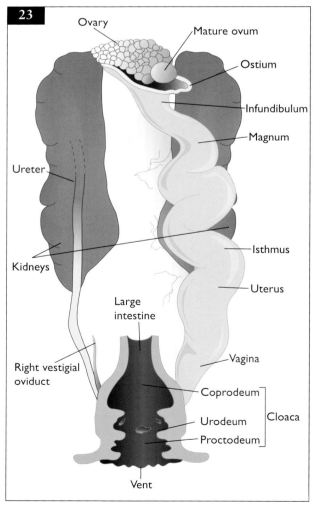

23 Ventral view of the female reproductive tract.

- Culmination phase. Ovulation and egg laying commences.
- Refractory phase. With egg laying completed, the ovary reduces in size.

Each follicle, containing an oocyte surrounded by the wall of the follicle, is suspended by stalk, which possesses smooth muscle, blood vessels and nerves. The wall of the follicle is very vascular and innervated with cholinergic and adrenergic fibres. Running across the surface is the stigma, a meridional band, which is less vascular and has no connective tissue or smooth muscle. Vitellogen or yolk, consisting of protein and lipid, is synthesized in the liver (vitellogenesis) and enters the follicle as it develops.

During ovulation the wall of the follicle splits along the stigma, releasing the yolk and oocyte. The follicle then shrinks to a thin-walled sac, which quickly regresses and is absorbed. No corpus luteum is formed, although the regressing follicle may secrete progesterone for the first 24 hours, affecting oviposition and nesting behaviour.

The oviduct can be divided into five regions: the infundibulum, the magnum, the isthmus, the uterus (shell gland) and the vagina.

The infundibulum resembles a funnel with a thin wall; its opening, an elongated slit, faces into the ovarian pocket formed by the left abdominal air sac. The infundibulum tapers rapidly into a tubular part (the chalaziferous region) with a thickened wall with higher mucosal folds. The infundibulum is reasonably motile, moving to envelop the developing follicle and capturing it as ovulation occurs. Fertilization occurs in the infundibulum before albumen (thick albumen immediately around the yolk, and the chalaza at each end of the yolk) is laid down by the chalaziferous glands in the tubular region. The egg passes through the infundibulum in 15 minutes.

From the infundibulum the developing egg passes into the magnum, the longest and most coiled part of the oviduct. This transition is marked by a sudden great enlargement of the mucosal folds. There are numerous tubular glands in these folds, which secrete albumen. Passage through the magnum takes three hours, during which time the egg acquires albumen, sodium, magnesium and calcium.

The next part of the oviduct, the isthmus, is short and reduced in calibre, with folds less prominent than those in the magnum. After a short band of demarcating tissue without glands, the wall of the isthmus has tubular glands similar to those of the magnum. Passage through the isthmus is slow, taking 75 minutes, during which protein is added to the albumen and the shell membranes (inner and outer) are added.

There is no distinct separation between the isthmus and the uterus (shell gland). This part is relatively short, but divided into two areas, the initial short, narrow 'red region' and a larger pouch-like region. In the uterus the longitudinal folds are transected by transverse furrows, forming leaf-like lamellae. The egg stays in the uterus for 20 hours: plumping (the addition of watery solutions) occurs in the first eight hours, and then the egg shell is formed and calcified over another 15 hours.

The vagina, S-shaped due to smooth muscle and connective tissue, is separated from the uterus by a sphincter. The mucosal folds of the vagina are thin and low and it has a thick muscle wall. There are no secretory glands; however, near the sphincter are the spermatic fossulae, crypts that act as a storage site for sperm for up to several weeks. Immature birds have a membrane covering the entrance of the vagina into the cloaca; tearing of this membrane can account for the presence of blood on the shell of the first egg laid.

The oviduct is suspended from the dorsal wall of the coelom by the dorsal mesosalpinx. A ventral mesosalpinx extends ventrally from the oviduct, but has a free margin. Smooth muscle in both ligaments is continuous with smooth muscle layers of the oviductal wall and caudally the smooth muscle in the ventral ligament condenses into a muscle chord fused with the ventral surface of the uterus and vagina. These ligaments may help to move the egg along the oviduct, especially in the magnum.

As with the ovary, there is marked seasonal growth and differentiation of the oviduct under the influence of the neuroendocrine system.

Egg

Lying on the surface of the yolk is the germinal disc containing the blastoderm (if fertilized) or the blastodisc (if unfertilized). Underlying the germinal disc is the 'white yolk' or latebra, which is less dense than the yellow yolk and therefore will always be uppermost regardless of the orientation of the egg. It is made up of protein (two-thirds) and fat (one-third). The yellow yolk (two-thirds fat and one-third protein) is encased in four layers of yolk membrane, which, while mechanically strong, forms a water- and salt-permeable membrane between the yolk and albumen.

Albumen is less viscous than yolk and it contains protein (ovomucin). The amount of ovomucin determines whether it is dense or thin albumen. There is a dense chalaziferous layer around the yolk, which is continuous with the chalazae at each end of the egg that merge with the shell membranes. The chalazae therefore suspend yolk in the middle of the egg (**24**). Beyond this chalaziferous layer are three more layers of albumen: thin inner and outer layers, and a dense layer between them. Albumen contributes to the aqueous environment of the embryo, has antibacterial components, and is a source of nutrition for the embryo.

The egg shell has three layers: the shell membranes, the testa and the cuticle. There are two shell membranes, each composed of several layers of fibre. The inner layer is fused to the chalazae as described above. The outer layer is fused to the testa. They separate at the blunt end to form the air cell. The testa is made up of an organic matrix of fine fibres and an inorganic solid component of calcite (crystalline calcium carbonate). The organic matrix is made up of a thin inner mamillary layer, containing conical knobs embedded in the outer shell membrane, and a thick outer spongy layer. The inorganic component has a thin inner layer corresponding to the mamillary layer and a thick outer palisade layer corresponding to the spongy layer. Pores run through all the layers, through which gaseous and water exchange occurs. Surrounding the entire shell is the outer cuticle, a continuous organic layer that reduces water loss and is somewhat resistant to bacteria. It also has a water repellent effect. Not all species have a cuticle on their shells.

MALE REPRODUCTIVE TRACT

Like the female embryo, the male embryo initially develops a larger left testicle. Unlike the right ovary, however, the right testicle does not regress, so that while the left testis is often larger than the right in the immature bird, this changes after maturity so that both are similarly sized. Suspended by the mesorchium, the testicles are surrounded, but not cooled, by the abdominal air sacs. The bulk of the testis is made up of thousands of convoluted seminiferous tubules with numerous anastomoses. There is no lobulation as is seen in mammals, as there are no septa present. The size of the testicle increases with sexual activity due to increased length and diameter of the seminiferous tubules and a greater number of interstitial cells. The testicle is covered in the tunica albuginea, but there is no pampiniform plexus. The seminiferous tubules are lined by spermatogenic epithelium made up of germ cells and sustentacular cells (Sertoli cells), which provide mechanical support for the germ cells, produce steroid hormones and may have a phagocytic role. Between the tubules are the interstitial cells (cells of Leydig), which produce androgenic hormones, especially testosterone. There may also be melanocytes present in the interstitial spaces of some species, giving the testis a black coloration.

There are three phases of spermatogenesis: the multiplication of spermatogonia; their growth into primary spermatocytes; and then the maturation of primary spermatocytes into secondary spermatocytes and then spermatids, which then develop into spermatozoa. These mature spermatozoa detach and pass through a short straight tubule into the rete testis, a thin-walled irregular channel on the dorsomedial aspect of the testis, adjacent to the epididymis. (The rete testis is not present in all species.)

The epididymis lies on the dorsomedial side of the testis and is relatively small compared with that in mammals. It enlarges during sexual activity, but has no distinct head, body and tail because the efferent ductules, arising from the rete testis, enter along its entire length. They lead into connecting ductules and finally into the epididymal duct.

The ductus deferens runs from the epididymis to the cloaca, entering the cloaca at the urodeum (**25**). At the urodeum it enters the receptacle of the ductus deferens, a spindle-shaped dilation embedded in the cloacal muscle. In passerines the caudal end of the ductus deferens forms a mass of convolutions called the seminal glomus. This enlarges in the breeding season to push into the cloaca, forming the cloacal promontory, which pushes the vent caudally. This is the main site of spermatozoal storage in these birds.

REPRODUCTIVE PHYSIOLOGY

Most birds are seasonal breeders, with substantial variation between species in their reproductive strategies. This variation is based on the environmental cues used to trigger reproduction, the developmental stage of the chick at hatch and the extent of parental care.

Mechanisms controlling this breeding seasonality are both endogenous and exogenous. Endogenous factors are poorly understood, but are reflected in the fact that many captive birds held in constant environmental conditions still show seasonality, as do

24 Cross-sectional diagram of the egg.

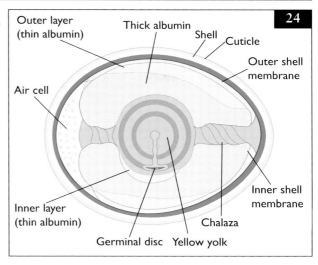

Outer layer (thin albumin)
Thick albumin
Shell
Cuticle
Outer shell membrane
Air cell
Inner shell membrane
Inner layer (thin albumin)
Germinal disc
Yellow yolk
Chalaza

25 Ventral view of the male reproductive tract.

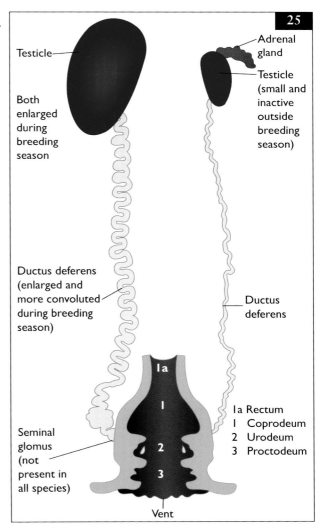

Testicle
Adrenal gland
Testicle (small and inactive outside breeding season)
Both enlarged during breeding season
Ductus deferens (enlarged and more convoluted during breeding season)
Ductus deferens
Seminal glomus (not present in all species)
1a Rectum
1 Coprodeum
2 Urodeum
3 Proctodeum
Vent

migratory birds going through a wide range of environmental changes and tropical birds with little variation in photoperiod. Exogenous factors are better understood. They can be either ultimate factors, which select for individuals that will breed when there are optimum conditions for offspring survival (e.g. food availability), or proximate factors that vary from year to year. These proximate factors are further broken down into:

- Initial predictive factors that initiate gonadal development in anticipation of breeding (e.g. photoperiod).
- Essential supplementary factors that supplement the initial predictive factors and initiate final stages of gonadal development. These include social cues (e.g. breeding plumage, mate availability, courtship behaviour), territorial behaviour, climate (e.g. rainfall) and nutrition (in particular an increase in fat and sugars in the diet).
- Synchronizing and integrating factors that regulate the sequence of breeding behaviour (e.g. social interaction between a pair).
- Modifying factors that can disrupt the breeding cycle (e.g. loss of a mate or disturbance of the nest site).

All of these factors have hormonal modulators. Their input into the hypothalamus has an effect on the release of gonadotrophin releasing hormone (GnRH), which in turn stimulates the pituitary to release follicle stimulating hormone (FSH) and luteinizing hormone (LH). In the hen, FSH supports ovarian and oviductal growth, gametogenesis and steroidogenesis, while LH also supports steroidogenesis. This steroidogenesis sees the release of oestrogen, which has effects on follicular and oviductal growth, calcium metabolism and vitellogenesis. Some female secondary behaviours are also influenced by oestrogen (e.g. courtship and nesting behaviours). In males FSH initiates growth of seminiferous tubules and results in increased spermatogenesis, while LH promotes development of the testosterone-producing cells of Leydig. This in turn gives rise to secondary male characteristics such as plumage changes, nesting activity, courtship behaviour and territorial behaviour.

Progesterone is produced by granulosa cells in the large follicles as they develop under the influence of LH. This in turn causes a surge in LH production from the pituitary just before ovulation. This surge of LH stimulates the production of prostaglandin (PG) F2α from ovarian follicles, causing the follicular stigma to rupture and allowing ovulation. Progesterone inhibits further ovulation and induces behavioural and physical changes associated with incubation and brood care.

PGF2α and PGE (1 and 2) are released by the F1 (first generation of follicles produced during ovulation) and postovulatory follicles. PGE2 and PGF2α bind at specific sites in the shell gland and vagina; PGF2α binds preferentially at the shell gland, allowing PGE2 to potentiate its effects and to allow relaxation of the vagina during oviposition. Therefore, PGE (1 and 2) allows relaxation of the uterovaginal sphincter, while PGF2α stimulates shell gland contractions. Uterine contractility stimulates AVT release from the pituitary, which stimulates further contractility and release of uterine PGs.

Eggs are successively laid until a clutch is formed: indeterminate layers continue to lay if eggs are removed, while determinate layers will only lay a set number of eggs. Incubation is performed by the hen only (in 25% of species), shared (54%), by the males only (6%) or by mixed strategies. Plasma prolactin levels are elevated in both sexes during incubation, which then has an inhibitory feedback on GnRH release.

ENDOCRINE GLANDS
PITUITARY

Also known as the hypophysis, the pituitary gland is attached to the ventral surface of the diencephalic part of the brainstem (the hypothalamus) immediately caudal to the optic chiasma. It has two components: the adenohypophysis, arising from embryonic stomodaeum; and the neurohypophysis, arising from the diencephalon.

The adenohypophysis has only two components; there is no pars intermedia as in mammals. The pars tuberalis is the smaller part of the adenohypophysis and covers part of the neurohypophysis, carrying portal vessels from there to the pars distalis. The pars distalis makes up the bulk of the adenohypophysis, lying ventral and rostral to the neurohypophysis. Seven types of secretory cells have been identified: alpha, beta, gamma, delta, epsilon, eta and kappa. They secrete at least seven hormones:

- FSH (beta cells). Stimulates ovarian follicular growth and secretion of oestrogen by the ovary; in males stimulates tubular growth of the testes and spermatogenesis.
- Thyroid-stimulating hormone (TSH) (delta cells). Controls the thyroid gland; under the control of thyrotropin releasing hormone (TRH).
- LH (gamma cells). Causes ovulation; in males stimulates interstitial cells to produce androgens. Controlled by luteinizing hormone releasing hormone (LHRH).

- Prolactin (eta cells). Causes broodiness (perhaps by suppressing release of the gonadotrophin hormones FSH and LH). Prolactin increases with norepinehprine, serotonin and histamine; it also produces hyperglycaemia and stimulates hepatic lipogenesis. Broodiness can be terminated by oestrogen (chickens) suggesting that oestrogens prevent release of prolactin from the pituitary.
- Somatotropic hormone (STH) (alpha cells). Regulates body growth. Also known as growth hormone.
- Adrenocorticotrophic hormone (ACTH) (epsilon cells). Regulates adrenal corticosteroid production. Presumably released when corticotropin releasing factor (CRF) is released. Stimulates adrenal cortical cells to produce and release corticosterone and other glucocorticoids.
- Melanotropic hormone (MSH) (kappa cells). Function unknown.

Releasing factors are formed in the hypothalamic nuclei and travel to the median eminence in some of the axons of the hypothalamohypophyseal tract. From there they enter the primary capillary plexus and, via the portal vessels, enter the secondary capillary plexus in the pars distalis and cause these cells to release their hormones.

THYROID

The paired thyroid glands are located on either side of the trachea on the ventral–lateral aspect of the neck just above the thoracic inlet and adhering to the common carotid artery just above the junction of the common carotid with the subclavian artery. They are medial to the jugular vein.

The gland is encapsulated by reticular connective tissue. Its follicles are composed of a single layer of endodermal epithelium of varying height, depending on the state of activity (secretory rate). Depending on the secretory state, the follicles may be filled with, or completely devoid of, colloid, which is a homogeneous fluid of protein gel composed of an iodinated protein, thyroglobulin (TG) (the storage form of thyroid hormones). During activity the amount of colloid is reduced and the secretory cells become taller. Between the follicles are connective tissue stroma, interfollicular cells and a rich blood supply.

The avian thyroid is unique in its lack of calcitonin cells; they are located separate from the thyroid gland in the ultimobranchial gland. Doves and pigeons appear to be exceptions, and are similar to the rat, with calcitonin cells found within the follicular epithelium.

Thyroid hormones (T_3 and T_4) are synthesized in a process similar to that in mammals. Iodide is concentrated within the thyroid, the so-called iodide trap. A peroxidase system within the thyroid converts the iodide to iodine and a second enzyme system is responsible for combining the iodinated tyrosines within the polypeptide chain of TG to form T_3 and T_4. Thyroid hormones are released from the thyroid as the predominant amino acid T_4. Once in the blood they are bound to protein. Both T_3 and T_4 are bound to serum albumin, and the binding affinity of albumin for T_3 and T_4 is the same. There is no thyroxine-binding globulin in avian species as there is in mammals. This binding of T_4 to albumin is evidently weak compared to that in man, resulting in more free T_4 in avian blood than in human or most mammalian blood. The half-lives of T_3 and T_4 are very short (measured in hours) and almost identical for both forms. The principal route of excretion of T_3 and T_4 is via bile and urine.

The function of the thyroid is governed by the concentration of the circulating thyroid hormones and their effects on the hypothalamic-controlled pituitary release of TSH. A decrease in the amount of circulating thyroid hormones to a level below metabolic requirements prompts the neuroendocrine-controlled anterior pituitary to increase the release of TSH. TSH stimulates the thyroid and produces both hypertrophy (increased cell size) and hyperplasia (an increase in cell numbers), together with accelerated formation or secretion of T_4.

Thyroid hormones play a major role in regulating the oxidative metabolism of birds and thus regulate heat production in response to changes in environmental temperature. Any pronounced alteration in thyroid function is reflected in an altered metabolic rate. Seasonal profiles of circulating T_4 and T_3 in birds suggest that T_4 seems to be associated with reproduction and moult, whereas T_3 is associated with calorigenesis and lipogenesis, especially during migration.

The size of the thyroid is influenced by several variables such as age, sex, climatic conditions, diet, activity, species and hypophysectomy. An iodine deficiency produces goitre (enlargement) due to cellular hyperplasia as a result of TSH stimulation. Low environmental temperatures increase thyroid activity and thus thyroid size. In primary hypothyroidism there is a loss of follicles resulting either from thyroiditis or atrophy, while in secondary or tertiary hypothyroidism the thyroid follicles are distended with colloid and the lining epithelial cells become flattened. In hyperthyroidism a diffusely hyperplastic epithelium may be observed, with little or no colloid present and possibly with lymphocytic infiltration.

PARATHYROID GLAND

In the chicken there are four parathyroid glands slightly caudal to the thyroid. A pair of glands is found on each side of the midline. Each pair represents an anterior and posterior lobe, which are often fused. The cranial gland is usually slightly larger. In the chicken the left parathyroid gland is not in contact with the thyroid gland, while the right-sided cranial lobe lies next to the thyroid gland.

Each parathyroid is encapsulated by connective tissue and is composed mainly of chief cells (very similar to those of the rat). Oxyphil cells are absent in many avian species. It may be assumed that the parathyroid chief cell in avian species is responsible for synthesis, packaging and secretion of parathyroid hormone (PTH).

PTH plays a major role in the regulation of blood calcium. It is secreted in response to hypocalcaemia and its effects appear to target the kidney and the bones. The initial response (within 30 minutes) is to decrease calcium excretion through the kidneys by increasing tubular reabsorption of calcium. It also causes an increased excretion of urinary phosphate. Renal tubular secretion appears to play a role in the response, although decreased tubular reabsorption of phosphate also plays a part, at least in the laying hen.

A third renal effect is the activation of vitamin D3 through the conversion of 25-hydroxycholecalciferol to 1,25-dihydroxycholecalciferol. Vitamin D3 elevates plasma calcium and inorganic phosphorus by increasing small intestinal absorption of these minerals. It also works with PTH to increase bone resorption and decrease calcium excretion.

ULTIMOBRANCHIAL GLANDS

The left and right ultimobranchial glands lie caudodorsal to the caudal lobe of the parathyroid gland. They are small, flattened, irregularly shaped and unencapsulated glands. They have four major components:

- C cells. Eosinophilic cells arranged in scattered groups and chords.
- Parathyroid nodules. Encapsulated accumulations of parathyroid tissue. Cords of parathyroid tissue grow from these nodules, penetrate between the C cells, and link up with the vesicles.

- Vesicles. Large proportion of the gland. Lined by secretory epithelium. They accumulate a carbohydrate–protein secretion in their lumen.
- Lymphoid tissue. Foci of lymphoid cells and thymus tissue.

The C cells secrete calcitonin, which blocks the transfer of calcium from bone to blood. However, in contrast to its action in mammals, calcitonin does not induce a hypocalcaemia in normocalcaemic birds. It appears, rather, to control hypercalcaemia and to protect the skeleton from excessive calcium resorption. Its mode of action is still unclear.

ADRENAL GLANDS

The paired avian adrenal glands are located anterior and medial to the cranial division of the kidney. They are flattened and lie close together, even fusing in some species. Their arterial blood supply comes from branches of the renal artery, and each gland has a single vein draining into the posterior vena cava. There is evidence in some species, including the domestic fowl, of an adrenal portal system between the glands and the muscles of the lateral abdominal wall. Sympathetic nerves reach the cranial and caudal ganglia on the pericapsular sheath of the adrenal glands. Nonmyelinated fibres originate from these ganglia and penetrate the gland. Each fibre innervates up to three chromaffin cells.

In birds, adrenal zonation is less clear than in mammals, with two zones, a subcapsular zone and an inner zone. Cortical and chromaffin tissue is intermingled in birds, with clusters or strands of chromaffin cells distributed throughout the cortical tissue. The adrenal cortical tissue is divided into a subcapsular zone, which is about 20–40 cells thick and produces aldosterone, and the more extensive inner zone, which produces corticosterone. Cortical tissue accounts for 70–80% of the avian adrenal gland. The cortical cells are arranged in numerous cords, with each being composed of a double row of parenchymatous inter-renal cells. The cords radiate from the centre of the gland, branching and anastomosing frequently, and loop against the inner surface of the connective tissue capsules. The arrangement of specific cell types along the cords results in some structural zonation. The cortical cells release primarily corticosterone and a smaller amount of aldosterone, along with some cortisol and cortisone (the levels of both decline as the bird reaches maturity). As in mammals, the secretion of corticosterone is primarily regulated by ACTH (corticotropin) that is released from the pituitary gland in response to CRF or AVT. The control of aldosterone secretion in birds is believed to be similar to that of mammals (i.e. via the renin–angiotensin system), although some control via the hypothalamus and pituitary gland is believed to occur. Renin is released from the juxtaglomerular cells of the kidney in response to various stimuli including low sodium concentrations and reduced blood volume. The renin acts on angiotensinogen to form angiotensin I, which is converted to angiotensin II. Aldosterone secretion is in turn stimulated by angiotensin II. In contrast to mammals, birds do not release aldosterone in response to elevated extracellular potassium concentrations. Therefore, aldosterone increases when blood volume decreases, sodium increases or under the influence of ACTH. Avian adrenocortical hormones may have both mineralocorticoid and glucocorticoid properties and play important roles in regulating metabolism, stress responses, reproduction, moulting and electrolyte homeostasis.

Chromaffin tissue constitutes about 15–20% of adrenal tissue. The chromaffin cells are in close association with blood spaces and appear to be more abundant in the middle of the gland. Two distinct types of chromaffin cells exist in the avian adrenal, releasing epinephrine and norepinephrine, respectively. These can be differentiated cytochemically and ultrastructurally, the latter including differences in the size and shape of the cytoplasmic neurosecretory granules. Chromaffin cells store and release the catecholamine hormones, either epinephrine or norepinephrine. The release, and presumably also the synthesis, of epinephrine and norepinephrine are separately controlled by the cholinergic innervation of the avian adrenal gland; in addition, hormones such as ACTH, corticosterone and aldosterone influence their synthesis and release. Their effects include changes to carbohydrate and lipid metabolism, cardiovascular parameters and the release of other hormones.

PANCREAS

The anatomy of the pancreas has been discussed earlier (see p. 17). Like pancreatic tissue in all other vertebrates, most (99%) of the organ is devoted to the synthesis and secretion, through well formed ducts, of digestive enzymes. The remaining 1–2% of the pancreas is endocrine and has no functional association with the pancreatic ducts. An extension of the ventral pancreatic lobe, which runs from the most superior portion of the lobe to the side of the spleen, is frequently referred to as the splenic lobe. This portion of the pancreas represents about 1–2% of the total wet weight of the organ and is without an exocrine duct. The majority of the pancreatic islet cells are in the splenic lobe. These islet clusters synthesize and release their peptide products directly into the bloodstream. Pancreatic hormones (released in response to absorbed nutrients, to cholinergic input and probably to hormonal stimulation) include insulin, glucagon, pancreatic polypeptide (PP) and somatostatin.

Two types of endocrine islets have been described. The larger (and more numerous) islets appear to be composed predominantly of the glucagon (A cell) type, but also contain some B, D and PP cells. D cells (somatostatin) frequently occupy a central position within the glucagon islets. The smaller (and less numerous) islets, documented to be predominantly B cells that synthesize and release insulin, are scattered throughout the pancreas, although B islets residing in the splenic lobe are very large compared with the those found elsewhere in the pancreas. Distribution of PP cells appears to be without preference for any single lobe. Thus, they are fairly uniformly distributed in islets, as PP cell clusters and as single cells throughout the entire acinar pancreas.

The proportion of cell types varies between species: in carnivorous birds the proportions are approximately 70% B cells, 20% A cells, 9% D cells and 1% PP cells; in granivorous birds the proportions have changed to 37% B cells, 50% A cells, 12% D cells and 1% PP cells.

A islets, containing predominantly glucagon-secreting cells, secrete glucagon, which is a powerful hepatic glycogenolytic agent. Glucagon levels in avian plasma have been reported to be at least 10–80 times higher than in mammals, and pancreatic tissue glucagon concentrations are two to four times higher in the various avian species studied. It therefore appears to be the dominant pancreatic hormone in granivorous birds. It is a powerful catabolic hormone, stimulating gluconeogenesis, glycogenolysis and lipolysis. Its release is triggered by free fatty acids, cholecystokinin and somatostatin, while insulin inhibits it. The insulin:glucagon ratio is usually 1:2, thus favouring catabolic reactions and ensuring a continuous supply of energy to sustain higher metabolic rate.

Insulin is synthesized within the B cell. Once in the bloodstream this hormone acts primarily as an anabolic agent to increase the availability of glucose transport carriers, allowing easier transfer of glucose into the cell. It inhibits gluconeogenic processes and may be involved in lipogenesis. Insulin is not antilipolytic in birds as it is in mammals, and it is known to decrease glucagon secretion in birds. Avian plasma levels of insulin are much higher than in mammals. Its secretion is not triggered by glucose; rather, it appears to be more sensitive to cholecystokinin, glucagons and a mixture of absorbed amino acids. Carnivorous birds are thought to be more insulin dependent than granivorous species, although it is still important in granivorous birds.

The PP cell is identified as the sole source of avian pancreatic polypeptide (APP). Circulating levels of APP in the well-fed bird approximate 6–10 ng/ml, a level that decreases about 50% after an overnight fast. These values are 40–60 times greater than those found in mammals, including man. In addition to inhibiting gastrointestinal motility and secretions, APP exerts certain metabolic effects in birds; it stimulates gastrin release and mobilizes liver glycogen, but has no effects on plasma glucose levels. It is primarily involved in lipogenesis, having an antilipolytic effect. Its levels rise sharply after a meal and it induces a sense of satiety.

Somatostatin is synthesized and secreted by the D cells. The D cell represents almost 30% of the cell population of dark (glucagon) islets, but only half of this population in insulin islets. The possibility exists that neural elements, with which the D cell appears to be well endowed (in the chicken), play a major role in regulating somatostatin release. Somatostatin depresses glucagon secretion and may act as the regulator of glucagon and insulin, 'fine tuning' their release. It also slows the absorption of nutrients, especially glucose and lipids, and inhibits lipolysis.

Growth hormone, thyroid hormones, prolactin and catecholamines are also involved in carbohydrate metabolism.

In many ways, carbohydrate metabolism in birds is similar to that in mammals. Differences include the hormonal control in granivorous birds, the absorption of glucose and gluconeogenesis. The end-product of digestion is glucose, which is then absorbed (usually passively) across the gut wall and either utilized locally by the enterocytes or enters portal circulation. It is then metabolized, aerobically or anaerobically, to produce adenosine triphosphate (ATP), which is used for energy. Glycogenesis (the formation of glycogen from glucose) occurs when there is excess glucose to body needs. Glycogen is synthesized in the liver and then stored in liver and muscle. This is controlled by glucagon (which controls liver glycogen stores) and epinephrine (which affects liver and muscle).

Gluconeogenesis is the formation of glucose from other molecules (usually lactate or glycerol) when there is insufficient intake of glucose. This occurs primarily in the liver, although there may be slight renal involvement. The transition to gluconeogenesis is rapid, usually beginning several hours postprandially. Carnivorous birds may exhibit continuous gluconeogenesis from amino acids, regardless of whether fed or not. This allows carnivorous birds to eat less frequently than granivorous birds.

Fasting or starvation induces catabolism; insulin levels are low while the glucagon levels are high. The glucagon stimulates lipolysis, as fat is preferentially mobilized during starvation. Glycogenolysis is also stimulated; hepatic glycogen is utilized first, but may be all gone within hours. Skeletal muscle stores are then used, especially in carnivorous birds. At this time blood glucose levels start to fall, stimulating gluconeogenesis, which begins after several days. Blood glucose levels then rise again. (In carnivorous birds, constant gluconeogenesis means that hepatic glycogen stores are usually untouched.) If the starvation continues, gluconeogenesis induces more protein catabolism to produce the amino acids needed for the process.

Hypermetabolism occurs when there is an increased demand for nutrients (e.g. sepsis, trauma, severe illness, surgery, pain, hypotension), leading to an associated increase in metabolic rate due to effect of catecholamines, glucocorticoids and glucagon, but at the same time there is a reduction in food intake or absorption. In this situation fat oxidation cannot meet demands for energy requirements and so body proteins are broken down for gluconeogenesis. This results in increased susceptibility to disease, delayed healing and wound dehiscence.

ORGANS OF THE SPECIAL SENSES
EYE

The size of eye is extremely large in relation to the head, particularly when compared with that of mammals; in many birds the two eyes together outweigh the brain. Large eyes equal a large image projected on the retina, which contributes to visual acuity. The globe can be one of three basic shapes. Flat globes are found in the majority of diurnal birds with narrow heads. The short distance between the cornea and the retina means that the image thrown onto the retina is relatively small, with corresponding low visual acuity. Globular globes are found in diurnal birds with wider heads, such as insectivorous wing-feeders, crows and diurnal birds of prey. The cone-shaped eyeball results in greater visual acuity. Tubular globes are found in nocturnal birds of prey; the elongated shape gives the greatest visual acuity.

The lower eyelid is thinner, more extensive and more mobile than the upper lid. In most species the eyelids only close when sleeping, therefore the nictitating membrane, lying beneath the eyelids on the nasal side of eye, is responsible for blinking. Tears are produced by the Harderian gland and the lacrimal gland, which is present inferior and lateral to the globe. The tears drain into the conjunctival sac on the bulbar surface of the lower lid and then exit via the inferior and superior nasolacrimal puncta at the medial canthus. Meibomian glands are absent in birds. In budgerigars and others, a nasal or salt gland lies in the orbit dorsomedial to the globe and the duct of this gland pierces the frontal bone and enters the nasal cavity. Hyperplasia of this gland may occur in waterfowl given drinking water high in salt. Modified feathers (filoplumes) are present near the eyelid margin and have a protective and tactile function.

The cornea is small compared to the rest of the eyeball. It is small in underwater swimmers and more extensive and more strongly curved in species such as eagles and owls with globular or tubular eyes. It consists of five layers: an anterior (outer) stratified squamous epithelium; an anterior (outer) limiting lamina (Bowman's membrane), not always differentiated in birds and not found in mammals; the substantia propria, consisting of bundles of collagen fibres, which forms the great bulk of the corneal wall; a posterior limiting lamina (Descemet's membrane); and a posterior (inner) layer of simple cuboidal epithelium.

The sclera is reinforced by a continuous layer of hyaline cartilage which, in the zone nearest the cornea, is modified into a ring of 10–18 small, roughly quadrilateral, overlapping bones called the scleral ossicles. The ossicles strengthen the eyeball and provide attachments for the ciliary muscles. In large eyes the scleral ossicles can be pneumatic. In many species, including falcons, hummingbirds, woodpeckers and passerines, the scleral cartilage around the optic nerve is ossified, forming a U-shaped bone called the os nervi optici. The scleral venous sinus (canal of Schlemm) is conspicuous in some species, but small or almost invisible in others; it lies at the limbus (junction between the cornea and sclera). The trabecular reticulum, or pectinate ligament, in this region (a wide-meshed plexus of connective tissue fibres) joins the limbus to the iris and to the ciliary body. The spaces between these fibres form the spaces of the irido-corneal angle (spaces of Fontana) through which the aqueous humor drains into the scleral venous sinus.

The uvea, the vascular part of the eye wall, consists of the choroid, the ciliary body and the iris. The choroid is a thick, highly vascular, darkly pigmented layer coating the retina. A tapetum lucidum is only found in a few nocturnal species. The choroid continues as the ciliary body and the iris. The ciliary body suspends the lens by the zonular fibres; it also forms small folds (ciliary processes), which are pressed against the rim of the lens by the ciliary muscles. The iris is dark in most species, but highly coloured in some. It forms a round aperture in most species. The ciliary muscles and the sphincter and dilator muscles of the iris are striated muscles, in contrast to the smooth muscle of mammals.

The retina arises as a direct continuation of the brain. It consists of an external, nonsensory single layer of cuboidal epithelium containing pigment (pigment epithelium) and an internal transparent and thicker neuroepithelium (sensory retina) containing several types of neurones and glial cells. Rods and cones are present in birds, serving similar functions as in mammals. The retina is thick compared to other vertebrates, and contains an array of photoreceptors and several possible combinations of areas and foveas specialized for more acute (and often stereoscopic) vision. It is completely devoid of blood vessels and derives its nutrients from both capillaries within the choroid, external to the pigment epithelium, and the well vascularized pecten with the vitreous body.

Areas are circumscribed thickenings of the sensory retina involving thinner and longer visual cells that improve the resolving power and are, therefore, associated with improved visual acuity in birds. There is almost always one central area, but often two or even three distinct areas (a circular lateral area and a horizontal linear area) are present. Foveas are depressions within either a central or lateral area or both. Not all areas have foveas, but foveas are only found within an area. Visual cell density is greater in the fovea than elsewhere in an area, and its shape acts to magnify the retinal image and increase its resolution. Although some species have no fovea, most have one or two. The location, depth and relative position of these foveas exhibit considerable variation depending on the species. The presence of three distinct retinal areas (central, lateral and linear), two of which (central and lateral) possess a fovea, is a unique avian adaptation that permits the formation of three separate and distinct visual fields (visual tridents), two lateral monocular fields (one for each eye) and a central binocular field.

Birds are able to detect a spatial frequency much higher than that of mammal: 160 frames/second compared with 60 frames/second in humans. This higher spatial frequency can cause problems under artificial light, which has a frequency of 100–120 frames/second and can therefore produce a stroboscopic effect, which may attribute to some behavioural disorders. High-frequency lights are therefore recommended for indoor birds.

The pecten, unique to birds, arises from the site of exit of the optic nerve and projects a variable distance into the vitreous body in the ventral and temporal quadrant of the fundus. It consists almost exclusively of capillaries and extravascular pigmented stromal cells; there are no muscular or neurological tissues. It can be conical, vaned or pleated. The pleated pecten is the most common structure, arising as a single accordion-pleated lamina held in place at its free (apical) end by a more heavily pigmented crest or bridge of tissue. The mass, shape, number and arrangement of pleats, their extent of pigmentation and their relationship to the ventral ciliary body varies considerably in different birds. The size of the pecten and number of pleats do not coincide with size of eye, but seem to be related to the behaviour of the bird towards illumination and its general level of activity. Active diurnal birds with a high visual acuity and monocular vision have a larger and more pleated pecten, while those nocturnal species with poor vision usually have a smaller pecten of simpler morphology. It may play a number of roles: nutrition of the retina; secretion of glycosaminoglycans and other products; regulation of intraocular pressure through the secretion of fluids; light absorption, which would reduce internal reflections that may possibly interfere with the production of a clear image; the perception of movement; and perhaps orientating birds in space by acting as a sextant, casting a shadow upon the retina to permit the latter to estimate the angular position and movement of the sun.

The lens of birds is much softer than that of mammals due to a fluid-filled lens vesicle between the annular pad and the body of the lens. This softness allows rapid accommodation. The lens is optically clear, rendering ultraviolet radiation visible. An annular pad runs around the equator of the lens, adjacent to the ciliary processes. This is well developed in diurnal predators, but reduced in nocturnal species and flightless species. It has extensive equatorial thickening for contact with the ciliary body. Contraction of the ciliary muscles thrusts the ciliary body inward against the annular pad, transmitting the stress directly to the softer lenticular centre. This occurs evenly along the entire extent of the equatorial lens, and allows for flexible accommodation and focuses light directly onto the retina. The transparency of the avian lens allows the passage of a broader spectrum of light than mammals, allowing birds to see not only blue, green and red, but also ultraviolet and fluorescent.

Both the anterior and posterior chambers of the eye are filled with aqueous humor, which is responsible for regulating intraocular pressure and maintaining the proper shape and rigidity of the eyeball. It is continually secreted into the posterior chamber by the ciliary body and then circulates through the pupil and into the anterior chamber. It then drains into the scleral venous sinus through the spaces of Fontana at the iridocorneal angle (**26**).

The attainment of exceptional avian visual abilities is the result of both the structure and function of the eye. The positioning of the eyes allows, in many birds, a wide field of vision. The large size of the eye permits the formation of a large retinal image. The actions of the cornea, lens and aqueous humor provide a superb accommodative apparatus, increasing the depth of focus. The retina acts as a parabolic reflector, allowing all round visual acuity, unlike mammals, which only have central vision acuity. And finally, the presence of elaborate and diverse retinal areas and foveas provide a high degree of acute monocular and binocular vision.

EAR

Birds have a keen sense of hearing and a high degree of equilibration. Their excellent voice production and remarkable ability to imitate sounds has inferred an exceptional degree of sound analysis (pitch

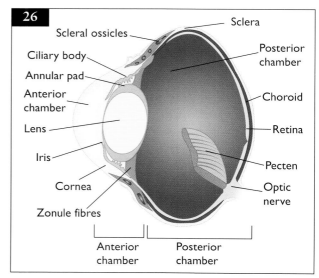

26 The eye.

discrimination) within a wide range of auditory frequencies. Their aerial mode of life demands sonic acuity, in addition to a well coordinated balance and position sense. In many ways the avian ear closely resembles the mammalian ear, but it is simpler in structure and reptilian in design. It includes three separate but contiguous anatomical segments (the external, middle and inner ears). These develop completely independently and from different embryonic primordia and then combine to form a synchrononized functional unit.

The external ear collects sound waves from the outside air and conducts them to the middle ear. It consists of a collecting device, the external acoustic meatus (a small aperture, nearly always circular, which opens externally on the side of the head), and a simple conducting tube. It terminates medially as a partition, the tympanic membrane (eardrum), completely separating the external ear from the middle ear. It is covered by specialized contour feathers (the ear coverts) in most birds; the width of the feathers is related to sound localization and their fine structure varies in accordance with auditory efficiency. The coverts lying on the rostral aspect of the meatus reduce the drag caused by turbulence in flight and thus diminish the masking of sound by noise generated from turbulence in the external ear; the barbs of these ear coverts lack barbules; the sound waves are not obstructed. On the caudal aspect of the meatus these specialized feathers combine into a tight funnel, which is particularly enlarged in songbirds, parrots and falcons.

The middle ear is an air-filled, ossicle-containing space (tympanic cavity) that receives the sound waves as mechanical vibrations of the tympanic membrane in its lateral wall and transfers them in an amplified form to the inner ear at its medial wall. It is directly continuous with the pharynx via the pharyngotympanic tube (Eustachian tube), which enters the pharynx at the interfundibular cleft. The middle ear also communicates with a large group of accessory air cavities occupying the surrounding skull bones and then extending into the mandible and beak in some species. The right and left tympanic cavities communicate with each other via interconnecting air sinuses; this has been implicated in the transference of pressure fluctuations emanating at the round window.

In contrast to mammals, birds transfer sound with a single skeletal element, the columella, which extends medially across the tympanic cavity to form a direct connection between the tympanic membrane and the fluid within the inner ear. The columella is homologous to the mammalian stapes; the mammalian incus and maleus are homologous to the avian quadrate and articular bones, respectively. The tympanic membrane and columella function as a mechanical transformer that matches the impedance of air and inner ear fluid, facilitating the transfer of sound energy. The tension in the tympanic membrane is altered by the columellar muscle, which attaches to the columella and to the tympanic membrane itself. Vibrations of the tympanic membrane are carried to the perilymph of the inner ear by the extracolumella cartilage in contact with the tympanic membrane and the rod-like bony columella, which is implanted medially in the vestibular window. The cochlear (round) window lies near the vestibular window; it is in contact with the scala tympani of the inner ear.

The inner ear is responsible for the initial analysis and characterization of the sound vibrations and for maintaining equilibrium. It consists of two very complex, fluid-filled components or labyrinths, one membranous, the other bony. The membranous labyrinth includes several nonauditory receptive areas composing the vestibular labyrinth and a single organ of hearing, the cochlear labyrinth. The vestibular labyrinth is a series of canals and ducts filled with endolymph and surrounded by perilymph. It is then encased within the bony labyrinth. The cochlea is a relatively short and slightly curved tube containing the cochlear duct (scala media) filled with endolymph. It ends at the lagena, which contains a group of sensory cells; afferent nerve fibres from this area appear to end in the auditory centres of the medulla.

Movement of endolymph within the vestibular labyrinth provides the bird with its proprioception. Vibrations carried through the cochlear duct are detected in the brain as sound.

CHEMICAL SENSES

The olfactory capabilities of birds have been controversial for years. Research conducted over the last two decades has indicated that birds possess olfactory systems whose complexity and development vary widely among species. They possess nasal conchae, but lack a vomeronasal (Jacobsen's) organ. The turbinates of the third nasal conchae possess olfactory epithelium; the peripheral terminals of the olfactory nerves lie in this epithelium and communicate with the olfactory bulbs of the brain. The sense of smell is well developed in kiwis, New World vultures, albatross and petrels; it is moderately developed in poultry, pigeons and most birds of prey; and poorly developed in songbirds. It is possible that development of a sense of smell is related to food sources (e.g. vultures are carrion feeders that are led to the general area of food by olfaction; once in the general area they rely on vision to find the food source).

The function of a sense of taste (gustation) is to encourage ingestion of nutrients, to discriminate among foods that are available and to avoid toxic foodstuffs. As such, gustation in a particular species can be expected to complement digestion, metabolism and the dietary requirements of that species. Taste receptors (buds) are found in close association with the salivary glands at the base of the tongue and the floor of pharynx. Some are found in other areas and the number of buds and their distribution may change over time. The glossopharyngeal nerves innervate posterior buccal and pharyngeal areas. Cutaneous and taste information is carried by both nerves. The relationship between the number of taste buds and taste behaviour is not clearly defined; the relatively poor taste acuity in birds may be related to the small number of sensory cells.

Most avian species demonstrate little or no interest in common sugars except for parrots, hummingbirds and nectar feeders. These birds will actively select sugar solutions. While many birds kept on salt-free diets will actively pursue salt when offered, few will drink salt water at a concentration greater than its kidney can handle; many will die of thirst rather than drink. In parrots the salt threshold appears to be 0.35%. There is a wide range of tolerance for sour tastes, as there is for bitter foods. The temperature of the food is an important factor; many birds will reject food that is significantly higher than their body temperature.

The common chemical sense is relatively primitive; the senses of taste and olfaction are later differentiations. The major component of the common chemical sense is the trigeminal system. Irritants such as ammonia and acids stimulate free nerve endings of the nasal chamber, mouth and eyelids. It differs between species. For example, pigeons are indifferent to strong ammonia that can affect other birds and parrots can consume capsicum peppers that other birds cannot.

THE IMMUNE SYSTEM

The major lymphoid organs found in birds are the thymus and bursa of Fabricius and, to a lesser extent, the spleen and disseminated lymphoid tissue. Other than some waterfowl, birds do not have discrete lymph nodes.

The thymus is found in the neck, often in multiple sites extending from the angle of the jaw to the thoracic inlet. It consists of lobules of epithelial cells, each covered by a connective tissue capsule. Each lobule has an outer dark cortex and an inner light medulla. Lymphocytes are most dense in the cortex, while thymic corpuscles (islands of reticular tissue known as Hassal's corpuscles) are present in the medulla. The thymus is at its largest in the sexually immature bird. It serves as the source of T lymphocytes, which are the circulating cells responsible for cell-mediated immune responses. Approximately 65% of the mononuclear cells in the spleen and 80% of the mononuclear cells in blood of chickens are T cells.

The bursa of Fabricius is a dorsal median diverticulum of the proctodeal region of the cloaca. It contains a central cavity that forms a single large cavity opening into the proctodeum. The internal wall of the bursa is folded and covered by simple columnar or pseudostratified columnar epithelium. Lymphoid nodules are located between these epithelial folds. Each nodule has a cortex and a medulla, separated by a basement membrane and epithelial cells. Lymphocytes, plasma cells and macrophages are found in the cortex, while lymphoblasts and lymphocytes are found in the medulla. In the embryo the medulla is the first lymphoid organ to produce immunoglobulins. Mature B lymphocytes, responsible for humoral immunity, migrate from the bursa to peripheral/secondary lymphoid tissue. This occurs as early as day 17 of incubation. It also produces a hormone, bursapoietin, which stimulates the movement of B cells from the yolk sac to the bursa, and induces maturation of bone marrow cells. The bursa involutes as the bird ages; in psittacines this may take as long as 18–20 months, compared with chickens where the bursa has involuted by 2–3 months of age.

The spleen is found on the right side of the junction between the proventriculus and the ventriculus. It varies in size and shape; it may be round, elongated or slightly triangular, depending on species of bird. There are no well-defined trabeculae; instead there is a basic network of reticular fibres and cells. Lymphoid tissue, known as white pulp, surrounds the arteries and is responsible for lymphopoiesis. Numerous venous sinuses are present, surrounded by lymphocytes, macrophages and elements of circulating blood. This red pulp is responsible for the phagocytosis of aged erythrocytes. Both white and red pulp contribute towards antibody production. The spleen does not function as a significant blood reservoir.

Disseminated lymphoid tissue is found in the Harderian gland in the third eyelid, throughout the alimentary tract (caecal tonsils, oropharynx, small intestine, and caudal oesophagus) and as solitary nodules in all organs and the bone marrow. It responds to antigens similarly to the spleen.

The immune system serves two primary purposes; it clears infection from the body and it then develops a pathogen-specific resistance to protect the bird from future infections. It does this through a combination of nonspecific defences (including barriers such as the skin and mucosa, and the innate immune system — macrophages, heterophils, thrombocytes and complement) and specific defences, including humoral (B cells) and cell-mediated immunity (T cells).

Macrophages (in tissue) and monocytes (in blood) identify and consume damaged cells and foreign materials. They are attracted to sites of inflammation by lymphokines produced by damaged cells. Once this phagocytosis is complete, more lymphokines are released by the macrophages/monocytes, which attract B and T cells.

B cells produce antibodies (proteins that coat and neutralize an invading pathogen and 'mark' infected cells so that the immune system can identify and destroy them). An antigen, usually a protein on the pathogen, may activate a B cell directly or initially bind an accessory cell that leads to the activation of T and then B cells. Either way, the B cell then differentiates into the antibody-producing plasma cell.

Antibody response can be either a primary response, stimulated the first time the body is infected with a specific pathogen, or a secondary response to subsequent reinfections. A primary response is characterized by a lengthy (1–2 week) latent phase during which immunocompetent cells are activated, leading to a progressive increase in circulating antibody. This initial antibody is usually IgM; it declines after reaching a peak. A secondary response is characterized as a shortened latent period, with a peak of antibody production, usually IgG (although some species utilize IgY), occurring earlier and at higher levels. Young birds originally passively derive both IgM and IgG (IgY) from the egg yolk and albumen, but an active humoral system begins to develop approximately two weeks after hatching, reaching maturity at 4–6 weeks of age.

Following the humoral response is the cell-mediated response. T cells originate in the thymus, and therefore cell-mediated immunity is dependent on the normal development of the thymus. Lymphokines (chemotactic factor, thrombocyte migratory inhibitory factor, interleukins 1 and 2, several types of interferons and lymphocytotoxin) attract both B and T cells to an area of inflammation. There are three types of T cell: T helper cells, which release chemical signals controlling other cells involved in the immune response; T cytotoxic cells, which destroy infected and damaged cells; and T suppressor cells, which modulate the effect on the immune system, preventing over-stimulation and autoimmune damage.

FURTHER READING

Jones MP (1994) Avian immunology: a review. In: *Proceedings of the Annual Conference of the Association of Avian Veterinarians*, pp. 333–336.

King AS, McLelland J (1984) *Birds: Their Structure and Function*, 2nd edn. Baillière Tindall, London.

Korbel RT (2002) Avian ophthalmology: principles and application. In: *Proceedings of the World Small Animal Veterinary Association Congress 2002*.

Whittow G (ed). (1999) *Sturkie's Avian Physiology*, 5th edn. Academic Press, San Diego.

CHAPTER 2
THE PHYSICAL EXAMINATION

UNDERSTANDING THE MASKING PHENOMENON

A common misconception held by many bird owners (and many veterinarians) is that birds are not very resistant to illness. To the novice it often appears that birds show signs of illness one day, are at the bottom of their cage the next, and dead the day after. This misconception has stemmed from two sources.

Firstly, many of the birds seen in practice are only a few generations descended from wild birds. As such, they still retain many of the protective instincts inherited from their forebears. As many of the species kept as companions are relatively low on the food chain, quite a few of these instincts have been developed to avoid drawing the attention of predators. One such instinct is often known as the masking phenomenon. Predators are naturally drawn to prey that looks or behaves differently from others. Unusual colouring, weakness and lameness can single out a bird and make it a draw card for a predator. A

natural instinct is therefore to avoid looking 'different': a sick bird will make a determined effort to look healthy, even when there are no predators around (**27**). The classical 'sick bird look' signs we usually associate with illness (fluffed up, eyes closed, lethargic) only develop when the bird is incapable of masking these signs (**28**). Many of the patients presented to veterinarians are well past the initial stages of their illness and are now decompensating rapidly.

There are many subtle changes in a bird's behaviour or appearance, however, that are indications of a health problem. While these signs are often discernible by experienced owners and veterinarians, they are just as often overlooked by those with less experience. Missing these early signs, when combined with the bird's efforts to mask obvious clinical signs, invariably leads to the late detection of illness and the presentation of the bird *in extremis*. It is important that veterinarians learn to recognize these early signs of

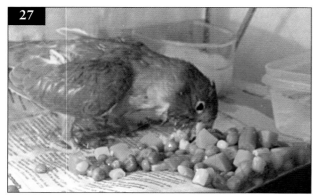

27 The 'masking phenomenon'. This bird was eating just minutes before it died.

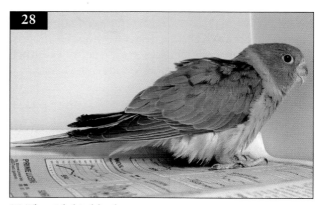

28 The sick bird look.

illness, and then educate their clients so that illnesses can be detected before becoming too advanced.

The masking phenomenon and the ease with which early clinical signs can be overlooked highlight the importance of regular health examinations for the companion bird. Long-standing conditions such as malnutrition can be detected and corrected before the bird begins to decompensate and show signs of overt illness.

EXAMINATION ROOM EQUIPMENT

Appropriate equipment for use in the examination room includes:
- A supply of freshly laundered towels of different sizes (or paper towels) for restraining birds.
- Scales capable of weighing in grams, preferably with a detachable T-perch (to allow birds to perch on while being weighed), and a container in which to weigh smaller birds.
- A training perch for the bird to perch on while being examined.
- Clinical equipment such as a stethoscope, a focal light source, magnifying loupes, needles and syringes, blood collection bottles and culture swabs.
- Alcohol for wetting feathers down for a closer examination of the skin and underlying fat and muscle.
- Treats to reward pet birds and make the experience more enjoyable (or at least, less stressful).

The use of gloves to catch and restrain birds should be discouraged. With these gloves on, the clinician cannot be sensitive to small movements of the bird, and can easily hurt or even kill the patient.

Ensure the room is escape-proof, and that clinic staff do not enter the room unexpectedly. Avoid stressful sights and sounds such as dogs, cats and other potential predators.

HISTORY TAKING

The collection of an accurate and thorough history of a patient is as crucial to making a diagnosis as the physical examination and appropriate diagnostic testing. A good history can alert the clinician to likely problems and allow him/her to focus on likely possibilities and refine the rest of the diagnostic approach. History taking can be divided into:
- Background history:
  - Signalment.
  - Origin of the bird.
  - Husbandry.
  - Nutrition.
- Behaviour.
- Previous medical history.
- Presenting problem.

SIGNALMENT
The first step in obtaining a history is to gain as much information about the bird itself as possible. A good receptionist or technician can often obtain such information, but the clinician needs to be familiar with birds in general, as often clients are not aware of some basic facts about their bird (such as species, sex and age). Things that need to be ascertained include:
- The species of bird. The clinician needs to be able to recognize common species and have access to literature that will enable him/her to identify other species. Be aware of local names that may differ from those in the literature. Knowing the species, its behaviour and its dietary requirements can offer the clinician vital clues to likely problems.
- The age of the bird can offer other clues. As a general rule, juveniles are more likely to suffer from infectious diseases and nutritional deficiencies, while adult birds are more likely to suffer from neoplasia, chronic malnutrition and degenerative conditions.
- The sex of the bird. Many psittacids are sexually monomorphic and require DNA or surgical sexing. Do not accept the owner's assertion of their bird's sex, unless they have proof of sex identification (e.g. a history of egg laying or a certificate of sex identification that can be correlated with this bird). Knowing the sex of a bird can be vital, as many conditions, including behavioural problems, can be linked to the bird's sex. For example, abdominal hernias are almost nonexistent in male birds, while being relatively common in females; yolk-related peritonitis is obviously only seen in hens; cocks do not become egg-bound.

ORIGIN OF THE BIRD
- How long have the clients owned this bird? Birds that have been in the owner's possession for many years, with no recent exposure to other birds, are less likely to have infectious diseases. Recently obtained birds are more likely to have been in close contact with other birds and, as such, have possibly been exposed to infectious diseases.
- Where did the owner obtain the bird? With experience, the clinician will be able to identify 'problem sources' of birds in the local area (e.g. a certain breeder or a pet shop). Developing

a working knowledge of the quality of the sources of pet birds in your area can be a key element of patient evaluation in your practice.

- Is the bird aviary bred or wild caught? Wild-caught psittacids, although less common in recent times, still appear occasionally in the pet market. The behaviour and diseases of such a bird may well be linked to its source.
- Is the bird hand reared or parent reared? The health of juvenile birds is dependent to a large extent on the health and nutrition of the parents. Hand-reared birds have two additional factors to be aware of, namely the quality of the hand-rearing formula being fed and the skill of the person doing the rearing. Parent-reared birds tend to be more difficult to tame, unless they are handled on a regular basis before fledging. Hand-reared birds on the other hand, while usually more closely bonded to people, often have behavioural disorders associated with poor socialization skills, especially if reared in isolation. If a large number of chicks from different sources are reared in the one facility, there is a higher probability of the spread of diseases such as polyomavirus and *Chlamydophila*. All of these factors need to be assessed during the history collection, especially when examining juvenile birds.

HUSBANDRY

- How has the bird been managed? Is it an aviary bird, a companion bird or a zoological specimen? An assessment of a companion bird's husbandry must include the cage, the environment around the cage and the bird's interaction with its environment (**29, 30, 31, 32**).
- Ascertain whether the cage in the examination room is the bird's permanent cage or simply a transport cage. If the latter, ask the owner to describe the permanent cage or to bring along photographs or video images.
- Where is the cage located in the house? Is it exposed to toxins such as burning Teflon®, cigarette smoke or household plants? Does the bird get any privacy? Is it kept isolated, away from family activities? Does it get a good night's

sleep or is it forced to stay up with its owner watching television all night? Does the bird get access to direct, unfiltered sunlight on a daily basis? If the bird is kept outside, is it safe from predators and from vectors of diseases such as *Sarcocystis*?

- Does the bird come out of its cage? How long does it have outside the cage each day? Are its wings clipped? Is it supervised when out of the cage? Does it interact with other animals and birds?
- Does the client have other birds? Any other pets?

NUTRITION

Underlying many health problems in pet birds is a common thread of malnutrition. For many generations bird owners have accepted as fact that birds eat seed, and that is all they need (**33**). Birds, as with many other animals, have a preference for high-fat diets. Given a choice between seed, vegetables, formulated diets and fruits, nearly all birds will consume the seed first. Given this preference, it is not surprising to hear many bird owners state, 'All he will eat is the seed, so that is all that I give him.' See **34** and **35**.

It is therefore important to ascertain:

- What does the owner feed the bird and what does the bird actually eat? The clinician needs to be aware that there are major species differences in dietary requirements with, for example, some species having a higher requirement for fat than others. There is no one diet to suit all avian species, any more than there is one diet to suit all mammalian species.
- How much food is being consumed? (Some birds on an excellent diet will still eat too much and gain excessive weight.)
- Is the food prepared fresh daily?
- Are dishes cleaned each day?
- Does the bird dunk food into its water dish, creating a nutrient-rich broth ideal for bacterial contamination?
- Does the bird get any treats such as food off their owner's plate?
- Are vitamin and mineral supplements being offered?

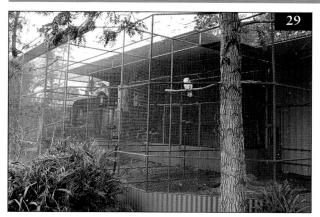

29 Full flight aviaries allow for greater movement in all directions and provide a more 'natural' environment. However, if not managed well, parasitic ova and eggs can accumulate on the floor, adding internal parasitism to the list of potential husbandry issues.

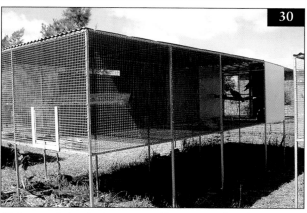

30 Suspended aviaries are usually parasite free, but it can be argued that they limit the birds' ability to exihibit normal behaviours.

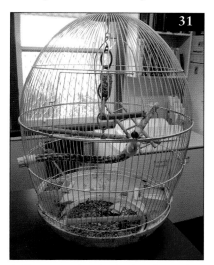

31 Inappropriately sized and poorly cleaned cage.

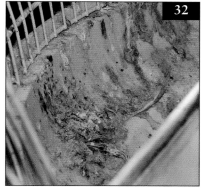

32 The floor of the cage in 31.

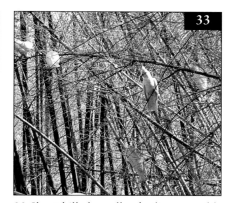

33 Short-billed corellas feeding on wild bamboo. Contrary to popular belief, wild birds eat a wide range of foods, not just seed.

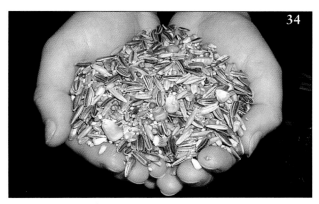

34 Typical high-fat seed diet.

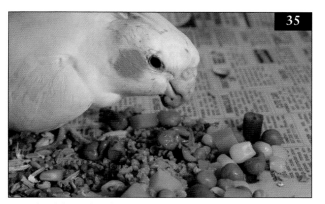

35 A healthier diet for pet birds incorporates formulated foods, vegetables and sometimes a small amount of seed.

Paediatric cases open another spectrum of questions. What hand-rearing formula is being used? How is it prepared? Are the manufacturer's recommendations being followed? Has anything extra been added to an already balanced diet? At what temperature has it been fed? How much has been fed, and how often? How has the chick been fed: syringe, crop tube or spoon? How are these utensils cleaned and disinfected?

BEHAVIOUR

A behavioural history is becoming increasingly more important as pet birds move out of their cages and more into their owners' lives. Just as countless dogs and cats are euthanased every year because of behavioural problems, many birds suffer the same fate, or are transferred from household to household, for the same reasons.

As psittacine behaviour is determined to a large extent by the interaction between the bird, its owners and its environment, questioning must focus on these areas:
- How many hours per day does the bird spend alone?
- What does the bird see and hear when it is alone?
- Does the bird spend time with other birds or other pets?
- Are toys provided for the bird? Does it utilize those toys?

It is important to clarify the bird's interaction with its owners (human flock):
- Who is the primary caretaker?
- Who does the bird seem to prefer?
- Does the bird dislike anyone?
- How tame is the bird?
- Does it readily step up on to a proffered hand?
- Does it always try to move up on to a person's shoulder? Is this allowed or encouraged?
- Does the bird talk?
- Does it like to be petted? Where?
- How does it react to different family members?
- How does it react to strangers?

PREVIOUS MEDICAL HISTORY

It is important to ascertain the patient's medical history. Has the bird been ill before? Who saw it, what did they diagnose, and how was it treated? Has it had remedies supplied by pet shops or breeders? Is the bird being presented for a second opinion or a specialist referral? If appropriate, permission to obtain copies of medical records from the previous (or referring) veterinarian should be requested.

PRESENTING PROBLEM
- What exactly is the problem? This needs to be clarified with the client, as confusion often exists between owners and veterinarians over the precise description of clinical signs.
- When did it start?
- Is this the first time it has happened?
- Have other treatments been tried? Who prescribed these treatments? Did they work?
- Is this condition progressing or static, or perhaps even improving?
- Are other birds affected?

The history taking described above is not a comprehensive review of every possible question that can be asked of the owner. As the process continues, areas of interest will become apparent and more questions may be needed to clarify these areas. The clinician must take care to ensure that he/she does not dominate the conversation; rather, ask short questions and listen carefully to the client's reply. However, the clinician must be prepared to guide the discussion, as otherwise some clients may become distracted and lose track of the original question!

THE DISTANT EXAMINATION

Although the history taking should be done before the bird is handled, the clinician should be using this time to gain some insights into the bird and its health by careful observation of the bird, its cage and its droppings.

THE BIRD
- Most birds, no matter how ill they are, will make an effort to mask their clinical signs when first brought into the examination room. This effort will rarely last long, usually only a minute or two. Avoid disturbing the bird until it has settled, otherwise valuable clinical signs may be overlooked.
- Watch the bird's breathing. Once the bird has settled in its cage in the examination room, there should be no open-mouth breathing, marked tail bobbing or marked respiratory effort. There should be no audible respiratory noise. The presence of these signs should alert the clinician to the likelihood of respiratory compromise and great care must obviously be taken with handling such a patient.

- Look at the bird's posture. Many sick birds become hypothermic and attempt to conserve body heat and energy by fluffing their feathers, sitting still and sleeping more. These signs are often referred to as the 'sick bird look', but not all sick birds will display these signs. Evidence of a wing droop, lameness or reluctance to bear weight on one leg indicates a musculoskeletal problem. Spinal deformities can often be detected by an abnormal positioning of the tail. An upright position with a wide-legged stance may indicate egg-binding or a similar space-occupying lesion in the coelom. Birds holding both wings away from their body and panting are usually heat stressed.
- Examine the plumage. Normally it should be sleek and well groomed, and should be clean. Untidy or dirty plumage can indicate either that the bird is not grooming itself for some reason or that there is a feather dystrophy of some description. Discoloured feathering can reflect a variety of problems, such as psittacine beak and feather disease (PBFD), chronic liver disease, excessive handling with oily hands or malnutrition.
- Examine the beak and toenails. Overgrown or flaky beaks or overgrown and twisted nails can be associated with PBFD, poor husbandry, chronic liver disease or malnutrition.
- Watch the bird defecate. Look for signs of straining or discomfort and listen for any accompanying flatulence.
- Observe the bird's behaviour, assessing how tame the bird is and whether it is showing any overt sexual display towards the owner or other people present in the room. Look at how the owner interacts with the bird, as this can give valuable clues to relationships at home.

THE CAGE

- Is the cage large enough to allow the bird to extend and flap its wings and to turn around without damaging feathers (36)?
- Is it constructed of materials that are safe for the bird and appropriate for the size and power of the bird's beak?
- Is the floor of the cage solid or wire? Is it covered in grit, sand or wood shavings, which becomes soiled quickly, is not changed frequently enough and may be ingested, leading to gastrointestinal obstructions. Newspaper is an appropriate lining, as it is nontoxic, readily available and cheap, and therefore more likely to be changed frequently as it becomes soiled.
- Many cages are sold with plastic or wooden dowel perches. These are rarely suitable, as the smooth, unchanging surface and diameter offer little exercise for the feet and toes. If these perches are present, the bird should be checked for pododermatitis. The positioning of the perches is also important; can the bird defecate and urinate into its own food and water?
- Dishes should be constructed of a material appropriate to the species using them, and free of contaminants such as the lead solder often seen on cheap galvanized dishes. They should be cleaned daily and positioned where they are unlikely to be soiled. Food and water dishes should not be placed alongside each other, as many birds will drop their food into the water, producing a broth within a few hours.
- Toys should be appropriate for the bird and not overcrowding the cage. Cheap toys, especially bells, are a common source of lead. Toys should be made of natural materials such as rope and wood and should be replaced as soon as they become frayed.
- Is the bird offered the opportunity to bathe, or at least be misted, on a daily basis?

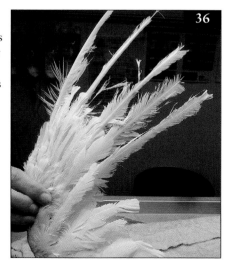

36 These primary feathers have been badly damaged by striking the bars of the cage.

FAECAL EXAMINATION

Birds' droppings are made up of three components: faeces, urates and urine (37). In a healthy bird the faecal portion should be formed and homogeneous, with little odour (except for poultry, waterfowl and carnivorous birds). The colour should range from brown to green. The urates should be a crisp white and slightly moist. Old droppings will have greenish urates as biliverdin leaches out of the faeces. The urine should only extend a couple of millimetres past the dropping. True polyuria should not be confused with so-called 'excitement polyuria', the excess urine produced by an excited or nervous bird. Lorikeets, due to their liquid diet, will produce large amounts of urine, which should not be mistaken for pathological polyuria. A close examination of the droppings is a valuable starting point to a clinical examination.

Some abnormalities commonly encountered include:

- Diarrhoea. Unformed faecal portion.
- Undigested food in faeces (38).
- Very bulky droppings indicate maldigestion, malabsorption, reproductively active hens, abdominal growth or pelleted diets (39).
- Melena or very dark droppings can indicate anorexia or intestinal haemorrhage (40).
- Malodorous droppings are often associated with bacterial/fungal overgrowth.

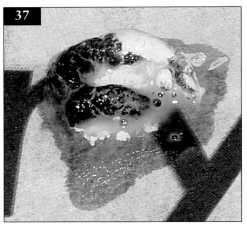

37 Normal droppings.

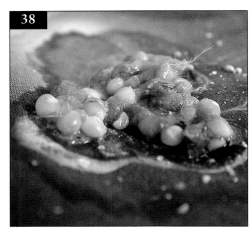

38 Whole seed in droppings.

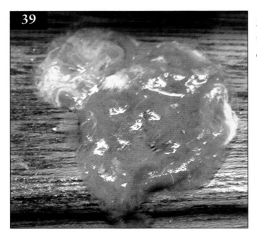

39 Bulky, unformed droppings.

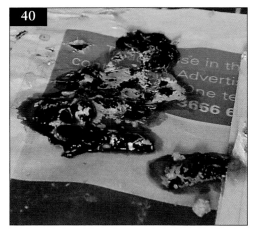

40 Melena.

- Green urates (biliverdinuria) are often indicative of liver disease (**41**).
- Pink/red urates (haematuria/haemoglobinuria) are seen in cases of renal disease often associated with lead poisoning, especially in Amazon parrots and galahs (**42**).
- Yellow urates can be associated with anorexia.

- Orange urates indicate that a vitamin B injection may have been given in the last few hours.
- Thick, pasty urates are seen in dehydrated birds.
- Polyuria.
- Anuria.
- Discoloured urine: similar causes to discoloured urates (**43**).
- Fresh blood indicates either a cloacal problem or oviductal disease.

THE PHYSICAL EXAMINATION

A thorough, systematic physical evaluation of the patient is essential to obtaining clues about the bird's problem and diagnosis. Clinicians should develop a thorough examination protocol that they are comfortable with, and use it for every patient regardless of the reason for presentation.

HANDLING AND RESTRAINT

At some time during every examination the veterinarian must handle, and sometimes restrain, the patient. Traditionally, it was considered acceptable to put on a heavy pair of gloves, pin the bird to the tabletop or the side of the cage and then drag it, struggling and screaming, into a position where it could be better examined. Undoubtedly this stress, imposed on an already compromised patient, contributed to the myth that birds were 'soft' animals, prone to dying while just being examined!

Just as it is inappropriate to muzzle and grapple with every dog and cat that comes into a veterinary surgery, it is inappropriate to use heavy-handed restraint on a companion bird. Many of these birds have learnt to trust humans and regard them affectionately. Destroying this trust through aggressive catching and handling techniques can adversely affect the bond between owner and bird. This relationship must be preserved at all costs, and handling techniques for closely bonded birds should emphasize minimal stress and fear.

As the oils on human skin can be detrimental to the feathers of many species, a light dusting of talcum powder on the clinician's hands is appropriate before beginning an examination. This is particularly necessary for those birds that do not produce powder down (e.g. Amazons, eclectus parrots and lorikeets). Handled frequently without talcum powder, the green feathers on these birds begin to acquire a black discoloration that can become quite unsightly.

If the bird is presented in a cage or carrier, it is often more appropriate to ask the owner to remove the bird from its cage. Doing so will often relax the bird in a

41 Green urates.

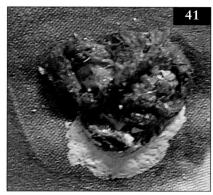

42 Haematuria.

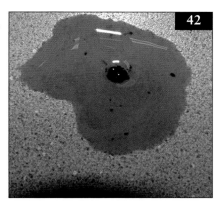

43 Biliverdinuria and polyuria, highly suggestive of liver disease.

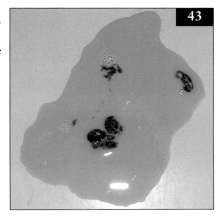

new environment. If the owner is unwilling (or unable) to do so, the clinician should firstly offer the bird the opportunity to step out of the cage by itself. If it is unwilling to do so, an attempt should be made to bring the bird out on the clinician's hand (if the cage door is large enough). A hand is slowly and gently introduced into the cage, with the back of the hand to the bird. If there is no aggression, the forefinger or hand is extended and placed under the bird's chest. A tame bird will usually step on to the finger or hand. If possible, one toe is restrained by gently pressing on it with a thumb against the finger, keeping the bird steady, and it is gently brought out of the cage. During this procedure the clinician should keep talking to the bird, praising it and maintaining eye contact. When the bird is out of the cage, one should continue to talk to it and praise it, scratch its ear and generally make a fuss of it.

If the bird will not step on to a hand, it is best to use a small hand (or paper) towel to gently envelop and then restrain the bird. The bird is shown the towel and allowed to get used to it. If possible, the clinician should slowly envelop the bird in the towel from below; an approach from above is potentially a very intimidating experience for a pet bird. The clinican should keep talking in a friendly voice and maintain eye contact.

Birds that are not tame can be caught using a towel as described above. These birds will rarely stay still during capture, so a quick capture is the best approach. A few seconds spent removing obstacles in the cage (food and water containers, perches, toys) is a worthwhile endeavour, as it will reduce the bird's opportunities to avoid capture.

Once the bird has been removed from the cage, the next step will be determined by how tame it is. Very tame birds can be placed on a T-perch for further examination and weighing; less tame birds may need to be examined while restrained in the towel.

At all times the clinician must be aware of the bird and how it is handling the stress of restraint and examination. As many birds are presented for evaluation of an illness, and they have been ill for some time, even being restrained can add extra burden to an already overburdened body. Collapse and death are, unfortunately, not uncommon with critically ill birds. (If the bird appears critically ill when first presented, it is often worthwhile having oxygen and mask on hand to assist with resuscitation if the bird collapses.) If there is any doubt as to the bird's ability to cope with the stress, it should be immediately returned to a perch or the cage and be allowed to regain its composure before proceeding.

Once the examination is complete the bird can be gently replaced in its cage the same way it was removed. The whole procedure should be conducted with a minimum of stress, noise and excitement.

WEIGHT RECORDING

A vital aspect in avian medicine is the accurate recording of the patient's weight. All birds should be weighed on each visit to the veterinarian and each day while hospitalized. An accurate weight record allows the clinician to quantify the bird's body condition (if normal weights for that species are known), to accurately calculate drug dose rates and to monitor the patient's response to therapy (if it is weighed daily). Over a period of time the clinician will also develop a working knowledge of expected body weights for different species.

Weights should be recorded to the nearest gram. As such, a veterinary practice dealing with birds will need to invest in a good quality digital scale, readily available in many electronics or kitchenware stores.

Once practised, the weighing of an avian patient is relatively easily performed. Larger birds can be weighed by having them stand on a T-perch mounted on the digital scale (**44**). Smaller birds such as budgerigars, canaries and finches may be placed inside a metal or plastic container similarly mounted on the scale.

The patient's weight must be recorded on its medical records in order to demonstrate to clients

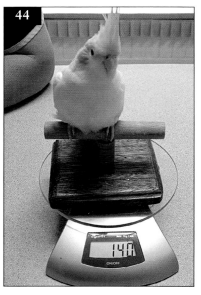

44 Using a T-perch on a set of scales allows for easy weighing of most pet birds.

their pet's weight gain or loss, and to provide part of that patient's minimum database.

AUSCULTATION

When to auscultate is the prerogative of the clinician, but it may be better performed before the bird is handled for too long. The heart rate is usually rapid, although that of some larger pet birds (e.g. cockatoos) can be surprisingly slow compared with wilder birds. Murmurs, arrhythmias and bradycardia are occasionally detectable.

Lung and air sac noises can be auscultated and, occasionally, friction rubs associated with air sacculitis can be detected.

BODY CONDITION

Traditionally a bird's body condition was determined by palpation of the pectoral muscles and allocating a body score based on the muscle and fat coverage of the sternum. This technique fails to take into account that most birds do not store fat in their pectoral region and they can be carrying significant fat deposits while still having an apparently good body score. Wetting the feathers over the abdomen and flanks with alcohol allows visualization of subcutaneous fat deposits, seen as yellow fat under the skin rather than pinkish-red muscle.

The combination of bodyweight recording, pectoral muscle palpation and examination of subcutaneous fat allows for a more accurate assessment of body condition than just palpation.

SKIN AND PLUMAGE

The bird's skin and feathering should be examined in detail. Attention should be paid to the following areas:

- Colour of the feathers. Abnormal coloration of feathers can be due to a multitude of causes. PBFD can cause green feathers to turn yellow and blue feathers to turn white. It will also lead to a generalized dirtiness of the feathers, especially in cockatoos. Chronic liver disease and/or malnutrition can cause darkening of feathers. Frequent handling of green birds by the owner can leave a deposit of oil on the feathers, which then encourages fungal overgrowth. This causes a black discoloration on these feathers. This is not seen in birds with powder down, presumably because the powder keeps the feathers clean.
- Tidiness of the plumage. Birds generally keep their plumage well groomed and tidy. If the plumage is untidy, with no immediately obvious

cause (e.g. recent handling), the clinician should suspect that either the bird is unable to groom itself properly, or a generalized feather dystrophy (e.g. PBFD) is present.
- Evidence of feather damage. Chewed and/or broken feathers should lead the clinician to suspect overgrooming, self-mutilation or malnutrition. Saw-toothed edges can indicate a failure to moult normally, hence old, worn feathers are being retained. It should be noted in cases of feather picking whether the feathers have been bitten off level with the skin or plucked out, or if the shaft has been chewed.
- Evidence of feather dystrophies. Retained feather sheaths, retained pulp, haemorrhage in the shaft of feathers, strictures of the calamus and twisted feathers are indicative of feather dystrophies, often of viral origin (e.g. polyomavirus, circovirus).
- Wing clipping (if present). The wings should be examined to determine if the bird's wings have been clipped and, if so, if that clip is appropriate to the species of bird. The quality of the clip should be examined to determine if the cut ends of feathers could be bothering the bird (45).
- Absence or presence of powder down. Powder down is produced by the powder down feathers on the thighs of many species of birds, particularly cockatoos and African grey parrots. It is easily recognized by the presence of a fine

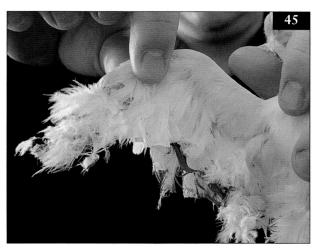

45 Excessive wing trim resulting in injury.

white powder on the clinician's hands and clothing after handling the bird. A lack of powder down leads to staining of the feathers and a shiny appearance of the beak and feet. The most common cause of a loss of this powder is PBFD.

- Moulting patterns. Most birds will typically moult heavily twice yearly, in spring and autumn, the so-called 'prenuptial' and 'postnuptial' moults. Outside of these annual moults there is a steady and progressive turnover of old feathers. Continual heavy moults or the sudden loss of many feathers is abnormal, as is the failure to moult (seen as the retention of worn and broken feathers).
- The presence of stress lines. Stress or disease at the time a feather is growing will lead to a transverse 'break' in the vane of the feather. The presence of many feathers with such stress lines is indicative of a problem in the bird's recent past. The black marks left on green-coloured birds by human skin oils (see above) should not be confused with stress lines.
- The condition of the skin. The presence of erythema, excessive scale or areas of skin trauma should be noted. This can be done by parting the feathers with a cotton bud or gently blowing on the feathers.
- Areas of trauma. The skin should be thoroughly examined for areas of trauma, especially on the wing tips, sternum and axillae.
- Flexibility of the feather. The feather of a healthy bird on a good diet should flex, rather than bend, when the tip is drawn down towards the base, and then spring back to a normal position when released.
- Parasites. The presence of parasites on the feathers should also be noted. Microscopic examination may be needed.

It is important that changes in feathers and skin be recorded in a detailed manner. Veterinarians should familiarize themselves with the descriptive terminology used for the external anatomy of a bird, and use that when describing lesions. In addition, it is important that lesions be described accurately (e.g. whether feathers are been stripped, chewed, plucked or bitten off). Such precise terminology is essential when describing a case to other veterinarians and can assist in developing a clearer picture for all concerned.

The uropygial (or preen) gland is located on the dorsal base of the tail. It is bilobed and is not present in all species (it is absent in many Columbiformes and psittacids, but prominent in budgerigars and waterfowl). It should be assessed for evidence of impaction, enlargement, inflammation or trauma.

HEAD

- Look for asymmetry arising from sinus swellings, exophthalmos, enophthalmos and trauma.
- Loss of feathers on the head can be due of a variety of conditions. Some cockatiel mutations, especially lutinos, have a bald spot behind the crest. Feather loss in other species can be associated with fungal dermatitis, *Cnemidocoptes* infection, PBFD or excessive grooming by a cage mate. Feather loss around the eyes can indicate facial rubbing associated with conjunctivitis or sinusitis.
- Matting of the feathers over the crown and nape can indicate that the bird has been vomiting (**46**).
- The conformation of the beak should be assessed for the presence of congenital or acquired abnormalities such as scissor (wry) beak, prognathism and bragnathism. Trauma to the beak or localized sinus infections can result in localized anatomical abnormalities (e.g. longitudinal grooves in the keratin). Excessive keratin flaking of the beak can reflect poor nutrition or simply a lack of opportunity to rub the beak on a suitably abrasive surface (such as a cement perch). Overgrowth of the beak can occur with PBFD, *Cnemidocoptes*, malalignment of the upper and lower beaks, chronic liver disease or malnutrition. It is rarely the result of a lack of

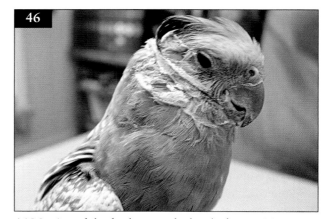

46 Matting of the feathers on the head of a vomiting cockatiel.

objects to chew on. (It is important to note that some species such as the long-billed corella naturally have elongated beaks. This should not be mistaken for an overgrown beak.) Underrunning of the ventral surface of the rhinotheca is commonly seen in cockatoos with PBFD.

- The cere, the fleshy skin at the top of the beak, is not present in all species. In the budgerigar cere colour can be used to sex the bird, with cocks having a blue cere and hens a brown cere. However, this will vary with the age of the bird, the colour mutation and the degree of health. Cere hypertrophy, a thickening of the brown cere in the budgerigar hen, may reflect a hyperoestrogenic state.
- The nares, the openings into the sinuses located at the top of the beak, should be symmetrical and dry. They should be open and the presence of keratin plugs (rhinoliths) is abnormal. Blockage of the nares may result in a subtle movement of the skin over the infraorbital sinuses. This may be the only clue that a blockage exists. Discharge from the nares, often seen as staining and matting of the feathers dorsal to the nares, may be an indication of upper respiratory disease. Previous or chronic episodes of sinusitis may be seen as asymmetrical enlargement of the nares, sometimes associated with a longitudinal groove in the keratin of the beak.
- The eyes should be bright and clean. Ocular discharge and loss or matting of the feathers around the eyes indicates either conjunctivitis or sinusitis. Conjunctival hypertrophy is common in chronic conjunctivitis, especially in cockatiels with *Chlamydophila* infection. Focal light, magnification and fluorescein dye are needed for a detailed ocular examination.
- Examination of the oropharynx can be accomplished by using gauze bandage or metal gags to open the mouth. The choana (the slit on the roof of the oropharynx) should be free of excessive mucus or discharge, and fringed with well-defined papillae. There should be no abscesses or diphtheritic membranes present.
- The ears can be examined by parting the ear coverts with the handle of a cotton bud or similar appliance. The ears should be open and free of discharge or erythema. Visualization of the tympanic membrane is difficult in most species without the use of an endoscope.

CROP

The crop can be palpated in most birds at the base of the neck, just cranial to the thoracic inlet. It should be carefully and gently palpated to assess if:

- Food is present (i.e. is the bird eating?).
- It feels doughy or fluid-filled, indications that crop stasis may be present.
- Ingluvoliths or other foreign objects are present.
- The crop mucosa feels thickened.

Care must be taken in critically ill birds not to force fluid or ingesta back up the neck into the oropharynx, as aspiration and death can result.

BODY

Palpation of the skin over the trunk occasionally reveals the crackling of subcutaneous emphysema. While this is normal in species such as pelicans, in most species it is often the result of trauma or infection rupturing air sacs and allowing the escape of air under the skin.

The abdomen in the normal bird is concave between the end of the sternum and the pubic bones. The clinician needs to distinguish between internal and external distension of the abdomen. Internal distension of the abdomen can be due to fat, organ enlargement, ascites, neoplasia or the presence of an egg. External distension can be due to subcutaneous fat, neoplasia (especially lipomas) or hernias. Radiography and ultrasonography may be required to distinguish between internal and external abdominal distension, and between different aetiologies of both. Abdominal pain or discomfort can occasionally be elicited by careful palpation.

The back should be carefully palpated for evidence of scoliosis, lordosis or kyphosis. As the thoracic and lumbar vertebrae are predominantly fused, flexibility of the spine cannot be assessed in the same way as it is in dogs and cats.

The carina of the sternum should be palpated for evidence of distortion, trauma or congenital defects such as splitting. Distortion of the carina, often indicating a history of rickets or other metabolic bone disease, should lead the clinician to recommend radiographic evaluation of the rest of the patient's skeletal system.

The cloaca can be assessed externally for enlargement and dilation (often indicative of reproductive behaviour in a hen), prolapse, ulceration or inflammation around the mucocutaneous junction, and the presence or loss of sphincter tone. Gently everting the cloaca can give a cursory examination of the mucosa, possibly revealing papillomas in susceptible species. Suspicious areas can be painted with dilute acetic acid; blanching indicates the presence of a papilloma. A more thorough evaluation of the cloaca requires endoscopy.

The area between the cloaca and the tail should be assessed for splitting of the skin. This is commonly seen in pet psittacids and is associated with a poor diet and a poor wing clip. The wing clip causes the bird to land awkwardly, pushing its tail up as it does so. Malnutrition causes the skin to lose its elasticity. The result is that the skin in this area splits, leading to bleeding and feather picking in this area. It is also a common area for hernia in hens, often containing the oviduct or even cystic ovaries.

WINGS

Each wing should be carefully extended and flexed to assess mobility and compared with the other wing. The bones and joints should be palpated for swelling or crepitus. Recent trauma may be evident as greenish discoloration of the soft tissue. This is bruising, and should not be mistaken for infection or tissue death. If the cause of a wing droop is not detectable after careful palpation, radiography is required to assess the pectoral girdle. The bones of this girdle are covered in strong muscles, and fractures are often not detectable by palpation alone. The patagium should be evaluated for loss of elasticity, trauma or scarring and for the presence of a tattoo (indicating the bird has been surgically sexed).

LEGS

Each leg should be carefully palpated to detect abnormalities such as fractures, swelling (**47**) and bruising, healed calluses and angular deformities of the long bones. Each joint should be extended and flexed to assess mobility and range of movement. Joints should also be examined for swelling and deposition of chalky white uric acid crystals (i.e. articular gout). Each leg should be compared with the other in all aspects (e.g. symmetry, length, swellings).

The toes should be examined for abnormalities including:
- Missing digits or nails.
- Annular constrictions (**166**).
- Swelling of interphalangeal joints, occasionally with the deposition of uric acid crystals.
- Avascular necrosis.
- Excessive thinness, especially in neonates.
- Abnormal position and conformation of the toes.
- Excessively long or twisted nails.

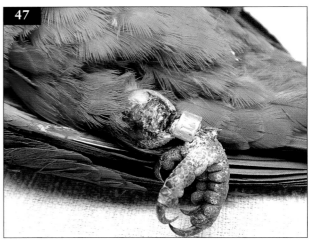

47 Leg band constriction.

The plantar surface of each foot should be examined and the condition of the metatarsal pad and digital pads noted. Abnormalities seen here include loss of definition of the epidermis (seen as a shiny, reddened surface), swelling, erosions, ulcers and scabs. Pododermatitis (bumble foot) is common in raptors, but can be seen in any bird where a unilateral lameness causes more weightbearing on the unaffected leg. This in turn can lead to pressure necrosis, infection and subsequent pododermatitis. Consequently, in cases of a unilateral lameness, the opposite leg should always be closely examined.

Occasionally, due to the nature of the injury or the disposition of the bird, a full examination may require general anaesthesia. If this is the case, radiographs can be taken at the same time, minimizing handling of the conscious (and therefore stressed) patient.

NEUROLOGICAL ASSESSMENT

Birds presented for any of the following problems require a thorough neurological assessment:
- Abnormal posture or behaviour.
- Abnormal mentation.
- Paresis or paralysis of any or all limbs.
- Fractures of limb bones.
- Weakness or inability to grip with one or both feet.
- Other neurological abnormalities.

The assessment should be performed methodically and logically. The order in which the assessment is performed depends on the clinical condition and cooperation of the patient. The degree of cooperation should be considered when interpreting responses to neurological tests.

The first part of the neurological assessment is to step back and observe the bird's posture, mentation, flight, gait and behaviour. The bird is then caught and examined physically. In particular, the tone of the wing and leg musculature is evaluated. Muscle atrophy is suggestive of reduced innervation. The skeletal system is palpated for evidence of crepitus or other abnormalities.

A systematic evaluation of the nervous system is then conducted.

Cranial nerve assessment

- The menace response, evaluating cranial nerves II and VII, can be provoked by bringing the hand towards each eye. Normal responses include eye-blink, pulling away of the head or aggressive action of the beak.
- The pupillary light response evaluates cranial nerves II and III. It is often considered unreliable in birds because, although there is complete decussation of the optic nerves at the chiasma, and therefore no consensual pupillary light response, the thin bones of the avian skull can allow a light shone in one eye to stimulate a response in the other eye.
- Pupil size. The pupils should be symmetrical. If not, consider intraocular inflammation, ocular structural lesions or sympathetic neuropathy affecting cranial nerve III.
- A symmetrical eye blink normally occurs when the cornea is gently touched with a moist cotton swab. If not, consider an abnormality affecting cranial nerves V and VII.
- A symmetrical eye-blink should be elicited by touching each side of face or the lateral canthus. This evaluates cranial nerves V and VII.
- The tongue should be positioned and move normally. Abnormal tongue movement or a deviated tongue indicates damage to cranial nerves IX to XII.
- Reduced beak strength when biting or eating indicates possible damage to cranial nerves V, IX, X, XI and XII.
- Nystagmus, the periodic, rhythmic, and involuntary movement of both eyeballs in unison in either a vertical, horizontal or rotary direction, indicates damage to cranial nerve VIII, a cerebellar lesion or increased intracranial pressure.

- Strabismus, an involuntary deviation of one eye, can occur with damage to cranial nerves III, IV or VI and vestibular lesions.
- Horner's syndrome. Enopthalmos, upper eyelid ptosis, slight elevation of the lower lid, piloerection of feathers on the affected side of head, pupil constriction and narrowing of the palpebral fissure. Has been reported with intracranial lesions or lesions affecting the cervical sympathetic tract or brachial plexus. Note that miosis and third eyelid protrusion are not as obvious in birds as in mammals because of the presence of striated muscle.
- Torticollis, cervical muscle contraction producing neck torsion, has been seen with lesions involving cranial nerve XI.

Peripheral nerve assessment

Spinal reflexes, although difficult to assess objectively in birds, can help determine if a lesion is centrally or peripherally located. In most situations determining if a reflex is present or absent is sufficient, and symmetry of response should receive particular attention. Spinal reflexes require reflex arcs only to be intact; no other parts of the central nervous system (CNS) are involved. Spinal reflex tests include:

- Body balancing. With the wings held into the body, suspend the bird vertically and head down, then quickly rotate up to a horizontal position and observe fanning of the tail feathers. Dip the bird forward again, back to the vertical position, and observe the tail flick up. This reflex functions to maintain balance.
- Wing withdrawal. Lightly touch a wing and observe it being pulled away. This is a segmental reflex which, if present, indicates that the reflex arc and associated spinal cord segment in the cervicothoracic cord are intact. Damage may still exist higher in the CNS.
- Leg withdrawal. Lightly touch a leg and observe it being pulled away. This is again a segmental reflex; if present it indicates that the reflex arc and associated segment in the thoracolumbar spinal cord are intact.
- Vent reflex. Touch the vent mucosa with a fine object and observe it close tightly. This is also a segmental reflex that indicates that the reflex arc and associated lumbosacral spinal cord segment are intact.

Reactions require reflex pathways (ascending and descending fibre tracts in the spinal cord and higher centres). It is important to look closely for subtle asymmetrical deficits.

Comparison of spinal reflexes and reactions helps to localize lesions. If a reflex exists, but its corresponding reaction does not, a lesion exists within the CNS rostral to the segment involved in the reflex arc. Reactions include:

- Proprioception (wings). Note the resting wing carriage. Pull one wing out of its resting position and note the time taken for its return. Only normally innervated wings will correct displacement.
- Proprioception (legs). Observe the bird at rest. Knuckling of the foot is quickly corrected in normal birds.
- Unilateral and bilateral wing fanning should be assessed while the bird is moved up, down and from side to side, while the feet and lower back are restrained. Forceful, rhythmic, fanning out of the wings should be evident and, in the bilateral test, wing movements should be simultaneous. Unilateral wing fanning will occur only in the normally innervated wing, while in the bilateral test a lesion causing loss of afferent stimulus on one side will be compensated for by afferent stimulus from the other side and normal wing movements may occur.
- Placing. With wings held into the body and the legs free, approach a horizontal surface (such as a desk top). As soon as any part of the foot touches the surface, both feet should swiftly position themselves accurately on the surface in order to support the bird's weight.

- The differentiation between pain perception and withdrawal reflex is critical. Movement of a pinched limb does not indicate that the patient is able to feel the stimulus. Some type of conscious recognition of the stimulus is required (e.g. vocalization, attempts to escape or bite). This part of the examination is best kept till last, so as not to influence the patient's behaviour to other segments of the neurological examination. Loss of pain perception is a poor prognostic sign. Deficits in a particular wing may only be obviously detected if its counterpart is restrained.

FURTHER READING

Clippinger TL, Bennett RA, Platt SR (1996) The avian neurologic examination and ancillary neurodiagnostic techniques. *Journal of Avian Medicine and Surgery* **10**(4):221–247.

Doneley B, Harrison GJ, Lightfoot TL (2006) Maximising information from the physical examination. In: *Clinical Avian Medicine, Vol 1*. GJ Harrison, TL Lightfoot (eds). Spix Publishing, Palm Beach, pp. 153–212.

Greenacre CB, Lusby AL (2004) Physiological responses of Amazon parrots (*Amazona* species) to manual restraint. *Journal of Avian Medicine and Surgery* **18**(1):12–18.

Platt SR (2006) Evaluating and treating the nervous system. In: *Clinical Avian Medicine, Vol 1*. GJ Harrison, TL Lightfoot (eds). Spix Publishing, Palm Beach, pp. 493–518.

CHAPTER 3
CLINICAL TECHNIQUES

DIAGNOSTIC TECHNIQUES

The limited range of responses to disease that is available to birds, and their relatively small size, has increased the requirement for diagnostic testing in order to better diagnose disease and provide an appropriate treatment. The full gamut of testing available in small animal medicine is also available for avian practitioners. However, before any diagnostic test can be interpreted, it is vital that the clinician understands how to, and be able to, collect quality samples and position the patient correctly for diagnostic imaging.

BLOOD COLLECTION AND HANDLING

There are a number of haematological, biochemical, serological and polymerase chain reaction (PCR) tests available for avian veterinarians to utilize in the care of their patients. The basic requirement for these tests is to collect a sufficient volume of nonhaemolysed blood without endangering the patient. Secondary requirements include storing the collected sample correctly and making fresh blood smears without damaging the relatively fragile nucleated erythrocytes.

Blood can be collected from the right jugular vein (48) (the left jugular vein is accessible, but much smaller), the basilic vein (on the medial aspect of the elbow) or the median tibiotarsal vein (in large birds) (49). The right jugular vein is usually preferred in companion birds because of the relatively easy access; it lies under an apteryla and, with practice, a sole operator can both restrain the bird and perform the venipuncture. It must be remembered that avian veins have thin walls and tear easily. Coagulation in birds usually relies on extrinsic clotting pathways requiring tissue thromboplastin, rather than the intrinsic clotting pathways utilized by mammals. Care must therefore be taken to prevent accidentally tearing the vein wall, which can lead to a rapidly fatal haemorrhage. It is advisable to apply digital pressure to the venipuncture

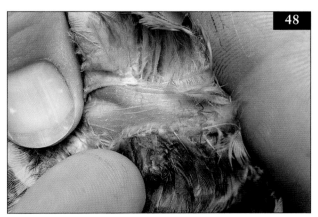

48 The right jugular vein can be found under an apteryla on the right side of the neck.

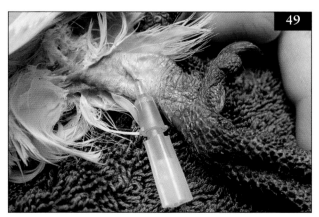

49 An intravenous catheter placed in the medial tarsal vein of a cockatoo.

site for 30–60 seconds to minimize haematoma formation. Using a 25–29-gauge needle minimizes the iatrogenic trauma to the vein, but the smaller the needle bore the more likely haemolysis is to occur during collection. Once the needle has entered the vein, avoid using excessive pressure to draw back; this will prevent both collapsing the vein and haemolysing the sample. It is sometimes advantageous to use a heparinized syringe for blood collection (50).

A toenail clip, once advocated as a means of blood collection in birds, is the least desirable method of blood collection because of contamination with debris, increased incidence of clotting of the sample, increased incidence of abnormal cell distributions and the pain it causes the patient.

Many clients (and veterinarians) are surprised at how much blood can be safely collected from a bird. The blood volume in any given bird is approximately 10% of its bodyweight. Given that 10% of this blood volume can usually be safely collected for diagnostic testing or other purposes, an amount of blood equal to 1% of a bird's bodyweight can be safely collected (i.e. 1 ml of blood can be collected for each 100 g of bodyweight). With the modern laboratory equipment available in both external and in-house laboratories, this is usually a sufficient sample to run both haematological and biochemical assays.

Biochemistry testing is best performed on blood that has been collected into lithium heparin. If testing is likely to be delayed for anything more than a few hours, it should be centrifuged and the plasma decanted and submitted. The use of plain tubes that allow the blood to clot and serum to come off it is not advisable. Although serum collected in this manner has no anticoagulant in it, it has been in contact with haemolysing red blood cells for a significant time, which causes more artefactual changes. (Serum is lower in total protein, albumin and glucose; it is higher in uric acid, potassium, calcium, magnesium and phosphorus.)

Haematology, on the other hand, is usually best performed on blood that has been stored in sodium EDTA. (Note that some labs prefer lithium heparin for haematology; the clinician should consult with their local laboratory for preferences.) Fresh blood smears should always be made before the blood is placed into any anticoagulant. There are several techniques used for preparing blood smears:

- The traditional glass slide angled 'push' method: often results in significant cell lysis.
- The angled slide 'drag' method: the angled slide is used to drag, rather than push, the blood film along the preparation slide. Cell lysis is much less common than with the previous technique.
- The coverslip method: place a 2 mm diameter drop of blood between two coverslips, allow the drop to spread close to the edges, then slide the coverslips apart horizontally. The dried coverslips can then be stained and mounted face down on a glass slide using mounting medium, immersion oil or a drop of adhesive.
- The coverslip on slide method: a drop of blood is placed on the glass slide and the coverslip is then placed on the drop. Once the blood has spread to the edges of the coverslip, it is then drawn horizontally along the slide. If not done gently, significant cell lysis can occur.

MICROBIOLOGY

Microbiology is an essential tool in avian medicine (51). It can begin with a Gram stain to determine if bacteria or fungi are present in an area or organ of interest, and in what proportions. The sample is collected, rolled on to a slide, air dried and then heat-fixed with a gentle flame. Excessively thick smears should be avoided. The staining procedure for Gram stain is as follows:

- Apply crystal violet solution for 60 seconds, rinse gently with water.
- Apply Gram's iodine solution for 60 seconds, rinse gently with water.
- Decolorize with acetone or ethanol for 2–5 seconds, rinse gently with water.
- Stain with 0.1% basic fuchsin solution for 60 seconds, rinse gently and dry.

Gram-positive organisms and yeast stain deep violet and gram-negative organisms stain red. Gram-negative bacteria are predominantly rod- or coccobacilli-shaped

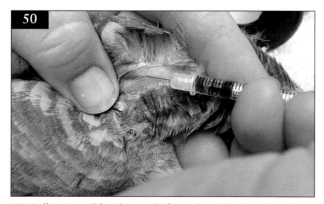

50 Collecting a blood sample from the right jugular vein.

and are usually much smaller than gram-positive rods in birds. Spirochaetes are gram-negative spiral bacteria.

Samples collected for culture and sensitivity are collected with sterile swabs, placed in a transport medium and sent to the laboratory. Common sites cultured in live birds include the cloaca, choana, crop, eye, ear and skin. Less commonly sampled sites include the sinuses, the trachea, joints, air sacs and the oviduct.

Swabs used to culture the choana, crop or cloaca should be premoistened with either sterile saline or transport medium to minimize iatrogenic damage to mucosal surfaces (**52**, **53**). Cloacal swabs are preferred to faecal swabs, as there is less chance of environmental contamination. The owners should be advised that after the swab has been collected from this site the next few droppings may have blood on them. This is common and rarely of concern.

Choanal cultures are similarly collected with a premoistened swab. Some clinicians prefer to flush the nares with 1–2 ml of sterile saline immediately prior to swabbing the choana; this reduces oral contamination and gives a more representative sampling of the nasal cavity. A mouth speculum or gauze strips are used to hold the mouth open. The swab is gently inserted into the anterior choana.

It must be noted that the sinus and nasal cavity anatomy is such that a choanal culture may not represent the pathology occurring in the sinus. In cases of sinusitis it is therefore usually preferable to culture a sample from a sinus aspirate. This is done by inserting a 22–27-gauge needle, attached to a 3–5 ml syringe, midway between the commissure of the beak and the medial canthus of the eye, under the zygomatic arch. The sinus is more easily entered if the mouth is held open with a speculum during this procedure. Care must be taken to avoid iatrogenic trauma to the eye.

Culture of joints is indicated when bacterial or fungal infection is suspected based on cytology. The bird should be anaesthetized unless it is severely depressed. The skin over the joint is prepared aseptically and joint fluid aspirated using a small needle. The sample is expressed on to a swab, placed in transport media and sent to the laboratory.

Tracheal washes are useful for evaluating birds with suspected lower respiratory tract disease. The procedure can be performed on a conscious patient, but care must be taken with birds in respiratory distress. In many cases, however, anaesthesia reduces the chances of undue stress in an already compromised patient, iatrogenic trauma and contamination of the sample. A sterile catheter, long

51 Culture plate.

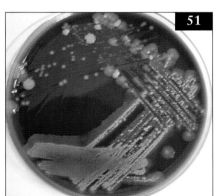

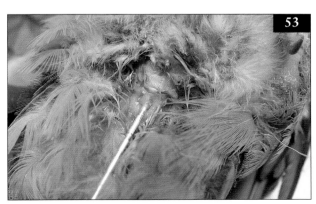

52 Use of a moistened swab reduces iatrogenic trauma to the cloaca.

53 Swabbing the cloaca.

enough to reach the tracheal bifurcation, is introduced through the open glottis, taking care to avoid contamination through indirect contact with the mouth. Once the catheter is in position, sterile 0.9% saline (0.5–1.0 ml/kg) is quickly infused and immediately re-aspirated. (The lower dose rate should be used in larger birds and those with severe respiratory compromise.) Approximately 25–50% of the volume infused should be recovered and can be processed for both culture and cytology.

CYTOLOGY

Cytology is a useful tool in avian medicine. Antemortem samples can be collected from the choana, pharynx, sinuses, joints, skin, feather follicles, trachea, lungs, the crop, the cloaca, the coelom and the bone marrow. Collection techniques for the most part are similar to those described above.

Abdominocentesis is indicated in the presence of ascites or other abnormal abdominal fluid. (Often these birds present with dyspnoea, so care should be taken when handling.) The ventral midline is aseptically prepared and a 21–25-gauge needle attached to a syringe is inserted on the midline immediately caudal to the sternum, directed to the right side of the coelom to avoid the ventriculus.

Bone marrow cytology is useful for the evaluation of haematopoiesis. Under anaesthesia the proximal cranial tibiotarsus is aseptically prepared. A small incision is made over the cnemial crest; a spinal or bone marrow needle is inserted into the shaft of the tibiotarsus with a gentle, twisting pressure, the stylet is removed and the sample is aspirated with a syringe and expelled on to a slide. A smear is then made in a manner similar to making a blood smear. For the best evaluation of the bone marrow, a peripheral blood sample collected the same day should also be submitted to the laboratory.

Fluid samples collected for cytology are often dilute, with a low cellularity; they must therefore be concentrated before being examined. It is preferable to use a gravity-based cell concentration method that avoids cell distortion. Centrifugation can be used, but often causes variable degrees of cellular distortion.

PARASITOLOGY

External parasitism can be diagnosed by direct examination of the patient and its feathers. The characteristic 'honeycomb' appearance of cnemido-coptic mite infection is unmistakable, but a gentle skin scraping can be used to confirm the diagnosis. Other mites such as *Dermanyssus* spp. can be difficult to diagnose, but can usually be found after a careful examination. Close examination of the feathers may reveal lice eggs (nits) and the lice themselves. Examination of the feather shaft under magnification may be needed to diagnose quill mite (*Syringophilus* spp. and others).

Internal parasitism can be assessed by a combination of crop wash aspirate and faecal examination. Motile protozoa such as *Trichomonas* spp., *Spironucleus* spp., *Cochlosoma* spp. and *Giardia* spp. are best detected by immediate examination of a fresh crop wash aspirate or faecal material suspended in 0.9% saline solution. Protozoan oocysts and nematode eggs are sometimes detected by this method, but may require concentration methods such as faecal flotation using hypertonic solutions (zinc sulphate, sodium nitrate or sugar solutions) or faecal centrifugation.

It has been suggested by some researchers that faecal centrifugation consistently detects more parasitic ova than standard faecal flotation techniques. The technique can be performed in most veterinary clinics:

- Mix 2–5 g faeces with 10 ml faecal flotation solution and shake well until dispersed.
- Strain this fluid into a 15 ml centrifuge tube until a slight positive meniscus forms at the top.
- Place a coverslip on the tube and centrifuge it in a swinging head centrifuge at not less than 1200 rpm for five minutes.
- Let it stand for ten minutes before examination under the microscope.

Note that if a fixed head centrifuge is used, the tube should not be completely filled with the faecal solution, nor should a coverslip be applied. After centrifugation the tube is placed in a vertical rack and filled with fresh flotation solution until a meniscus forms. A coverslip is applied and the tube left to stand for ten minutes.

It should be noted that cestode infections can be difficult to detect by any of the above means, as proglottid sections are often too heavy to float and may be missed on a fresh faecal smear.

DIAGNOSTIC IMAGING

Radiography is a valuable diagnostic tool in avian medicine; unfortunately much of its value is lost due to incorrect technique and equipment. The advent of digital radiography may go a long way towards overcoming these deficiencies, but the basic principle of do it right the first time remains.

Good avian radiography requires both short exposure times (to minimize the effect of 'blurring' due to the patient's relatively rapid respiratory rate) and a combination of high-detail screens and films.

These requirements mean that a relatively powerful x-ray machine is needed, with the ability to produce a high mA with a short exposure time. Most x-ray machines used in veterinary practices will fulfill these requirements. Nonscreen film can be used but requires a higher exposure time. The screens that are used for radiographs of the extremities in man, cats and dogs are also excellent for birds. Mammography cassettes, screens and film are also very useful and give excellent detail, but processing the film is more critical than with other films.

Digital radiography is becoming more obtainable in many private practices. With the ability to obtain and manipulate high-definition images as well as storing them electronically, high-definition digital radiography offers major advancements in avian radiology.

Whether using conventional or digital radiography, positioning of the patient is absolutely vital for the accurate interpretation of an exposed radiograph. Correct positioning can usually only be obtained under anaesthesia, although very tame (or very sick) birds can often be positioned conscious in a plexiglass restraint device or similar restraints. (Often, however, anaesthesia is less stressful and therefore safer than manual restraint.) The lateral view is taken with the patient in right lateral recumbency, with the wings extended dorsally and the legs pulled caudally so that the acetabula are superimposed (54, 55). The ventrodorsal view is taken with the patient in dorsal recumbency with the wings laterally and the legs caudally alongside the tail, with the femurs parallel to the spine and each other. The keel should be superimposed over the vertebrae (56, 57).

Contrast studies can add greatly to the diagnostic value of radiography. Contrast media such as barium,

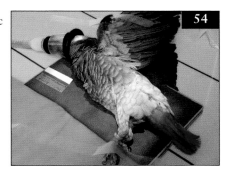

54 Radiographic position: lateral view.

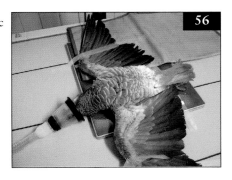

56 Radiographic position: ventrodorsal view.

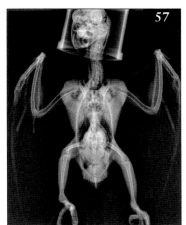

55 Lateral view: mature eclectus parrot. (Photo courtesy L Nemetz)

57 Ventrodorsal view: mature eclectus parrot. (Photo courtesy L Nemetz)

iohexol and diatrizoate have all been used in avian radiography. Gastrointestinal contrast studies utilizing iohexol are often comparable to those using the more routinely recommended barium sulphate. Diluted iohexol does not provide adequate contrast and should not be used.

Ultrasonography is less commonly used in avian medicine. The sonogram produced by the reflection of high frequency sound waves generated by a transducer is based on the unique echoes produced by different tissues. Bone completely absorbs the sound waves, while air reflects them (preventing passage through to deeper structures). The presence of air sacs therefore limits the usefulness of ultrasound in birds. However, it can be used to give some definition of the internal structure of tissues and organs including: examination of small organs such as the gall bladder, spleen and pancreas; examination of fluid-filled lesions; and to measure cardiac function. It is a valuable tool in assessing abdominal distension in avian patients. See *Table 1*.

A 7.5–10 MHz transducer with a small contact area (e.g. a paediatric scanner) is most commonly employed. The most common 'windows' used are the ventromedial abdomen and right lateral abdomen.

Table 1 Interpretation of ultrasonographic findings in birds.

Organ	Normal	Pathology
Liver	The parenchyma has a homogenous, finely granular appearance. The gall bladder, if present, lies to the right of midline	Blood vessels appear enlarged, with an increased wall density, with severe hepatomegaly Hepatic lipidosis produces hepatomegaly with a diffuse increase in echogenicity Neoplasia causes focal or diffuse changes in echogenicity Abscesses, granulomas or necrosis also produce focal or diffuse changes in echogenicity Haematomas produce focal, hypoechoic lesions
Spleen	Can be seen on the lateral approach. Its size and shape varies between species. It has a slightly more granular and echodense appearance than the liver	
Kidneys	Normal kidneys are difficult to visualize	Enlargement is readily seen. Neoplasia causes a nonhomogeneous parenchyma Renal cysts are clearly defined anechoic areas
Reproductive tract	Both approaches can be used. Inactive gonads are difficult to detect, while active follicles appear as anechoic areas	Egg-binding is easy to detect. Ovarian cysts and gonadal neoplasia are also detectable. Metritis and pyometra can be detected readily
Gastrointestinal tract	Structure and motility can be visualized	Proventricular dilation can be seen (e.g. proventricular dilatation disease [PDD], lead toxicosis). Thickening of wall can be seen with enteritis. Cloacal concretions, papillomas and dilation can be seen
Heart	Only B mode and Doppler flow have been used successfully in birds	Cardiomegaly and pericardial effusion are readily differentiated. Mitral valvular disease has been reported

With the patient restrained or anaesthetized, the feathers are parted or plucked and ultrasound gel applied to the skin. Stand-offs may be required for small patients.

Fluoroscopy uses an image intensifier that amplifies low-level ionizing radiation to allow capture of real time motion using a closed charge-coupling video imaging device. Anaesthesia is not required, and this technique is particularly useful for studying gastrointestinal motility, especially in diseases such as proventricular dilatation disease (PDD) (58).

Advances in diagnostic techniques such as computed tomography (CT), positron emission tomography (PET) and magnetic resonance imaging (MRI) are identifying areas in avian diagnostic imaging where these techniques can play significant roles.

CARDIOLOGY

Radiography plays an important role in the diagnosis of heart disease. In healthy, medium-sized parrots the maximum width of the cardiac silhouette in a ventrodorsal radiograph should be 35–45% of the length of the sternum, 51–61% of the width of the thorax and 545–672% of the width of the coracoid.

Electrocardiography is an underutilized tool in avian medicine. As knowledge of avian cardiology and cardiovascular disease increases, it is likely that the use

of this diagnostic modality will increase in practice. Electrocardiography may be useful for the detection of cardiac enlargement from hypertrophy of any of the four cardiac chambers, and it is indispensable for the diagnosis and treatment of cardiac arrhythmias.

The electrocardiogram (ECG) is a graphic record of sequential electrical depolarization–repolarization patterns of the heart, detected on the surface of the body by changes in electrical fields. These patterns are detected by attaching leads to both wings and both legs. In large or well muscled birds it may be necessary to attach the V electrode to the right or left of the sternum to provide greater amplitudes of all complexes. Needle electrodes placed subcutaneously are superior to alligator clips for use in avian patients. The Biolog® hand-held ECG machine has been used with one foot (lead) on the chest, one on the right wing and one on the right thigh, giving a lead II reading only. QRS complexes are larger than with standard machines, but they are comparable.

Different lead systems are used to record differences between different limbs. The standard lead system records leads I, II and III. The sequence of depolarization and repolarization is recorded as follows:
- Atrial depolarization is seen as a positive P wave on leads I, II and III.
- Ventricular depolarization is recorded as a negative QRS complex (unlike mammals). There is no Q wave in leads I, II and III.
- Ventricular repolarization is seen as a positive T wave on leads II and III; it may be positive, negative or absent on lead I. The T and P waves frequently overlap.

The rapid heart rate of many birds means that the recording paper needs to be run at 50 mm/second or greater. Heart rates can vary from 100–1,000 bpm and so some authors recommend paper speed of at least 100 mm/second and, for smaller species, up to 200 mm/second.

The determination and monitoring of blood pressure has recently been recognized as a valuable diagnostic tool in the avian patient. Systolic blood pressure is the pressure exerted against the blood vessel wall during systole. Direct arterial pressure measurement requires specific skills and is both invasive and expensive. Consequently, indirect blood pressure measurement techniques, based on the detection of blood flow beneath an inflated cuff, are more commonly used and have been found to correlate well with direct blood pressure measurements.

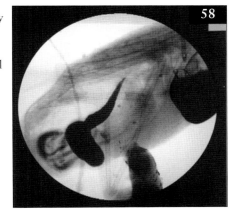

58 Fluoroscopy is a useful tool in assessing gastrointestinal tract motility.

The ultrasonic Doppler flow detector (Parks Medical Electronics Inc) uses ultrasonic waves to detect arterial blood flow distal to a blood pressure cuff and produce an audible signal (**261**). An appropriately sized cuff (depending on the size of the bird) is placed around the distal humerus or femur and taped in place. The Doppler probe is then placed above the radial carpal bone or tibiotarsal bone to detect arterial blood flow, and secured in place. The cuff is inflated until the Doppler signal is lost, and then slowly deflated. The pressure on the cuff when the first sound heard is marked and recorded as the systolic pressure. The blood pressure of various avian species under gaseous anaesthesia lies between 90 and 140 mmHg systolic.

Another useful tool for the diagnosis of cardiac disease is echocardiography. Probes with small coupling surfaces and frequencies of at least 7.5 MHz are necessary, and the ultrasound devices should be able to produce at least 100 frames/second. Evaluation is best performed via the subcostal imaging plane, viewing the heart through the liver. (If the patient has ascites or hepatomegaly, it is much easier to visualize the heart, due to the larger window these conditions provide.) A standard four-chamber view may be difficult to obtain in a normal bird, but this becomes easier with increasing heart size. Echocardiography is useful in the diagnosis of pericardial effusions, cardiac chamber enlargement, and vegetative endocarditis. The lack of normal values makes evaluation of contractility subjective, but these values are been developed.

ENDOSCOPY

Endoscopy, the examination of the interior of body organs, joints or cavities through an endoscope, had its beginnings in the early 1900s when lighted telescopes were first used to examine inside a human patient. In avian medicine, endoscopes were first used in the 1970s and 1980s to determine the sex of parrots, many of which are sexually monomorphic (i.e. there are no distinguishing physical differences between the sexes). Examination of the gonads, located between the lung and kidney, allowed a rapid and accurate identification of sex and revolutionized the breeding of many species. It was quickly realized that the unique avian anatomy, with its air-filled body cavities, made birds ideal candidates for endoscopy. Insufflation is not required, reducing the costs and technical difficulty involved. Techniques and instruments have been developed to take advantage of this, and endoscopy is now a widely utilized diagnostic tool in avian medicine around the world (59).

Several endoscopy packages are available for avian practitioners; all consist of the following items of equipment:
- Endoscope. Most practitioners use a 2.7 mm rigid endoscope with a 30° oblique view. This allows a much wider field of view than the more common 0° scopes. 1.9 mm endoscopes are available for smaller patients (<100 g).
- Light cable and light source. There are two types of light sources available, the tungsten–halogen and the xenon. Xenon light sources, while more expensive, provide a more intense, whiter and cooler light than tungsten–halogen. Not only does this give better illumination while viewing inside the body, it is essential if cameras and video documentation are to be used.
- Endoscopy camera. The use of an endoscopy camera and monitor provides better magnification of the operating field while being more ergonomic for the operator. A three-chip digital camera gives a high-quality picture, and is light and easily used while attached to the endoscope.
- Operating sheath and instruments. The Taylor Operating Sheath® (Karl Storz) provides three 5 Fr instrument channels to allow the introduction of a variety of 3 Fr endoscopic instruments including biopsy and grasping forceps, scissors and aspirating and injecting needles.

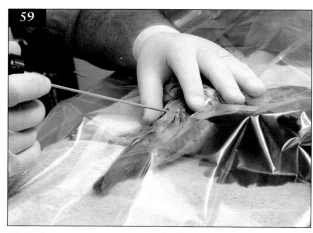

59 Endoscopic examination of a bird.

- Video documentation is desirable, as it allows better documentation of procedures and is a valuable tool for educating both veterinarians and clients.

The more commonly used endoscopic approaches are described in the following sections.

Tracheal approach

It is important to note that for anything other than a quick examination of the trachea and syrinx, the patient should have an air sac catheter placed to provide anaesthesia and respiratory support during the procedure. The approach to placing this catheter is the same as for abdominal endoscopy (see Coelomic approach, below). Under anaesthesia the patient is placed in either dorsal or ventral recumbency and the head and neck are extended. The endoscope is introduced over the tongue and through the glottis into the trachea. It is important to keep the trachea extended and straight and to ensure that the patient is in a surgical plane of anaesthesia in order to avoid iatrogenic trauma. It is also important to keep in mind that the tracheal cartilage in birds is a complete circle and, therefore, the trachea cannot be stretched from the inside. The lumen of the trachea narrows as it passes caudally to the syrinx. If the syrinx cannot be visualized, it is sometimes helpful to withdraw the endoscope, reverse the patient's positioning (i.e. dorsal to ventral and vice versa) and then reintroduce the endoscope.

Coelomic approach

The standard positioning is to place the patient in right lateral recumbency with the wings extended and restrained. The left foot is pulled forward and secured to the neck. The left flank behind the leg is then a septically prepared; it is rare to have to remove more than a few feathers (**60a, b**). The following landmarks are identified: the caudal rib, the flexor crura medialis muscle and the pubic bone. A 4 mm vertical incision is made in the skin where the flexor crura medialis muscle crosses the caudal rib. Curved haemostat forceps are then used to reflect the flexor muscle dorsally and then blunt dissect through the abdominal wall. If done correctly, the operator will feel a 'pop' as the haemostats enter the caudal thoracic air sac.

Once the coelom has been entered the haemostats can be withdrawn and the endoscope introduced. If entry has been performed correctly, the endoscope will now be in the caudal thoracic air sac. This can be confirmed by a clear view of the lung and ostium, with air sac membranes visible on the left and right view. The endoscope can be advanced to the lung and, in some patients, enter the lung through the ostium. The air sac membranes on either side of the caudal thoracic air sac can be penetrated either with endoscopic scissors or by placing the tip of the endoscope against the membrane and twisting sharply. Going to the left allows entry into the cranial thoracic air sac; to the right lies the abdominal air sac.

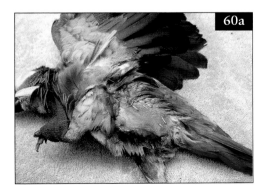

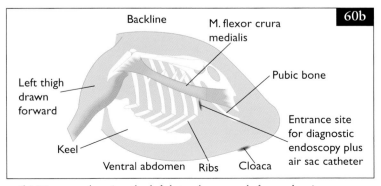

60 (**a**) Left lateral approach for coelomic endoscopy. (**b**) Diagram showing the left lateral approach for coelomic endoscopy.

Once the procedure is completed the endoscope is withdrawn. Tears in the air sac membranes heal well without any requirement for surgical closure. The muscle and skin incisions can be closed if the operator feels it is advisable, but are often left to heal by secondary intention, which occurs rapidly.

Choanal

Introducing the endoscope through the choanal slit allows visualization of the left and right nasal cavities and nasal turbinates. Saline can be flushed through the external nares to provide a better examination and to flush any foreign bodies out, or at least into the field of view. The patient must be intubated before this is performed.

Cloacal

Introducing the endoscope into the cloaca while insufflating it with water allows excellent visualization of the three chambers of the cloaca, the ureteral openings, the opening into the oviduct or the ductus deferens and, in young birds, the cloacal bursa.

Upper gastrointestinal tract

The oesophagus can be examined by passing the endoscope past the glottis in an anaesthetized patient. The crop can be examined in birds with crops (psittacines, pigeons, doves, gallinaceous birds and some passerines) by passing the tip of the endoscope through the cervical portion of the oesophagus. If possible, the bird should be fasted for several hours before the procedure in order to increase visualization. Insufflation of the crop with air or water will increase visualization. An ingluviotomy is needed to examine the proventriculus and ventriculus. The bird is anaesthetized, intubated and placed in dorsal recumbency. The cervical oesophagus or pharynx should be packed off with gauze swabs if possible. A small incision is made into the crop and the endoscope is passed into the thoracic oesophagus and into the proventriculus. The ventriculus may be entered by passing the endoscope through the proventricular–ventricular junction. Insufflation with water or saline will be necessary. When the procedure is completed the crop is closed with a two-layer closure.

TREATMENT TECHNIQUES

Once a patient's condition has been diagnosed, or the clinician is waiting for test results for a diagnosis, treatment can be given to both support the patient and to treat the causative problem. Supportive care, sometimes overlooked, is a critical part of the treatment for a patient that is often more ill than

many other species that are presented to veterinarians. Sick birds, on top of their original problem, are often hypothermic, dehydrated and hypoglycaemic. Obviously, sending such a patient home with some antibiotic powder to place in its drinking water is unlikely to help it much.

Because so many of the patients presented to veterinarians are in a critical condition, treatment (and diagnostic testing) has to be done carefully, in limited stages, to avoid 'overwhelming' the patient. Following a quick assessment to identify immediate life-threatening problems (e.g. uncontrolled haemorrhage or severe dyspnoea), it is often appropriate to commence supportive care before attempting diagnostic testing.

HEATING

Birds are particularly sensitive to hypothermia because of their small size and higher surface area to volume ratio. It is for this reason that sick birds sit still (to conserve energy) and fluff their feathers (to retain body heat). When presented with such a patient, it is prudent to provide exogenous heat before attempting any further treatment or diagnosis. As a general rule, ill birds should be maintained at a temperature of approximately 25–30°C, with a relative humidity of about 70%. Heat can be provided using an incubator, brooder, heat lamp (**61**), circulating warm water

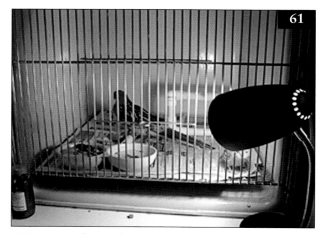

61 Keeping a hospital patient warm using an incandescent bulb.

blanket, hot water bottles or other device. The patient must be monitored carefully to prevent overheating or burns. Once the bird has regained its body temperature, as evidenced by increased activity, further treatment and diagnostic efforts can be attempted.

FLUID THERAPY

Most sick birds can be assumed to be at least 5% dehydrated, if not more. Signs of marked dehydration in birds include decreased skin turgor, sunken or closed eyes, dry oral mucous membranes and thick mucus in the pharynx. The clinician should aim to correct the calculated fluid deficit over 2–3 days, while at the same time providing maintenance fluids (50 ml/kg/day). A simplified calculation is to give 10% of the bird's bodyweight daily for three days, and then reduce this volume to 5%. The calculated volume should be divided into two or three doses, given over a 24-hour period.

In mildly dehydrated patients with a functional gastrointestinal system and the ability to withstand the necessary handling, replacement fluids can be given orally. Oral rehydration formulae or lactated Ringer's solution can be delivered by a crop needle or plastic tubing directly into the crop. Hypertonic liquids should be avoided, as these may exacerbate dehydration. A crop needle (a stainless steel needle with a stainless steel ball on the end) or plastic tubing is passed over the tongue and gently guided down the cervical oesophagus and into the crop (**62, 63**). Care must be taken not to inadvertently place the needle or tube into the trachea or to force it through the oesophageal/crop wall. Careful palpation of the crop can confirm the placement of the implement before giving the fluids. Care must be taken not to press on the crop while restraining the bird, to overfill the crop, or to fill it too quickly. If fluid appears in the pharynx or comes from the mouth while gavaging, the tube or needle should be immediately withdrawn and the bird placed back in its cage. As a general rule, the amount given by crop gavage should start initially at 5% of the bird's bodyweight. It can then be built up to 8–10%. It will typically take about 2–4 hours for the crop to empty completely.

Severely dehydrated patients, or those that cannot handle either oral fluids or physical restraint, can be rehydrated parenterally through subcutaneous, intravenous or intraosseous injections.

Subcutaneous fluids are not recommended for patients in shock due to concerns over absorption. They are, however, very useful for most ill patients. They may be given in the inguinal region or the interscapular region; the inguinal region allows for greater volumes to be given with less patient

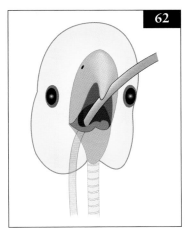

62 With the patient facing you and its head restrained, the crop needle is introduced into the bird's mouth on the left side, passed over the top of the tongue and directed to the right side of the oropharynx. It is then gently slid down the oesophagus, into the crop.

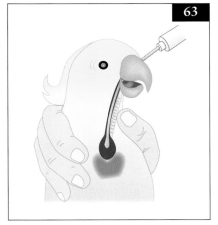

63 Correct placement of a crop tube into the crop.

discomfort (**64–66**). Volumes of 5–10 ml/kg can given two to three times daily in each site. If oedema is noted prior to subsequent administration, the fluid is not being absorbed (due to poor circulation, excessive volume administered or hypoproteinaemia) and additional fluid should not be administered by this route.

Fluids may be administered by constant infusion or slow bolus through an aseptically placed intravenous or intraosseous catheter. The jugular, basilic and medial metatarsal veins are suitable for this purpose. Intraosseous injections are considered equivalent to intravenous administration, with 50% of the fluid given intraosseously appearing in the

circulation within 30 seconds. Intraosseous catheters are most commonly placed in the proximal tibiotarsus and the distal ulna. A spinal needle is used to prevent the lumen plugging with bone and tissue, rendering the catheter useless. Care must be taken to insert the catheter correctly the first time, as subsequent attempts usually result in either a large hole or multiple holes in the bone at the entry site. Leakage will occur through each hole, resulting in discomfort from the deposition of the fluid or drugs into the soft tissues around the bone.

The needle is placed into the tibiotarsus in a manner similar to the normograde insertion of an intramedullary pin. The tibiotarsus is grasped, a small stab incision is made in the skin over the proximal cranial tibiotarsus, medial to the cnemial crest, and the needle is inserted into the marrow cavity with gentle pressure and a twisting motion of the needle. Following placement of the catheter, the stylet is removed and the catheter's position is evaluated to ensure it is within the medullary canal. In larger birds, aspiration will result in blood or bone marrow flash back. (If bone marrow is needed, it can be collected in this manner.) Alternatively, a small amount of saline can be injected and then re-aspirated. If the needle is in the medullary canal, this will usually yield blood-tinged fluid. A larger volume of fluid can then be

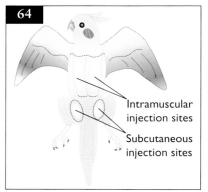

64 Sites for administration of intramuscular and subcutaneous injections.

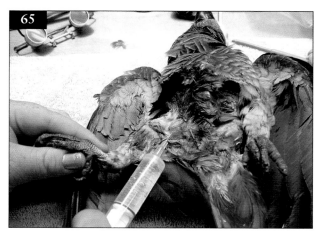

65 Administration of subcutaneous fluids into the inguinal area.

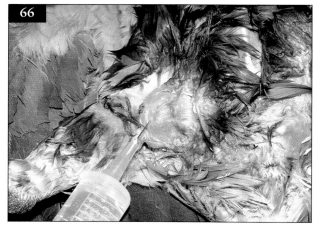

66 Administration of subcutaneous fluids causing the skin to bulge.

injected; if the needle is outside the bone, the soft tissues will swell. Once placement is confirmed, the catheter should be secured.

For placement in the ulna, the crest of the distal ulna is palpated with the carpus flexed. The needle is inserted between the distal ulna and the ulnar carpal bone and advanced into the medullary canal (**67**). The ulna is palpated with one hand during insertion to ensure that the needle is inserted at the proper angle. Again, aspiration, flushing and re-aspiration can be used to confirm correct placement. As the ulna in some birds is pneumatic, if air is aspirated the catheter should be removed and placed in the tibiotarsus. Infusion of a larger volume of fluids into a correctly placed ulnar catheter should result in a visible 'blanching' of the basilic vein as the fluid enters the circulation. Once correct positioning is assured, the catheter should be secured with a bandage.

As the bone is not distensible, and the rate that the fluid enters general circulation is a limiting factor, care must be taken to give intraosseous injections slowly in order to allow the fluid to enter the circulation without being forced. If the injection is forced, it will exit the insertion hole in the bone, again causing discomfort.

Infusion pumps and similar devices are most appropriate for constant infusion. While birds may be given up to 100 ml/kg/hours intravenously without

adverse effects, rates of between 3 and 10 ml/kg/hours are usually more appropriate. Fluid boluses of 20–30 ml/kg may safely be administered over a 2–3-minute period. If using this technique, the use of a butterfly catheter on the syringe and a luer injection port in the catheter can minimize handling of the bird.

Guidelines on the selection of the type of fluid to be given are similar to those for mammalian medicine. Crystalloids, colloids and whole blood are all used successfully in avian patients.

NUTRITIONAL SUPPORT

Sick birds often do not eat; birds that do not eat, die. It is therefore vital that anorexic or emaciated birds with a functional gastrointestinal tract should receive nutritional support. The procedure is identical to crop gavaging fluids; if this cannot be done for any reason, oesophageal and enterotomy feeding tubes can be used. Foods that will pass easily through a syringe and feeding tube are high in energy, easily digestible and have minimal residue are ideal. For these reasons, hand-rearing formulae are often used for short-term maintenance.

RESPIRATORY SUPPORT

Birds, with their high metabolic rates, have a higher oxygen demand than dogs and cats. Conversely, their gas exchange is more efficient; indeed, oxygen levels of 70–100% for 3–8 days have been shown to be toxic in birds. Birds with respiratory distress appear clinically to benefit from a 40–50% oxygen environment. Oxygen may be delivered by mask in the short term or in an oxygen cage.

In cases of tracheal obstruction (e.g. inhaled foreign body, *Aspergillus* granuloma, diphtheritic plaques) it may be necessary to provide an alternative airway by way of an air sac catheter. This is a 2 mm or larger plastic tube (e.g. a noncuffed endotracheal tube) placed into the caudal thoracic air sac. With the patient in right lateral recumbency, the left leg is drawn cranially, exposing the left flank. The following landmarks are identified: the caudal rib, the flexor crura medialis muscle and the pubic bone. A 4 mm vertical incision is made in the skin where the flexor crura medialis muscle crosses the caudal rib. Curved haemostat forceps are then used to reflect the flexor muscle dorsally and then dissect bluntly through the abdominal wall. If done correctly, the operator will feel a 'pop' as the haemostats enter the caudal thoracic air sac. The endotracheal tube or other catheter is then advanced through this incision into the caudal thoracic air sac, taking care not to advance it as far as the caudal border of the lung. Patency is determined

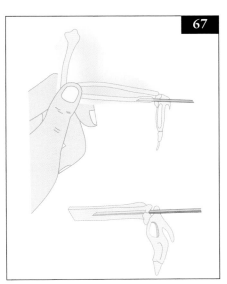

67 Intraosseous catheterization of the ulna.

by observing expired air moving a feather placed over the free end of the catheter. Once satisfied with the placement, the clinician can then use a 'Chinese finger-trap' suture to anchor the catheter to the skin. The free end of the catheter should be long enough so that powder down and feather dust are not freely inhaled; the author prefers to leave the catheter as long as the bird's tail, securing it to the tail feathers (**98**).

ADMINISTERING MEDICATIONS

Once a patient has been stabilized and diagnostic samples collected, medication can then be administered based on either a confirmed or suspected diagnosis. The route of administration is determined by a number of factors: the ease with which the patient can be handled; the patient's clinical condition; the pharmacodynamics and pharmacokinetics of the drug itself; and the clinician's experience and preferences. Commonly used administration routes include injection (intramuscular, intravenous or subcutaneous), oral dosing, topical application and nebulization. Some of these routes are discussed above and will not be repeated here.

The pectoral muscles are most commonly used for intramuscular injections because of their large size (**64**). Other muscles such as the quadriceps, caudal thigh muscles and gluteal muscles can be used in larger birds. Clinicians need to be aware that many drugs are, at best, tissue irritant when given intra-muscularly; caution needs to be taken to avoid giving repeated injections into one site.

Oral medications are often surprisingly easy to administer. In large birds, tablets can be placed directly into the oropharynx; for smaller birds, tablets can be crushed and suspended in either water or methylcellulose for administration with a syringe. When using a syringe, it should be placed over the tongue and the medication delivered in small quantities into the oropharynx. Care must be taken with screaming birds to ensure that the medication is not aspirated. In these birds, and with larger volumes of medication, crop gavage may be more appropriate.

While water-based or other drugs can sometimes be used topically in birds, topical application of oil-based medications is contraindicated. Their grooming behaviour usually sees the medication dispersed through the plumage, destroying the insulation and waterproofing capacity of the feathers. The thinness of the avian skin makes transdermal absorption of medication very easy. This can result in systemic absorption of toxic levels of a drug (e.g. use of topical corticosteroids invariably results in steroidal hepatopathy and other adverse effects).

Nebulization is often used in the treatment of respiratory disease, both to deliver medications directly to site where it is needed and to humidify the respiratory tract. The unique anatomy of the avian respiratory tract means that the nebulizer used should create droplets between 1 and 3 μm in size.

FURTHER READING

Campbell TW, Ellis CK (2007) *Avian and Exotic Animal Hematology and Cytology*, 3rd edn. Blackwell Publishing, Ames.

Divers SJ (2003) Modern endoscopy equipment and advanced endoscopy techniques in birds and reptiles. *Exotic DVM* 5(3):61–63.

Divers SJ, Hernandez-Divers SM (2004) Avian diagnostic endoscopy. *Compendium on Continuing Education for the Practicing Veterinarian* 26(11):839–852.

Fudge AM (2000) *Laboratory Medicine: Avian and Exotic Pets*. WB Saunders, Philadelphia.

Jaensch SM, Cullen L, Raidal SR (2001) The pathology of normobaric oxygen toxicity in budgerigars (*Melopsittacus undulatus*). *Avian Pathology* 30(2):135–142.

Krautwald-Junghanns ME, *et al.* (2004) Research on the anatomy and pathology of the psittacine heart. *Journal of Avian Medicine and Surgery* 18(1):2–11.

Krautwald-Junghanns ME, Pees M (2005) Ultrasonographic diagnosis of avian urogenital disorders. In: *Proceedings of the Annual Conference of the Association of Avian Veterinarians*, pp. 39–44.

Krautwald-Junghanns ME, Pees M (2006) Ultrasonography of the avian liver and gall bladder. In: *Proceedings of the Annual Conference of the Association of Avian Veterinarians*, pp. 53–58.

Nemetz L. (2006) Principles of high definition digital radiology for the avian patient. In: *Proceedings of the Annual Conference of the Association of Avian Veterinarians*, pp. 39–46.

Nemetz L. (2006) Application of high definition digital radiology for the avian patient. In: *Proceedings of the Annual Conference of the Association of Avian Veterinarians*, pp. 263–268.

Smith BJ, Smith SA (1997) Radiology. In: *Avian Medicine and Surgery*. RB Altman, *et al.* (eds). WB Saunders, Philadelphia, pp. 170–199.

Straub J, Pees M, Krautwald-Junghanns ME (2002) Measurement of the cardiac silhouette in psittacines. *Journal of the American Veterinary Medical Association* 221(1):76–79.

CHAPTER 4
INTERPRETING DIAGNOSTIC TESTS

CHOOSING WHICH TESTS TO USE

Veterinarians treating birds are faced with challenges often not encountered by their counterparts treating dogs and cats. Many birds are presented to veterinarians only when near terminally ill, and a quick answer is often the difference between life and death. Birds are often limited in their range of expression of clinical signs and many clinicians, through no fault of their own, lack the experience to conduct a thorough physical examination. The combination of these factors has led to an increasing tendency in avian medicine to conduct exhaustive diagnostic tests on patients, often with scant attention being paid to a complete history and a careful physical examination, and with little attempt to refine or focus the diagnostic efforts. The selection of diagnostic tests should be based on a solid understanding of the species in question, the results of a thorough history taking and physical examination, and a shortened list of probable differential diagnoses based on this work up.

Before proceeding with diagnostic tests, the clinician should first ask:

- Are the test(s) appropriate to the patient (e.g. species, age, sex) and its clinical signs?
- Has the test been validated to ensure that the result obtained is likely to be both accurate and meaningful?
- Are the physical risks to the patient and cost of the test(s) to the client justified by the likely clinical value of the results?

If the answers to these questions are 'yes', then diagnostic testing should proceed.

Diagnostic testing should be done in tiers, with each level focusing on the diagnostic effort of the next level. Where appropriate, the clinician should endeavour to start with low-cost, minimally invasive tests (e.g. faecal wet smears, faecal flotations and Gram staining) before moving on to more expensive and often more invasive tests. As each tier is passed, the information gained should allow the clinician to focus in on an ever-shortening list of differentials and concentrate efforts towards a final answer.

Clinicians also need to be familiar with the advantages, disadvantages and accuracy of the test(s) they are considering using. They need to be aware of the issues surrounding them. There is controversy and healthy debate within the avian medicine community on many of the tests currently in use. Examples include:

- Are faecal Gram stains an appropriate diagnostic test to use on healthy patients?
- Should the client's money be spent on assessing zinc levels in patients not showing clinical signs consistent with zinc toxicosis?
- Can a diagnosis of zinc toxicosis be made from a single blood level evaluation?
- Can aspergillosis be diagnosed in a patient based solely on serological tests?
- Can any disease be diagnosed solely on the evidence of a single positive DNA or PCR test?

Available diagnostic tests include:
- Haematology.
- Clinical biochemistries.
- Serology.
- PCR.
- Cultures and Gram stains.
- Cytology.

HAEMATOLOGY

The complete blood count (CBC) is an important test in determining many disease states in birds. A CBC involves assessing:

- The erythrocytes, through the determination and assessment of:
  - The haematocrit or packed cell volume (PCV).
  - Total erythrocyte count.
  - Haemoglobin concentration.
  - Erythrocyte morphology.
  - Reticulocytes.
- The leucocytes, through the determination and assessment of:
  - The total white cell count.
  - The leucocyte differential count.
  - The morphology of the leucocytes.
- Thrombocyte numbers.

ERYTHROCYTES

The PCV of most parrots lies between 0.4 l/l and 0.55 l/l. A low PCV (<0.35 l/l) can indicate blood loss, anaemia, shock or overhydration (68). A high PCV (>0.55 l/l) indicates dehydration or polycythaemia (primary or secondary). Primary polycythaemia may be seen in birds with bone marrow dysplasias. Birds kept at high altitudes, or those with chronic respiratory disease, may be polycythaemic secondary to low oxygenation of the blood.

Total red blood cell (RBC) numbers in birds are affected by age, sex, environment, hormonal influences and hypoxia. Because the erythrocytes are larger, red cell numbers are lower in birds than in mammals. RBC numbers tend to be lower in young birds and females. The normal RBC count in birds ranges from $1.5–4.5 \times 10^{12}$ cells/l.

The avian erythrocyte is elliptical in shape with a centrally located, oval nucleus. They are usually 10–15 µm in length, compared with the typical biconcave mammalian erythrocyte, which is 6–7 µm in diameter. Typically, healthy erythrocytes have a uniform colour and size when examined using a stained blood smear. They have a relatively short half-life (28–45 days) when compared with those of mammals, which results in a greater number of immature erythrocytes (reticulocytes) in the peripheral circulation. The cytoplasm of these immature erythrocytes stains more basophilic than that of mature erythrocytes, and the nuclear chromatin is less condensed than mature erythrocytes. In most healthy psittacines they represent approximately 1–5% of the total erythrocyte count. Reticulocytes are best seen with vital stains such as new methylene blue, which stains the characteristic clumps of residual cytoplasmic RNA. Reticulocytes can be measured as an indication of the response to an anaemia.

Morphological abnormalities seen in avian erythrocytes include:

- Excessive polychromasia. Polychromasia is an indicator of the patient's erythrocyte regenerative abilities. Although some polychromasia (1–5%) is normal, excessive polychromasia indicates a regenerative response to blood loss or anaemia.
- Reticulocytosis, especially when combined with increased polychromasia, is seen as a regenerative response to blood loss or anaemia.
- Anisocytosis. Variation in the size of avian erythrocytes is occasionally seen in peripheral blood smears as a normal finding. However, the number increases in response to anaemia.
- Poikilocytosis, or variable cell shapes, may represent artefactual error, but is also seen when severe systemic infections affect the bone marrow. Erythrocytes may appear round, elongated or irregular. The nucleus may vary in appearance, location and number. Erythrocytes that appear round with oval nuclei are indicative of accelerated erythropoiesis. Binucleated erythrocytes may also indicate abnormal erythropoiesis in association with severe, chronic inflammatory processes and neoplasia. Poikilocytes are susceptible to damage, and therefore have a shorter life.

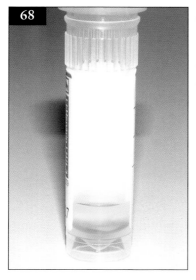

68 Centrifuged blood sample in lithium heparin, demonstrating a marked anaemia.

- Erythrocytic ballooning has been reported to be commonly associated with, although not pathognemonic for, lead toxicosis. It is also seen with 'conure bleeding syndrome'. There are bulges in the normal ellipsoid shape of the erythrocyte, often accompanied by areas of hypochromasia.
- Haemopararasites are occasionally seen in the erythrocyte cytoplasm of wild-caught birds or those exposed to biting insects.

Anaemia

Anaemia is usually the result of increased loss, increased destruction and/or decreased production of erythrocytes. It is classified as regenerative, nonregenerative, haemolytic or haemorrhagic.

Regenerative anaemia

This is characterized by the presence of polychromasia, reticulocytosis, macrocytosis and anisocytosis (**69, 70**). It is an indication of an appropriate bone marrow response. In order to distinguish between polychromasia and reticulocytosis the blood smear must be vitally stained with new methylene blue.

Nonregenerative anaemia

This is the most common type of anaemia described in birds. It arises due to a lack of appropriate bone marrow response combined with the relatively short life of avian erythrocytes. It is characterized by a lack of a regenerative response (i.e. little or no reticulocytosis, polychromasia or anisocytosis).

Possible aetiologies include:
- Acute, overwhelming infections: bacterial, viral (e.g. PBFD) or fungal.
- Chronic disease including chronic inflammatory conditions, chronic infectious diseases (tuberculosis, colibacillosis, salmonellosis, aspergillosis, chlamydiosis), some viral diseases, hypothyroidism and neoplasia.
- Toxicosis.
- Nutritional deficiencies.

Haemolytic anaemia

This is often regenerative in nature and is indicated by increased polychromasia, macrocytosis, anisocytosis and reticulocytosis.

Possible aetiologies include:
- Haemoparasites (*Plasmodium* spp. and *Aegyptianella* spp.).
- Bacterial septicaemia.
- Acute toxicosis (oil ingestion, lead, aflatoxicosis).
- Immune-mediated conditions.

Haemorrhagic anaemia

This results from blood loss due to trauma, gastrointestinal parasitism, coagulation disorders (as in conure bleeding syndrome), organ rupture or ulceration, aneurysms and some viral diseases.

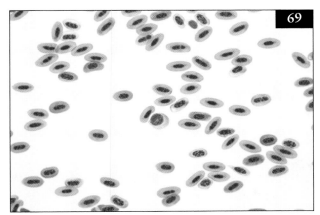

69 Mild regenerative anaemia showing polychromasia (variability in erythrocyte cytoplasmic colour) and anisocytosis (variability in erythrocyte size).

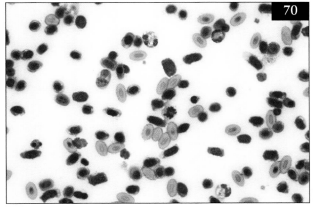

70 Pronounced regenerative anaemia; mitotic figures, poikilocytosis (variability in erythrocyte shape) and binucleate erythrocytes appear in the blood.

Following acute hemorrhage there is often a rapid response during which erythropoiesis increases dramatically. Healthy birds are remarkably adept at dealing with acute blood loss and haemorrhagic shock rarely occurs. Studies have shown that after the loss of even 50% of the blood volume, the PCV returns to normal within 3–7 days.

LEUCOCYTES

The white blood cell (WBC) count and differential are important tools in assessing a patient's response to disease or injury. The WBC count in birds can be determined using three testing methods:

- An automated count, which has recently become available in some laboratories.
- An estimated WBC count determined from a blood smear by counting all leucocytes in 10 high-power (40×) microscopic fields, dividing by the number of fields, and then multiplying this average by 2,000, giving a total WBC/μl.
- The Unopette method using phloxine B stain and a haemocytometer to count eosinophils and heterophils. This count is compared with the percentages of these cells in the differential and the WBC count is calculated using the formula: WBC = (Total Het + Eos) / (% Hets + % Eos) × 100. (Note: In late 2007 the Unopette system was discontinued by the manufacturer.)

Leucocytosis can be normal in young birds, but it can also be due to:

- Stress.
- Inflammation, often associated with bacterial and fungal infections.

Leucopenia can be due to:

- Chronic inflammation or disease, often with an acute decompensatory episode at the time of presentation.
- Overwhelming bacterial and viral infections (e.g. PBFD in juvenile parrots, especially young grey parrots).
- Artefacts resulting from poor sample handling (blood clotting) or technique.

White cell differential counts are best obtained from fresh blood smears, as cellular morphology can be affected by anticoagulants in blood collection tubes. A differential count is typically obtained by examination of stained smears under high magnification. Both the type and morphology of the white cells seen are recorded. In many cases the differential count and cellular morphology give more indication of a bird's health status than the total white cell count.

Heterophils

The heterophil is the avian equivalent of the mammalian neutrophil. While it has a similar function to the neutrophil, morphologically it appears quite different. The nucleus contains coarsely clumped chromatin and usually has two to three lobes. The cytoplasm contains eosinophilic, spherical, oval or spindle-shaped granules. It is, in most species, the predominant white cell. Heterophils lack lysozyme which is why birds form caseated, rather than liquid, pus. Abnormal changes seen with heterophils include:

- Heterophilia. Seen with inflammatory disease or stress and is considered normal in many young birds.
- Heteropenia. Seen with overwhelming septicaemia and certain viral diseases (e.g. PBFD in young African grey parrots). Poor smear preparation technique can 'smudge' many heterophils, causing an artefactual heteropenia.
- Toxic heterophils (increased cytoplasmic basophilia, vacuolization, nuclear degeneration, degranulation or abnormal granules) are seen with severe diseases that affect production and release from the bone marrow. As the severity of the disease increases, the toxicity of the heterophils may also increase as well.
- Immature (band) heterophils have a less distinctively lobulated nucleus and fewer granules, which are round and deeply basophilic. (Care must be taken not to confuse basophils with immature heterophils.) They are produced in response to bacterial or fungal infections, and indicate a depletion of mature bone marrow storage pool and therefore a poor prognosis.

Eosinophils

The eosinophil is a round cell with a slightly basophilic cytoplasm (in contrast to the colourless cytoplasm of the heterophil). The granules are usually rounded, although shape and colour may vary greatly between species. The granules are distinctly eosinophilic and brighter in colour when compared with the heterophil granules. The function of eosinophils is still largely unknown; eosinophilia in pet birds is rare, sometimes associated with parasitic infections or marked tissue damage.

Lymphocytes

Lymphocytes are second only to the heterophil in frequency in most species except Amazon parrots and some passerines (canaries) in which the lymphocytes appear to be the predominant leucocyte. Size and shape varies, with small, medium and large cells that may be round or moulded around neighbouring cells being seen in the same smear. They have a large, round, centrally located nucleus with densely clumped or reticulate nuclear chromatin. The cytoplasm is clear or slightly basophilic. Reactive lymphocytes (i.e. those responding to antigenic stimulation) usually have a more deeply basophilic cytoplasm, vacuoles in the cytoplasm, a clear perinuclear ring and scalloping of the cell edges. Occasional reactive lymphocytes are a normal finding in avian blood, but large numbers indicate marked antigenic stimulation as seen in severe infections (e.g. severe viral infections, chlamydiosis, aspergillosis, salmonellosis and tuberculosis).

Lymphocytosis is seen in:
- Chronic infectious or inflammatory conditions.
- Lymphoid leukaemia.
- Normal finding in Amazons and canaries.

Lymphopenia is seen in:
- Viral infections and diseases that cause bursal damage or bone marrow suppression.
- Relative to a marked increase in heterophils.

Monocytes

Monocytes are the largest of the mononuclear leucocytes, but are rarely seen in peripheral blood smears. They spend only a short time in circulation before passing into tissues and becoming macrophages. The eccentric nuclei are either round, elongated or indented, and the cytoplasm typically stains a blue–grey colour with a reticular or finely granular appearance, with occasional vacuoles. Care must be taken not to confuse them with large lymphocytes.

Monocytosis is most commonly associated with chronic granulomatous infections such as chlamydiosis, tuberculosis, mycoses and bacterial granulomatous diseases (e.g. mycobacterial infections). Because circulating numbers are usually so low, monocytopenia is not reported.

Basophils

Basophils are uncommon in peripheral blood smears of birds. They appear as small cells with clear cytoplasm and spherical basophilic granules. The nucleus stains a light blue colour. Care must be taken not to confuse them with immature heterophils. Basophilia has been reported in respiratory disease (e.g. air sac mite in canaries), chlamydiosis and tissue trauma more than 48 hours old.

THROMBOCYTES

Thrombocytes are small, oval, nucleated cells that can be differentiated from erythrocytes by their size (they are smaller than erythrocytes) and their nucleus, which is larger, more rounded and darkly basophilic-staining. The cytoplasm is colourless or a faint blue colour with one to two small basophilic inclusions at the poles. Total counts are difficult and not routinely performed as the thrombocytes tend to clump. However, there are typically 1–2 cells seen per high-power field. Their function is unclear; they contain little thromboplastin, so it is unlikely that they initiate clotting. With bacterial infections they tend to increase in numbers and become activated (pseudopodial formation and vacuolation) and tend to aggregate in clumps. They appear to have some phagocytic activity.

Thrombocytosis is rarely reported and may arise as in response to thrombocytopenia. Thrombocytopenia may occur due to bone marrow suppression or disease processes causing an excessive demand (e.g. viral diseases such as circovirus, reovirus or polyomavirus).

ASSESSING BLOOD CLOTTING

Vascular injury results in three events:
- The exposure of blood to tissue thromboplastin (factor III), which activates the extrinsic clotting pathway.
- The exposure of blood to subendothelium, which both activates the intrinsic pathway (which is weak or absent) and stimulates the adhesion and aggregation of thrombocytes to form a plug in the injury.
- Vasoconstriction, through various humoral and local mechanisms, which slows blood flow, reduces blood loss and allows time for thrombocytes to adhere to the injury.

Therefore, the extrinsic pathway is the major means of blood clotting in birds. Following vasoconstriction and thrombocyte adherence, the extrinsic pathway forms a fibrin clot over the thrombocytes and allows the vascular endothelium to begin repairs. This entire process can occur in as little as ten seconds.

Unfortunately there are no commercially available tests to evaluate the avian extrinsic pathway. Clinical tests for the assessment of coagulation in birds include:

- Thrombocyte evaluation. There should be 1–2 thrombocytes per oil immersion field. An estimated thrombocyte count/µl can be performed by counting the average number of thrombocytes in five high-power fields and then using the formula: estimated thrombocyte count per $\propto$l = (average number of thrombocytes / 1,000 × 3,500,000. The normal count is 20,000–30,000 per µl (20–30 × 10^9/l).
- Bleeding time has been used in poultry by pricking the comb with a needle. The normal bleeding time averages eight minutes.
- Whole blood clotting time, where whole blood is placed in a plain tube, incubated and then inverted until clot forms. This assesses the intrinsic and common pathway and blood will normally clot in 2–10 minutes. This time will be accelerated by contamination with tissue thromboplastin. An alternative technique is to place blood in capillary tubes and break the tubes until a clot forms, normally in less than five minutes.
- Prothrombin time (PT), which evaluates the extrinsic and common pathway, can be used but requires avian thromboplastin. Mammalian thromboplastin significantly prolongs PT.

CLINICAL BIOCHEMISTRY

Clinical biochemistry involves the measurement of specific groups of chemicals within the body and the interpretation of the results obtained (71). These chemicals include:

- Metabolites. Those chemicals that are produced as the end-products of various metabolic processes within the body.
- Tissue enzymes, which catalyse chemical reactions within the body without being altered themselves.
- Electrolytes, including sodium, potassium and chloride.
- Minerals, such as calcium, phosphorus and magnesium.
- Bile acids, produced in the liver from cholesterol and used in the emulsification of dietary fats.

The levels of these chemicals in the blood can be influenced by either physiological or pathological processes. Physiological variations can be due to age, sex, body fat to muscle ratio, nutritional status, reproductive status and species. However,

pathological processes, including cellular damage or abnormal function of an organ system (or systems), often produce significant changes in blood levels.

There are three major causes of abnormal clinical biochemistries:

- Normal variation between species and individuals.
- Artefacts.
- Pathology.

NORMAL VARIATION BETWEEN SPECIES AND INDIVIDUALS

There are over 9,000 species of birds, with major differences in anatomy, physiology, form and function. Some are carnivorous, some are nectivorous, some are granivorous and some are omnivorous. It is unrealistic to expect that they would all conform to a relatively narrow range of biochemical values.

Other variations arise between individuals of the same species. These variations occur because of differences in age, sex, diet, husbandry, etc. For this reason some clinicians recommend establishing a set of normal values for individual birds during annual health examinations, and then using these values as a comparison should the bird become ill.

ARTEFACTS

When interpreting a biochemistry analysis, care must be taken to distinguish between abnormal results due to disease, and abnormal results due to other factors. These other factors, referred to as artefacts, can occur for a variety of reasons, including:

- Physiological changes.
- Previous therapy.
- The clinical condition of the patient.
- The collection method.
- Storage and transport of the sample.

Physiological changes

Stress due to transport and handling of the patient can lead to a release of endogenous corticosteroids, resulting in changes in the haemogram and in blood glucose.

Lipaemia, while occasionally seen in diseases of the liver and reproductive system, can also occur naturally in the reproductively active female (72). Regardless of the cause, lipaemia can cause false elevations in bile acids, protein, calcium, phosphorus and uric acid. It may also falsely decrease amylase. Postprandial lipaemia is uncommon in pet birds, so fasting will not help; the clinician needs to check with the laboratory if the sample submitted was lipaemic before interpreting these biochemistries.

Previous therapy

Before interpreting biochemistries, the clinician should consider if any treatment given prior to the sample collection could have had an effect on the results. Therapy given by another veterinarian or in an attempt to stabilize a crashing patient can have marked effects. Parenteral fluids can dilute biochemistries; exogenous corticosteroids can markedly elevate aspartate aminotransferase (AST), creatine kinase (CK) and lactate dehydrogenase (LDH); intramuscular injections, particularly of irritant drugs, can do the same.

The clinical condition of the patient

Trauma, starvation and dehydration can all have marked effects on biochemistries, and need to be considered when interpreting results. Trauma can cause elevations in AST and CK and possibly glucose; starvation can lower glucose and also elevate AST and CK if protein catabolism has begun; dehydration can elevate uric acid.

The collection method

Ideally, sample collection should be performed in such a manner that it has minimal impact on the patient while providing an artefact-free sample suitable for analysis. This usually requires venipuncture to be performed on a minimally stressed patient. Inexperienced clinicians may need to consider gaseous anaesthesia in order to collect a good sample without the bird struggling.

Venipuncture should be performed on a large vein (e.g. the jugular) using a needle that is large enough to minimize haemolysis while being small enough to minimize trauma to the blood vessel wall. Haemolysis can cause elevations in bile acids, LDH, CK, alkaline phosphatase (ALP), potassium and phosphorus. Glucose and albumin may be decreased. Calcium may be elevated or decreased, according to the methodology used.

Toenail clipping should be discouraged. Not only is it unduly painful, but crush artefacts and contamination with uric acid and bacteria from droppings on the perch can cause elevations in uric acid and decreased glucose if testing is delayed long enough for bacterial growth to occur in the sample.

71 In-house testing assists in the rapid diagnosis of critically ill patients.

72 Lipaemia in birds is usually associated with high fat diets, liver disease, diabetes mellitus or reproductive activity.

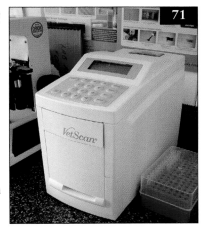
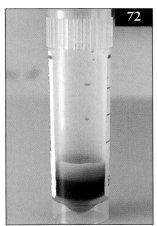

Storage and transport of the sample

Blood collected for biochemistry analysis should be placed immediately into a lithium heparin tube. Ideally, miniature tubes as used in medical paediatrics should be used. The sample should be gently rolled or rocked; clotting must be avoided, but haemolysis must be as well. If the analysis is to be performed in-house, it should be processed immediately. If a delay is likely, or if the sample is to be shipped to an outside laboratory, the sample should be centrifuged and the plasma harvested. Sending whole blood to an outside laboratory can result in decreased glucose (as cell metabolism continues) and haemolysis.

EDTA tubes are unsuitable for biochemistry analysis, but can be used for haematology, lead analysis and fibrinogen determination.

BIOCHEMISTRY ANALYSIS BY ORGAN SYSTEM
Liver

The detection of liver disease through biochemistry is complicated by the fact that there are no specific 'liver enzymes' that can be evaluated conclusively in each and every case. Liver disease can be broadly classified into three conditions: hepatocellular rupture, decreased hepatic function and cholestasis. These conditions can occur either separately or concurrently.

Hepatocellular rupture

This releases intracellular enzymes, which then reach elevated levels in the blood. These so-called 'leakage enzymes' include:

- Aspartate aminotransferase. This cytosolic enzyme is found in many tissues in the body, but the highest concentrations are found in skeletal muscle and liver. Significant elevations usually represent either muscular or hepatocellular damage. AST, therefore, must be interpreted alongside CK (released from damaged muscle) to distinguish between the two. In general, an elevated AST with a normal CK indicates hepatocellular rupture. However, CK has a much shorter half-life than AST; a single-point muscle injury (e.g. an injection) 4–7 hours before sample collection could duplicate this biochemistry pattern. Although AST is considered to be the most useful liver enzyme, it cannot be considered in isolation as an indicator of liver disease.
- Glutamate dehydrogenase (GLDH), a mitochondrial enzyme, is the most specific enzyme for the detection of liver disease, but its sensitivity is low. Because it is bound to mitochondria, extensive and severe liver damage is required before elevations are detectable.

- Lactate dehydrogenase is not specific to any tissue; its main advantage lies with a half-life shorter than CK. Persistent elevation in the presence of normal CK is strongly suggestive of liver disease.
- Alanine aminotransferase (ALT) and alkaline phosphatase are not considered useful in detecting liver disease in birds. ALT in birds is very nonspecific for the liver, and normal levels have been shown in cases with severe liver damage. ALP elevations are more commonly associated with bone disease in birds.

Decreased liver function

Decreased liver function can occur with any number of liver diseases, not all of which involve hepatocellular rupture. Chronic cirrhosis, amyloidosis and hepatic lipidosis can all have an adverse effect on liver function without causing any cellular damage. In these cases a 'liver function test' is necessary to detect the problem. Bile acids serve this purpose well. Produced in the liver, they are excreted in bile into the small intestine where they act to emulsify fat. Most of the bile acids are then resorbed in the small intestine, enter the portal system and are taken up by the liver to be recycled. Elevated levels occur when there is impairment of the liver's ability to remove bile acids from the portal circulation. A two- to fourfold increase in bile acids indicates a significant decrease in liver function. It needs to be noted though that a severely dysfunctional liver (e.g. end-stage cirrhosis) may not be able to produce normal levels of bile acids, leading to low to normal results. Total protein, especially albumin, may also be decreased with decreased liver function.

Cholestasis

Cholestasis occurs when the biliary system is partially or totally obstructed. This can be seen with biliary neoplasia, pancreatic disease or diffuse swelling of the entire liver. Gamma glutamyl transferase (GGT) is an enzyme found in the cell membranes of the bile ducts. Elevations can be seen in cholestatic disease (e.g. bile duct carcinoma), but it is considered to be a relatively insensitive test for liver disease in psittacines. Bilirubin is not produced in birds; they utilize biliverdin instead. There are no commercial assays for biliverdin.

Kidney

The end-product of protein metabolism in birds is uric acid. It is produced in the liver, enters the circulation and is then secreted by renal tubules (>90%) or filtered in the glomerulus (<10%). Significant loss of renal tubules will therefore result in elevations of uric acid. Dehydration is less likely to cause hyperuricaemia because glomerular filtration is relatively unimportant.

At first glance it would appear that uric acid offers a sensitive and specific test for renal disease. There are, however, several confounding factors. Firstly, species differences: carnivorous birds have higher normal uric acid levels than granivorous birds. Secondly, age: juvenile birds may have lower levels than adults. Thirdly, although significant elevations usually indicate renal disease, normal levels do not mean the kidneys are normal: mild increases could indicate early renal disease or dehydration (or both). There must be severe renal damage before uric acid levels begin to rise.

Because of this relative insensitivity of uric acid in detecting renal disease, levels are best interpreted alongside a determination of the bird's water intake and loss and a physical examination. To distinguish renal disease from dehydration, the patient's hematocrit, total protein and blood urea nitrogen (BUN) should be evaluated concurrently. Dehydration can lead to decreased glomerular filtration rates (GFRs), in turn leading to elevated levels of BUN; this same decrease in GFR can lead to elevations of uric acid without primary renal disease being present. It is therefore prudent, in cases of an elevated uric acid level, to rehydrate the patient over 2–3 days before definitively diagnosing renal disease. Persistent hyperuricaemia after fluid therapy, and with haematocrit, total protein and BUN returning to normal, confirms a diagnosis of renal disease.

Creatinine is generally accepted as being of little or no value in evaluating renal function in birds. Phosphorus elevations are usually not seen in birds with renal disease.

Reproductive system

Clinical biochemistries can tell the clinician little about the male reproductive tract; they can, however, reveal something about the activity of the female reproductive tract. Oestrogen, produced by developing follicles, induces the production of calcium-binding protein and vitellogenesis in the liver. The net result of this activity is an increase in circulating total protein, calcium and cholesterol. The serum may appear lipaemic. Radiographic evidence of hepatomegaly and increased long bone density can confirm reproductive activity. It should be noted, though, that normal calcium and protein do not reflect a lack of reproductive activity.

Gastrointestinal system

Gastrointestinal disease typically only gives nonspecific results with clinical biochemistry. Elevations of CK, AST and LDH are not uncommon, and are not specific to the intestinal tract. Electrolytes may give more information: sodium may be elevated with excessive water loss through vomiting or diarrhoea; chloride may be elevated with vomiting or regurgitation; and potassium may be decreased with vomiting/diarrhoea and elevated with dehydration. There are many other possible causes of electrolyte disturbance, and our understanding of avian electrolyte balance is still in the very early stages.

Amylase and lipase have been proposed as useful parameters in the detection of pancreatic disease. There is still considerable discussion of the incidence of pancreatic disease and the specificity of these enzymes. Significant elevations of these enzymes, when accompanied by clinical signs of gastrointestinal dysfunction (vomiting, ileus, diarrhoea, abdominal pain) should lead the clinician to consider pancreatic disease as a differential diagnosis. However, normal levels do not preclude a diagnosis of pancreatic disease, nor do abnormal levels confirm such a diagnosis.

Blood glucose

Glucose is an essential energy source for nearly every cell in the body. Blood levels are governed by its intake, absorption, the interactions of hormones controlling carbohydrate metabolism (insulin, glucagon and somatostatin), the body's metabolism, its ability to store glucose and its excretion. As disorders of glucose metabolism involve so many organ systems, it is treated here as a separate entity.

Hyperglycaemia may be a normal physiological process, (e.g. in juvenile birds). However, elevated levels are usually related to increased production or release (e.g. stress) or failure of tissues to take it up out of the blood (diabetes mellitus). Iatrogenic hyperglycaemia occurs when corticosteroids are administered or intravenous dextrose is given. Female reproductive disease may also elevate blood glucose, but this may be an indirect result due to inflammation affecting the endocrine pancreas.

Hypoglycaemia may result from poor handling of blood samples (i.e. it may be artefactual, rather than factual). However, it is seen in cases with decreased intake (starvation, anorexia), increased usage (septicaemias, neoplasia and multiorgan failure) or decreased production (liver disease).

SEROLOGY

Serological tests are designed to detect antibodies (usually IgG or IgM) in serum or plasma (73). The results can be affected by a range of factors:

- Host factors:
  - Persistence of antibodies postinfection. Serial tests, weeks apart, are needed to assess what is happening in the patient.
  - Lack of antibody postinfection. If test only assesses IgM, chronic cases with only IgG will be missed. Similarly, some animals that fail to seroconvert due to immunosuppression will test negative.

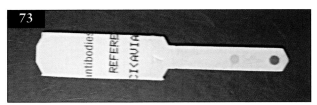

73 The Immunocomb *Chlamydophila psittaci* test is an in-house serological test.

- Changes in antibody titre. A single sample only indicates prior infection. Detection of active infections requires a measurement of rising titres (usually fourfold) over a 4–6-week period.
- Species-specific reaction to certain testing.
- Antigen factors:
  - Prepatent period. Usually 1–2 weeks. If testing during the prepatent period, a false negative may be obtained.
  - Antigen-specific reaction to certain testing methods.
- Assay factors:
  - Laboratory error.
  - Poor test selection.
  - Lack of reagents.
  - Cross-reaction between antibodies may cause false positives.
  - Sensitivity and specificity of test.

A variety of serological tests is available today (*Table 2*). The selection of the best test requires a clinician to have an understanding of the principles of immunology and the interaction between host and pathogen. He/she also needs to have an understanding

Table 2 Some of the available serological tests.

Test	Technique	Disease/pathogen	Advantages	Disadvantages
Enzyme-linked immunosorbent assay (ELISA)	Detection of antibody–antigen complex by use of a second enzyme-conjugated antibody that produces a colour change	Adenovirus in poultry, mycobacteria, *Chlamydophila*, paramyxoviruses, aspergillosis	Simple to operate, rapid, automated	Requires species-specific second antibody
Haemagglutination inhibition	Proteins present on the surface of some viruses cause agglutination of erythrocytes. By adding antibodies against these viral proteins, this agglutination is inhibited. Therefore, if agglutination occurs, no virus-specific antibodies are present, and *vice versa*. Titres are determined by serial dilution of the sample	Circovirus, paramyxoviruses, eastern equine encephalitis, avian influenza	Secondary antibodies not required, inexpensive, good sensitivity	Serum must be treated to clear nonspecific agglutination. Not all avian viruses cause agglutination

Table 2 Some of the available serological tests. (*continued*)

Test	Technique	Disease/pathogen	Advantages	Disadvantages
Complement fixation	Complement is needed to bind antibody and antigen. Detection of complement fixation demonstrates the presence of the antigen	Polyomavirus, psittacine herpesvirus, mycobacteria, aspergillosis, *Chlamydophila*	Quick, simple test; moderate sensitivity and specificity	Can have false positives. Does not work in all species. Usually only detects IgM
Virus neutralization	Serum is mixed with an antigen. If antigen-specific antibody is present in the serum, the antigen will be neutralized and will be incapable of causing cytopathic changes in a cell culture	Polyomavirus, psittacine herpesvirus	Very specific and sensitive. Detects both IgM and IgG	Takes up to 7 days to run; requires both cell culture and virus propagation. Nonspecific substances in the serum can give a positive result
Immunodiffusion assay	Antibody and antigen placed in agar gel diffuse towards each other. If an antibody–antigen complex forms, a precipitate develops that is visible as a white line	Adenovirus in poultry, reovirus in psittacines	Simple and cheap. Secondary antibodies not required. Moderate specificity	Low sensitivity. Difficult to quantify
Immunofluorescent antibody	Multiple dilutions of serum are incubated with cells infected with antigen fixed to plastic. A fluorescent-labelled second antibody is added. Positive results can be viewed with a fluorescent microscope	Avian influenza, *Chlamydophila*	Quick and simple. Moderate sensitivity and specificity	Requires species-specific second antibody. Requires a fluorescent microscope

of the types of tests available and the advantages and disadvantages of each.

USING SEROLOGY

Serology has several advantages that make it unlikely its use will ever disappear:

- PCR and other antigen-detection tests can sometimes be too accurate, detecting extremely low levels of antigen (or portions of antigen) that may not be significant. At other times the antigen may be extremely difficult to detect: it may shed only intermittently or at very low concentrations. In both these cases, serological evaluation of the bird (or birds) may better detect the presence of significant levels of antigen. Serological assays of a flock may be more sensitive in detecting a pathogen than more direct antigen-detection tests.

- Its relatively low invasiness. Direct testing for an antigen that is only intermittently shed (if at all) often requires the collection of a tissue sample, either by autopsy or biopsy. Serology, on the other hand, simply requires a blood sample. This is obviously much less invasive.
- Serological tests, especially when performed in large numbers, can be significantly cheaper than more direct pathogen-detection tests.

Although at first glance these appear to be almost overwhelming advantages, other factors play key roles in the selection of an appropriate serological test. These factors can be categorized into three groups, dicussed below.

The characteristics of the test

The selection of the test is of paramount importance. Is this test appropriate for this species? Has it been thoroughly validated for this disease? Antibodies are not necessarily consistent across species; a test that works well in poultry may not work well, or at all, in psittacines.

The sensitivity and specificity of a test will often determine its usefulness. Sensitivity is a measure of a test's ability to accurately detect antibodies in an infected bird. A highly sensitive test will hopefully detect most of the antibody-positive birds in a population. As such, it is useful as a screening test during the early days of a disease outbreak, where it is important to identify quickly potentially infected birds. Once these birds have been removed from a population, it becomes more important to be sure that the remaining birds that have tested negative are, in fact, not infected. At this time a highly specific test is desirable. Specificity is the proportion of truly noninfected birds that test negative. A clinician using a serological test should therefore be aware of the published sensitivity and specificity of a test.

Another test characteristic to be considered is its complexity to perform. The more complex a test, the more susceptible it is to operator error, leading to erroneous results. Errors can occur in the collection, storing and transport of the sample to the laboratory, and then again in carrying out the test; equipment can be faulty, the operator may be inexperienced or reagents may be out of date. There may also be error in the interpretation of the results, or even dissension about the significance of the results.

In some cases a test requires specific reagents, which may not be readily available (e.g. the haemagglutination inhibition test for PBFD requires specially prepared galah erythrocytes, readily available in Australia, but harder to obtain elsewhere). (Note: Goose erythrocytes can sometimes be used.) This limits its usefulness in the USA, UK and Europe.

The characteristics of the antigen and the disease

Some antigens/diseases are not readily detectable by some tests due to the behaviour of that antigen. Some viruses, for example, do not agglutinate erythrocytes, making haemagglutination inhibition tests unsuitable.

Some pathogens, such as viruses like the influenza A virus, undergo antigenic variance wherein the surface proteins of the virus change and prevent immediate detection. Other pathogens, such as *Mycobacterium* spp. and *Aspergillus* spp., seem not to provoke an antibody response in some patients for, as yet, undetermined reasons. In these situations, false-negative test results may occur.

From an epidemiological point of view, there will always be false-positive and false-negative results for any test. The clinician must therefore interpret results with care; if a disease is of a low incidence in a species or in a geographical area, is a positive result truly significant or even accurate? And *vice versa*? As with any laboratory test, the results must be interpreted as a part of the diagnostic test, not as a sole entity.

Host factors

Some clinicians seem to fall into the trap of forgetting that there is a patient attached to a laboratory test result. How the host is responding to the challenge of a pathogen has a major impact on the interpretation of a serological test (or any other test). The interaction between the host and the pathogen must be understood by the clinician in order to accurately assess the patient's status.

In the initial stages of infection (the prepatent period) there will be a delay while the immune system firstly recognizes the presence of an antigen and then mounts a response to it (usually in the form of IgM). In this prepatent period (usually 1–2 weeks), a serological assay that only detects IgG will give a false-negative result. On the other hand, direct antigen-detection tests may have a prepatent period of only 1–2 days, and are therefore more reliable in detecting early infection.

With appropriate treatment or an effective immune defence (or both) the host will inactivate/kill the pathogen and then clear it from the body. During this process there is a rising antibody titre. After the pathogen has been cleared, these titres should start to decline. The rate of this decline is dependent on many factors (e.g. the strength of the immune system, the persistence of the antigen, the degree of response to a specific pathogen). A single-point serological assay is unable to distinguish between rising and declining antibody titres; serial tests, 2–3 weeks apart, are needed to assess what is happening in the patient. For example, polyomavirus infection in a bird may result in detectable antibody titres for the life of the bird, even though the bird cleared the virus from its body after a few weeks or months. So while a single serological test may indirectly detect that a pathogen was/is present in the patient, it cannot (by itself) detect the ongoing presence of disease.

The serological detection of pathogens that are ubiquitous in the environment is fraught with error. Most birds, for example, are exposed to *Aspergillus* spp. at some time; relatively few develop aspergillosis. The detection of antibodies to *Aspergillus* does not, therefore, constitute a diagnosis of aspergillosis; rather, it indicates the patient has been exposed to the pathogen and has mounted an immune response to it.

Despite the presence of a pathogen actively causing disease, some birds fail to produce antibodies. This immunosuppression can be due to a number of factors. Concurrent disease frequently causes immunosuppression: viruses such as PBFD, polyomavirus, pox and herpes, bacterial and parasitic infections and aflatoxicosis have all been implicated in immunosuppressed patients. Certain drugs such as tetracycline, tylosin and gentamicin are known to decrease antibody production. Environmental stress (inadequate temperatures, humidity, noise, poor nutrition) is known to suppress both the bursa and the thymus, possibly through corticosteroid production by the adrenal gland. Immunosuppressed birds, for whatever reason, may give a false-negative result.

A final consideration is that antibodies produced in response to a particular pathogen may be difficult to distinguish from antibodies produced against another pathogen. Antibodies produced by vaccination may be indistinguishable from those produced by natural infection. In either case, false-positive results can be produced.

SCENARIOS INVOLVING THE USE OF SEROLOGY
Disease outbreaks
Serology is often employed in the face of an outbreak of an infectious disease. Serology has the advantages of being relatively simple (most labs can perform it), quick and cost-effective, particularly when compared with other (more direct) tests such as DNA/PCR and histopathology. Large numbers of birds can be tested quickly, giving an indication of the incidence of the disease in a given population. In the early stages of an outbreak, high sensitivity is needed; all infected (positive result) birds need to be identified as soon as possible. Sensitivity can be increased by using known high-sensitivity tests, increasing the sample size of the population being tested and parallel testing, using several different tests to increase the likelihood of an infected bird being detected.

Once the incidence of a disease has been determined, steps can be taken to control it. This will usually require the removal of birds that have tested positive and further testing of those that have tested negative. This introduces the problem of false-negative results (seronegative birds that are latent carriers of a disease). At this time highly specific tests are needed, and may require the employment of a different serological test or tests. As the incidence of a disease approaches zero, the detection of these latent carriers becomes even more difficult, and complete eradication may not be possible without complete culling.

Specific pathogen-free flocks
One of the cornerstones of successful farming is maintaining a disease-free flock. This is no different with birds, whether it is an intensive poultry flock, a zoological collection or an avicultural facility. The development of a specific pathogen-free (SPF) flock requires the testing of all members of that flock, preferably before they join it.

Veterinarians advising clients on a SPF protocol encounter similar problems to those faced when dealing with an outbreak of disease. No test can hope to be 100% sensitive and 100% specific. Therefore, parallel testing (several different tests, not necessarily all serological) and serial testing (repeated testing over a period of time) may help to detect those birds that are latent carriers and test negative the first time. While this can add considerably to the cost of new birds, it must be weighed up against the costs of remedying an outbreak of disease if it escapes detection and is introduced.

The individual bird
While serological tests are extremely useful in screening flocks, they often lack the sensitivity and specificity required for screening an individual bird. While relatively inexpensive, they may lack the accuracy of a more direct antigen-detection test. However, these more

direct tests only detect the presence of a pathogen, not necessarily the presence of a disease. Combining the two tests together can lead to a better screening of an individual. By looking for the pathogen, and the body's immune response to it, a better understanding of the bird's status can be achieved. When combined with ancillary tests such as haematology and biochemistry (which can reflect the effect the pathogen is having on the bird), a more complete picture of the host–pathogen interaction becomes apparent.

PCR TESTING

PCR is the amplification of a specific fragment of nucleic acid (DNA) from minute quantities of source DNA material. It is rapidly becoming one of the most widely used techniques in molecular biology because it is quick, inexpensive and simple.

Samples are first heated, which causes the DNA double helix strand to separate into single strands. Primers are then added to bind to these single strands (annealing) and the sample is allowed to cool. Each time this heating and cooling cycle is repeated, the amount of DNA present in the sample effectively doubles (amplification). Once the process has been completed the sample now contains numerous copies of specific DNA sequences. The reaction products are separated by gel electrophoresis. Depending on the quantity produced and the size of the amplified fragment, the reaction products can be visualized directly by staining with ethidium bromide or a silver-staining protocol or by means of radioisotopes and autoradiography.

The specificity of PCR depends on the primers used. As a general rule most PCR assays are highly specific, but a quantitative PCR assay may have variable degrees of sensitivity and may fail to detect very low quantities of DNA. In an attempt to increase the sensitivity of PCR, 'real-time PCR' has been developed. This assay allows the laboratory to view the increase in the amount of DNA as it is amplified by characterizing (through the use of fluorescent markers) the point in time during cycling when amplification of the target DNA is first detected, rather than the amount of target produced at the end of the assay. The higher the starting copy number of the nucleic acid target, the sooner a significant increase in fluorescence is observed.

While PCR is an accurate test for the detection of target DNA, results must be interpreted with caution. Firstly, the sensitivity and specificity of the test means that false positives can occur easily if the sample is contaminated during collection, processing or testing. Secondly, a problem sometimes arises with an overdiagnosis of a disease solely through the detection of a pathogen, without necessarily diagnosing the presence of a disease process. Clinicians must therefore exercise caution in the use of PCR, using it as a tool for obtaining a diagnosis, rather than as a diagnosis in its own right.

CULTURES

Over the last several decades there has been a quantum shift in thought about the significance of bacterial and fungal cultures taken from birds. The concept of bacterial and fungal infections being primary diseases has largely been replaced by a better understanding of how pathogens can take advantage of an immunosuppressed, malnourished patient. In other words, clinicians, instead of asking 'What infection does this bird have?', are now asking 'Why does this bird have an infection?' This change in thought has lead to better diagnoses, better treatments and better survival rates.

As part of this evolving thought process, clinicians have reviewed many of the tests that were commonly used to diagnose disease, and are questioning the correct use and interpretation of tests such as Gram stains and cultures. It is not appropriate to base a diagnosis of health or disease in a bird solely on a Gram stain and/or culture. Questions that need to be asked when selecting this test include:

- Does the clinical database (history, physical examination, haematology and biochemistries) collected on this bird suggest a bacterial or fungal infection?
- Is the site the sample has been collected from likely to give significant information about the patient's problem?
- What do the culture or stain results mean?

As veterinary skills and diagnostic equipment have improved, clinicians are now recognizing that many diseases in birds are not caused by infectious agents. Nutritional, metabolic, endocrine and traumatic conditions, amongst others, can all give rise to the classic 'sick bird look'. Neither bacterial cultures nor antibiotics are likely to assist in the diagnosis and treatment of these patients. A sound clinical database provides the clinician with the best information from which to direct further diagnostic and therapeutic steps.

While a Gram stain or culture from the faeces of a bird with gastroenteritis is likely to provide valuable information, it does not constitute a diagnosis in its own right. Nor will it assist in the diagnosis of a bird with a respiratory problem or a traumatic injury, or even an assessment on a bird that is otherwise normal and healthy. But there still persists a school of thought that insists a faecal Gram stain should be performed on all birds, regardless of why they have been presented. Cultures (**74**) and Gram stains are useful diagnostic tools, but the clinician must evaluate if their use is justified for each patient.

Normal faecal bacteria cultured from healthy birds include gram-positive bacilli (*Lactobacillus* spp., *Bacillus* spp., *Corynebacterium* spp., and *Streptomyces*) and gram-positive cocci (*Staphylococcus epidermidis, Streptococcus* spp., *Aerococcus* spp. and *Micrococcus* spp.). Older birds tend to have more *Corynebacterium* and less *Lactobacillus* than juvenile birds. *Escherichia coli* is commonly recovered from cockatoos, but less commonly in other species. Other gram-negative bacteria occasionally found in clinically normal birds include *Enterobacter, Klebsiella, Citrobacter, Pasteurella* and *Moraxella* spp. While some *Pseudomonas* spp. have been recovered from healthy birds, *P. aeruginosa* is rarely recovered from healthy birds. Isolation of *Proteus, Salmonella, Pseudomonas, Klebsiella, Listeria, Erysipelothrix* and haemolytic *Staphylococcus aureus* is clinically significant in sick birds.

Cultures from other sites (eyes, ears, choana) usually show similar results.

A heavy growth of a pure culture of any bacteria can reflect bacterial overgrowth and warrants further investigation.

Candida albicans is often detected by Gram stain in the droppings of birds eating yeast-containing feedstuffs (e.g. bread, biscuits). Unless the yeast are numerous and budding, or can be cultured in heavy numbers, they have little or no clinical significance. Development of pseudohyphae, seen on Gram staining, is significant and may indicate invasion of the intestinal mucosa by the yeast.

Culture of *Aspergillus* spp. or *Cryptococcus* spp. from a healthy bird is likely to reflect environmental contamination rather than infection.

CYTOLOGY

Cytological samples (**75, 76**) can be obtained from:
- Fine needle aspirates of masses or organs.
- Abdominocentesis.
- Sinus aspirates.
- Crop washes.
- Arthrocentesis.
- Tracheal and air sac washes.
- Contact smears from skin and internal organs.
- Scrapings from the palpebral conjunctiva, cornea, oral cavity or tissues that normally yield poorly cellular samples.

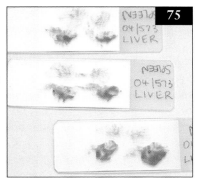

75 Smears of liver and spleen to be air-dried and then fixed in methanol. It is important to prepare more than one smear so that different stains can be applied. (Photo courtesy S Raidal)

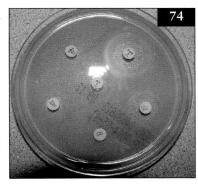

74 While sensitivity testing can indicate the most appropriate antibiotic to use, it does not answer the clinician's primary question, 'Why does this bird have an infection?'

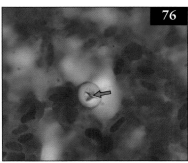

76 Artefacts can be confused with pathology. A talc crystal (arrow) from a disposable glove is seen in the liver of a lovebird. (Diff Quik, 100×) (Photo courtesy S Echols)

Assessment of a cytological sample requires the clinician to firstly identify both the cell types and the cellular response that is occurring in the sample.

CLASSIFICATION OF CELL TYPES

- Haemic cells are those cells found in the blood and the haematopoietic tissues.
- Epithelial cells typically exfoliate easily and are found in clusters or sheets. They vary in shape depending upon their origin and can be oval, cuboidal, columnar or polygonal. They typically have an abundant cytoplasm, small round to oval nuclei and distinct cytoplasmic margins. Cells from secretory epithelium may contain cytoplasmic granules or vacuoles.
- Mesenchymal cells tend to exfoliate poorly and normally occur as single cells. They have indistinct cytoplasmic margins. Fibroblasts are the most frequently encountered cell of this group.
- Nervous tissue cells are rare in cytological specimens. They may be seen as deeply basophilic, stellate cells with cytoplasmic projections.

CLASSIFICATION OF CELLULAR RESPONSES

The goal of cytology is to classify the cell response into one of the basic cytodiagnostic groups. These groups include inflammation, tissue hyperplasia, benign neoplasia, malignant neoplasia and normal cellularity.

Inflammation

A diagnosis of inflammation is made when an increased number of inflammatory cells is detected in the sample. The inflammatory cells of birds are heterophils, lymphocytes, plasma cells and macrophages. Eosinophils may be included in the list of inflammatory cells; however, eosinophilic inflammation is either extremely rare or difficult to detect based on routine cytological methods. Heterophils and eosinophils may be difficult to differentiate based on routine cytological methods. Avian inflammatory responses are classified as heterophilic, mixed cell or macrophagic:

- Heterophilic inflammation is present when heterophils make up >70% of the inflammatory cells and indicates an acute inflammatory response. Degenerate heterophils indicate a toxic microenvironment, usually caused by microbial toxins. If bacterial phagocytosis can be demonstrated, the cytodiagnosis of septic heterophilic inflammation can be made. If only extracellular bacteria are found, they may represent either normal flora or contaminants of the sample.

- Mixed-cell inflammation is represented by the presence of heterophils and mononuclear leucocytes. Heterophils usually make up at least 50% of the inflammatory cells. Mixed-cell inflammation usually represents an established, active inflammation.
- Macrophagic inflammation is indicated by the predominance of macrophages (>50%) in the inflammatory response. This type of inflammation does not necessarily imply chronicity, but may be suggestive of a number of aetiologies (e.g. intracellular pathogens). Macrophagic inflammation is common to certain avian diseases including tuberculosis, chlamydiosis, foreign body reaction, mycotic infections and cutaneous xanthomatosis. Multinucleate giant cell formation is often associated with macrophagic inflammation. Giant cells can appear within hours of the onset of some inflammatory responses and, unlike in mammals, their presence does not imply chronic inflammation.

Tissue hyperplasia or benign neoplasia

Tissue hyperplasia resulting from cellular injury or chronic stimulation is difficult to differentiate from benign neoplasia on cytology alone. Cells from hyperplastic tissue appear mature and do not exhibit much pleomorphism.

Malignant neoplasia

Malignant neoplastic cells show varying degrees of nuclear pleomorphism. There is an increase in nuclear size, which is reflected by an increased nucleus to cytoplasm ratio. Multinucleation may be present. The nuclei often have coarse, hyperchromatic chromatin and large or multiple (more than five) nucleoli. The cytoplasm shows increased basophilia, decreased volume and variability in the staining and it may have abnormal vacuolation or inclusions. There is often variation in cell margins. The cell types seen can be grouped into four basic classifications:

- Carcinomas: malignancies of the epithelial cells. Adenocarcinomas are frequently seen in birds. Cytological evidence of adenocarcinomas includes epithelial cells that tend to form giant cells, have cytoplasmic secretory vacuoles and tend to occur in aggregates.
- Sarcomas: malignancies of mesenchymal cells. Fibrosarcomas are the most frequently encountered sarcomas of birds. The cells tend to exfoliate poorly. They are abnormal appearing fibroblasts, which are spindle-shaped cells that typically exfoliate as single cells. Abnormal

fibroblasts show increased cellular size and nuclear:cellular ratios and nuclear and cellular pleomorphism. Other mesenchymal cell neoplasms such as chondromas, chondrosarcomas and osteogenic sarcomas may produce a heavy eosinophilic background material that can be seen on the microscopic sample.

- Discrete or round cell neoplasms: the only common neoplasm of this type is lymphoid neoplasia. Cellular features include a marked increase in the number of lymphoblasts, nuclear and cellular pleomorphism, an increase in cytoplasmic basophilia and mitotic figures and abnormal or multiple nucleoli.
- Poorly differentiated neoplasms produce cells having features of malignancy, but the cells are difficult to classify as carcinomas or sarcomas.

CYTOLOGY OF COMMONLY SAMPLED FLUIDS AND TISSUES
Abdominal fluids

Abdominal fluids can be classified as transudates, modified transudates, exudates, haemorrhage or malignant effusions.

Transudates are odourless, transparent fluids characterized by total cell count <1 × 10^9/l (<1,000 cells/mm^3), a specific gravity <1.020 and a total protein <30 g/l. Transudates do not clot. The cell types are primarily macrophages and occasional mesothelial cells. Transudates occur as a result of oncotic pressure changes or other circulatory disturbances. The common causes of abdominal transudates in birds include hepatic cirrhosis, cardiac insufficiency and hypoproteinaemia.

Modified transudates have total cell counts of 1–5 × 10^9/l (1,000–5,000 cells/mm^3). The mononuclear leucocytes predominate, with occasional mesothelial cells and rare heterophils. The mesothelial cells tend to be round or oval with increased cytoplasmic basophilia. Multinucleation, cytoplasmic vacuolation and mitotic activity are often associated with reactive mesothelial cells. Care should be taken not to mistake these cells for malignant neoplasia. Transudates and modified transudates are commonly found in the abdominal cavity of mynah birds suffering from haemochromatosis.

Exudative effusions are characterized by high cell counts, >5 × 10^9/l (>5,000 cells/mm^3), a specific gravity >1.020 and protein content >30 g/l. The majority of cells are inflammatory cells. Acute exudative effusions demonstrate primarily a heterophilic inflammatory response; however, macrophages quickly move into the fluid, creating a mixed-cell inflammatory response within a few hours of onset. Lymphocyte and plasma cells are often seen in long-standing exudative effusions. Lesions often associated with abdominal exudates include septic peritonitis, egg-related peritonitis and abdominal malignancies (77).

Haemorrhagic effusions are identified by the presence of erythrocytic phagocytosis. Thrombocytes usually disappear rapidly in haemorrhagic effusions. Iron pigment or haemosiderin crystals found in macrophages are also indicators of haemorrhagic effusions. Iron pigment appears grey to blue–black using Wright's stains. Haemosiderin appears as diamond-shaped, golden crystals within the macrophage cytoplasm.

Malignant effusions have features of either exudative or haemorrhagic effusions, but contain cells compatible with malignant neoplasia. Cystadenocarcinomas of the ovary are a common cause of malignant effusions in older females. These cells often form cellular aggregates of balls or rosettes and have cytoplasmic secretory vacuolation.

Urate peritonitis is a rare effusion that can occur when urinary fluids leak into the abdominal cavity. The acute lesion is poorly cellular, but it contains a marked number of sodium and potassium urate crystals. Urate crystals are spherical and have a spoke-wheel appearance. If the bird survives long enough, inflammatory cells will migrate into the fluid.

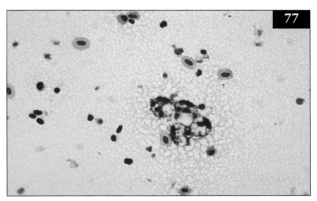

77 Egg yolk coelomitis in a budgerigar. (Diff Quik, 40×) (Photo courtesy S Echols)

Cytology of the alimentary tract
Oral cavity

The oral cavity is easily sampled when lesions are visible. Normal cytology of the oral cavity shows occasional squamous epithelial cells, varying amounts of background debris and extracellular bacteria represented by a variety of morphological types. The differential diagnoses for common oral lesions include septic stomatitis, candidiasis, trichomoniasis and squamous cell hyperplasia. *Alysiella filiformis*, a gram-negative small paired coccobacillus that forms ribbon-like chains, is normally associated with squamous epithelial cells.

- Smears made from a bacterial abscess reveal either a heterophilic or mixed-cell inflammation with bacterial phagocytosis.
- Candidiasis is evidenced by large numbers of typical organisms. *Candida* can be a normal inhabitant of the upper alimentary tract, so low numbers of organisms do not produce inflammation. An inflammatory response often occurs when the infection has involved the mucosa. The presence of hyphae formation suggests a potential systemic invasion by the yeast.
- Trichomoniasis is best diagnosed by observing the movement of the piriform flagellate protozoa in a wet mount preparation. It is important to recognize these organisms in a stained cytological sample if wet mount preparations are not part of the routine examination or if trichomoniasis is not suspected. Trichomonads appear as basophilic, piriform cells with flagella on Wright's stained smears (**78**). The cell nucleus usually stains more eosinophilic than most cell nuclei. An eosinophilic axostyle can often be seen as a straight line running from the nucleus to the opposite pole of the cell. An inflammatory response is usually found associated with trichomoniasis.
- Squamous cell hyperplasia and metaplasia lesions may grossly resemble bacterial, yeast or protozoal infections, but the cytological appearance is very different (**79**). Normally, squamous epithelial cells exfoliate as single cells or small sheets. With squamous hyperplasia associated with vitamin A deficiency, smears with large numbers of cornified squamous epithelial cells that exfoliate in large sheets or aggregates are common. The cytology resembles that of the vaginal cytology of a dog in oestrus. Inflammatory cells are not seen unless there are secondary infections with bacteria, yeast or protozoa.

Oesophagus and crop

Cytological evaluation of the oesophagus and crop is indicated in birds with clinical signs of regurgitation, vomiting, delayed crop emptying or other suspected oesophageal and crop disorders. Normal cytology reveals occasional squamous epithelial cells and a variable amount of background debris and extracellular bacteria. An occasional yeast is accepted as normal. Also, some foods contain yeast as a source of supplemental B vitamins, so this source of large numbers of nonbudding yeast must be ruled out. The presence of many bacteria represented by one morphological type, even without inflammatory cells, may indicate a problem. This may be a common finding in peracute ingluvitis.

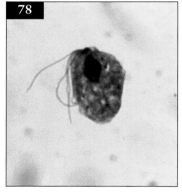

78 Bacterial pharyngitis associated with *Trichomonas* spp. infection. (Photo courtesy R Schmidt)

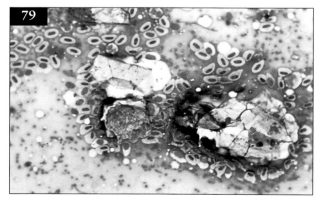

79 Squamous metaplasia with secondary bacterial invasion in an Amazon parrot with a vitamin A deficiency. (Photo courtesy R Schmidt)

A pH >7 is also suggestive of acute or peracute ingluvitis. *Capillaria* ova may be detected in cytological samples from the oesophagus or crop of some birds with capillariasis. These ova are double operculated and may not stain.

Cloaca

Cloacal cytology is indicated whenever a disorder of the lower intestinal tract, reproductive tract, urinary tract or cloaca is suspected. Normal cytology reveals a few noncornified epithelial cells, extracellular bacteria, background debris and urate crystals. Abnormal findings would include the presence of inflammatory cells, large numbers of yeast or a uniform population of bacteria.

Cytology of the respiratory tract
Nasal and infraorbital sinuses

Normal cytology reveals occasional noncornified squamous epithelial cells and low numbers of extracellular bacteria with little background debris. Evidence for periorbital sinusitis is provided by the presence of inflammatory cells in the aspirate. Lesions with a bacterial aetiology are indicated by a septic, heterophilic or mixed-cell inflammation. Mycotic lesions often reveal either a mixed-cell or macrophagic inflammation, with the presence of fungal elements such as yeast, hyphae or spores (80). Chlamydial sinusitis often reveals a mixed-cell or macrophagic inflammation. Chlamydial inclusions appear as small, blue-to-purple spherules, often in dense clusters, within the cytoplasm of macrophages when stained with Wright's stain.

Trachea

Normal cytology from a tracheal wash consists of a few ciliated respiratory epithelial cells and goblet cells.

Septic tracheobronchitis reveals inflammatory cells showing bacterial phagocytosis (81). Degenerative respiratory epithelial cells show a loss of cilia, cytoplasmic vacuolation and karyolysis. There is often increased mucin formation, which causes an increased thickness to the noncellular background. Mycotic lesions involving the trachea, syrinx and bronchi may reveal fungal elements on the tracheal wash. Aspergillosis is characterized by thick, septate hyphae that branch at 45° angles. Mycotic lesions usually reveal a mixed-cell or macrophagic inflammation (82).

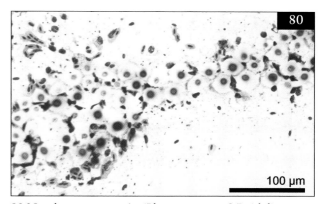

80 Nasal cryptococcosis. (Photo courtesy S Raidal)

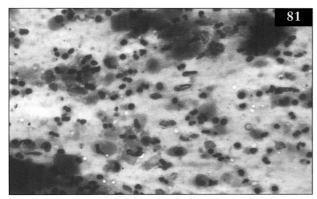

81 Purlent tracheitis in an umbrealla cockatoo. (Diff Quik, 40×) (Photo courtesy S Echols)

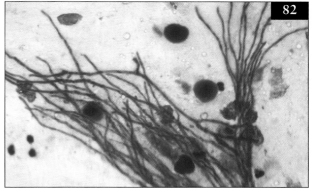

82 Fungal tracheitis in an Amazon parrot. (Diff Quik, 40×) (Photo courtesy S Echols)

Air sacs

Normal air sac samples are poorly cellular with the presence of a few noncornified epithelial cells. Bacterial infections show the typical septic inflammatory patterns. Chlamydial and mycotic lesions demonstrate mixed-cell or macrophagic inflammation with the presence of chlamydial inclusions or fungal elements, respectively. Neoplastic lesions of the respiratory tract of birds are rare.

Skin

Normal skin samples typically contain squamous epithelial cells, debris and extracellular bacteria.

- Bacterial infections involving the skin are usually associated with a heterophilic or mixed-cell inflammation (**83**) (bacterial phagocytosis must be demonstrated to detect a septic inflammatory lesion). Care must be taken not to confuse basophilic-staining powder down for bacteria or yeast.
- Cutaneous xanthomatosis is a unique condition of birds caused by an excessive accumulation of lipids in the skin. It is a macrophagic inflammatory response, with multinucleated giant cells and cholesterol crystals observed on the cytological specimen. (Cholesterol crystals appear as angular, translucent crystals that vary in size and shape.)
- Subcutaneous lipomas produce a cytological specimen that appears 'greasy' on the unstained slide. The cytology reveals numerous lipocytes, which vary in size. Fat droplets usually partially dissolve in the alcohol-based stains, but are easily seen in water-soluble stains such as new methylene blue. Special fat stains such as Sudan IV can be used to demonstrate the fat droplets.
- Feather cyst cytology may reveal RBCs and erythrocytosis in early lesions. More chronic lesions develop a caseous exudate with a mixed-cell inflammation.
- Cutaneous and subcutaneous malignancies are rare in birds. Lymphoid neoplasia produces a highly cellular sample of immature lymphocytes. Cutaneous melanosarcomas have also been found in birds.
- Avian poxvirus lesions reveal clusters of squamous epithelial cells that contain large eosinophilic cytoplasmic vacuoles. The large cytoplasmic vacuoles found in the affected squamous cell push the cell nucleus to the cell margin.

Cornea and conjunctiva

Normal conjunctival scrapings provide poorly cellular samples with little background material. The cells may contain intracytoplasmic pigment granules. Normal cytology of the cornea is also poorly cellular and consists of occasional noncornified squamous epithelial cells.

Inflammatory lesions involving the cornea and conjunctiva reveal inflammatory cells (**84**) and increased numbers of exfoliated epithelial cells. Chronic lesions may also reveal the presence of cornified squamous epithelial cells that are not normally found in the conjunctiva or cornea.

Synovial fluid

Normal synovial fluid is poorly cellular. The cells are mononuclear cells, representing either synovial lining cells or mononuclear leucocytes. The background of normal synovial fluid consists of a heavy, granular, eosinophilic substance representing the mucin in the fluid.

An increase in the inflammatory cells and change in the colour, clarity and viscosity of the fluid is indicative of inflammatory joint lesions. There may be a decrease in the granular eosinophilic background material, suggesting a decrease in mucin content. Erosion of the articular cartilage may result in the presence of multinucleated osteoclasts in the synovial fluid. Spindle-shaped fibroblasts suggest erosion into the fibrous layer of the articular capsule. Septic joint lesions may demonstrate bacterial phagocytosis by leucocytes. Traumatic arthritis also results in increased numbers of inflammatory cells.

Articular gout produces a cream–yellow-coloured deposit in affected joints. Cytology reveals numerous, needle-shaped crystals. Inflammatory cells are often present and the mucin content is often reduced, as reflected in the reduction in the amount of eosinophilic granular background.

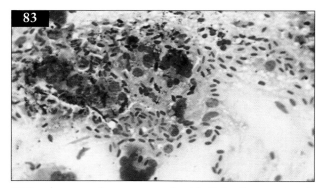

83 Erythrocytes, leucocytes and epithelial cells, associated with pododermatitis. (Photo courtesy R Schmidt)

Cytology of internal organs
Liver

Cytological samples are usually highly cellular, with a predominance of hepatocytes, erythrocytes and free nuclei. Hepatocytes are large epithelial cells that occur in sheets or clusters or as single cells. Normal haematopoiesis is occasionally found because the liver is a common location for ectopic haematopoiesis. Macrophages containing haemosiderin are occasionally seen.

Inflammatory lesions of the liver reveal numerous mature heterophils and an increase in the number of macrophages and plasma cells (85, 86). It is important not to confuse normal ectopic granulopoiesis with heterophilic inflammation. (If developing stages of the heterophils can be found, the cytology is representative of granulocytopoiesis. If the heterophils are mature cells, the cytology indicates inflammation.)

Avian tuberculosis produces a macrophagic inflammatory response in the liver. The cytology reveals numerous macrophages and multinucleated giant cells (87). The background of the smear and the macrophages may contain numerous bacterial rods that do not stain the waxy cell wall produced by mycobacteria.

Chlamydiosis often results in a mixed-cell or macrophagic inflammation in the liver, with a marked increase in the number of plasma cells. Small, blue–purple, intracytoplasmic inclusions suggestive of chlamydial elementary and initial bodies may be seen in macrophages.

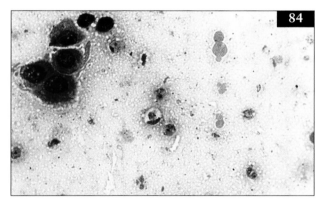

84 Conjunctival cytology showing epithelial cells, leucocytes and encapsulated yeast (*Cryptococcus* spp.). (Photo courtesy R Schmidt)

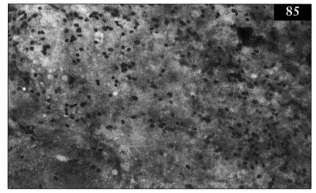

85 Hepatic necrosis in a grey parrot. (Diff Quik, 20×) (Photo courtesy S Echols)

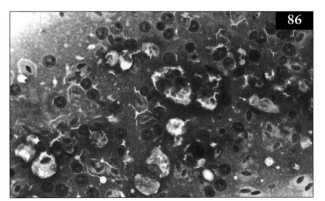

86 Granulomatous hepatitis in a grey parrot. (Diff Quik, 400×) (Photo courtesy S Echols)

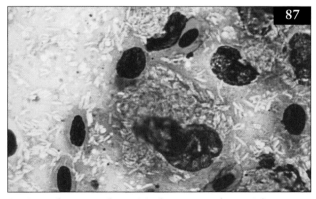

87 Granulomatous hepatitis due to mycobacterial infection in a bronze-winged pionus. (Diff Quik, 100×) (Photo courtesy S Echols)

Hepatic lipidosis reveals enlarged hepatocytes that contain round, cytoplasmic vacuoles (**88–90**).

Occasionally, parasites may be found on hepatic imprints. Those commonly seen are schizogony of *Haemoproteus* and *Leukocytozoon* and sporozoites of *Atoxoplasma* and microfilaria.

Spleen

Normal cytology shows a marked number of erythrocytes and lymphocytes, reflecting the cytology of a lymphoid tissue. Chlamydial infections often cause a marked increase in the number of splenic plasma cells. Macrophages often demonstrate intracytoplasmic chlamydial inclusions. See **91–94**.

Kidney

Normal kidney produces a highly cellular sample that contains numerous epithelial cells with an abundant, slightly basophilic cytoplasm and slightly eccentric, round-to-oval nuclei (**95**). Abnormal cytology (**96**) may include inflammatory cells or the presence of neoplastic cells:

- Epithelial cells from renal adenomas show increased cytoplasmic basophilia, slight pleomorphism and occasional mitotic figures.
- Renal adenocarcinomas produce epithelial cells having features of malignant neoplasia.
- Nephroblastomas produce poorly differentiated epithelial and mesenchymal cells.

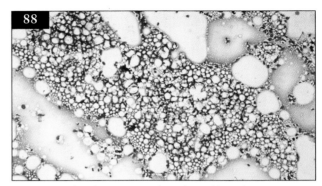

88 Hepatic lipidosis in a cockatiel. (Diff Quik, 10×) (Photo courtesy S Echols)

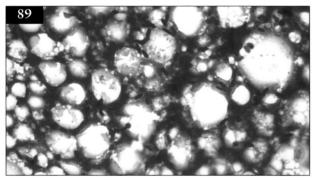

89 Hepatic lipidosis in a cockatiel. (Diff Quik, 40×) (Photo courtesy S Echols)

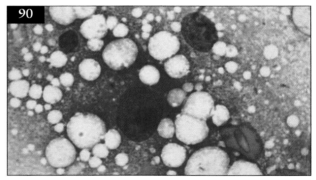

90 Hepatic lipidosis in an umbrella cockatoo. (Diff Quik, 100×) (Photo courtesy S Echols)

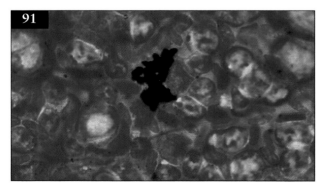

91 Haemosiderosis in the spleen of a pigeon with haemoparasitism. (Diff Quik, 100×) (Photo courtesy S Echols)

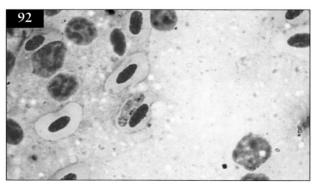

92 Reactive splenitis in a pigeon. Note the haemoparasite in the erythrocyte. (Diff Quik, 100×) (Photo courtesy S Echols)

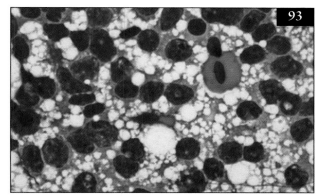

93 Splenic lipidosis in an umbrella cockatoo with hepatic lipidosis. (Diff Quik, 100×) (Photo courtesy S Echols)

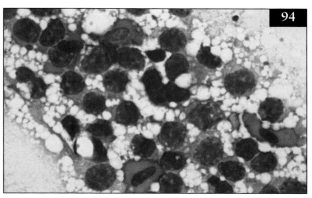

94 Splenic lipidosis in an umbrella cockatoo with hepatic lipidosis. (Diff Quik, 100×) (Photo courtesy of S Echols)

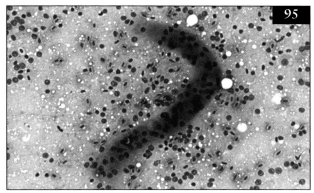

95 Normal renal tubule in an umbrella cockatoo. (Diff Quik, 20×) (Photo courtesy S Echols)

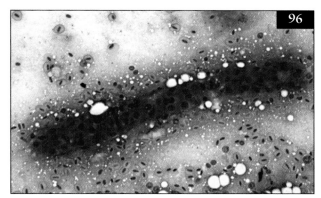

96 Renal tubule from an umbrella cockatoo with hepatic lipidosis. (Diff Quik, 20×) (Photo courtesy S Echols)

FURTHER READING

Campbell TW, Ellis CK (2007) *Avian and Exotic Animal Hematology and Cytology*, 3rd edn. Blackwell Publishing, Ames.

Fudge AM (1997) Avian clinical pathology. In: *Avian Medicine and Surgery*. RB Altman, SL Clubb, GM Dorrestein, K Quesenberry (eds). WB Saunders, Philadephia, pp. 142–157.

Fudge AM (2000) *Laboratory Medicine: Avian and Exotic Pets*. WB Saunders, Philadelphia.

Gerlach H (1994) Bacteria. In: *Avian Medicine: Principles and Application*. BW Ritchie, GJ Harrison, LR Harrison (eds). Wingers Publishing, Lake Worth, pp. 949–983.

Harr KE (2006) Diagnostic value of biochemistry. In: *Clinical Avian Medicine, Vol 2*. GJ Harrison, TL Lightfoot (eds). Spix Publishing Inc, Palm Beach, pp. 611–630.

Hochleithner M (1994) Biochemistries. In: *Avian Medicine: Principles and Application*. BW Ritchie, GJ Harrison, LR Harrison (eds). Wingers Publishing, Lake Worth, pp. 223–245.

Ritchie BW (1995) Diagnosing viral infections. In: *Avian Viruses: Function and Control*. Wingers Publishing, Lake Worth, pp. 83–104.

Samour J (2006) Diagnostic value of hematology. In: *Clinical Avian Medicine, Vol 2*. GJ Harrison, TL Lightfoot (eds). Spix Publishing Inc, Palm Beach, pp. 587–610.

CHAPTER 5
SUPPORTIVE THERAPY

Although obtaining an accurate diagnosis and then applying a specific treatment are essential components of avian medicine, the clinician must not overlook the importance of supportive care. It is usually far better to have a tentative diagnosis in a live patient than a confirmed diagnosis in a dead one! When the masking phenomenon, hiding signs of illness until the bird is decompensating, is combined with an owner's approach of 'waiting a few days to see if he gets better', the result is often a patient that is presented badly dehydrated, in hypothermic shock and in a catabolic state due to anorexia. Occasionally, some birds will present with severe respiratory compromise, either acute or chronic in onset. In some cases, especially trauma, the patient may be in pain or have experienced significant blood loss. The clinician must recognize the clinical signs of these conditions and deal with them aggressively, often prior to making any diagnostic attempts.

DEHYDRATION
Clinical presentation
Signs include sunken eyes, strands of mucoid saliva seen in the mouth when the beak is opened, and decreased capillary refill, seen by pressing on the basilic vein (medial side of the elbow) and assessing refill time. There may be wrinkling and/or tenting of the skin on the toes and torso, and decreased urinary output; urates appear thick and pasty.

Management
Fluid therapy may be given via the following routes:
- Orally, if the bird is not moribund or vomiting.
- Subcutaneously, if the bird is not in shock, hypothermic, hypoproteinaemic or has poor circulation.
- Intravenously or intraosseously. Can be difficult to maintain for extended periods in an alert, active patient.

The volume to be given can be simply calculated as follows:
- 10% of the bird's bodyweight in grams = the volume (in ml) to be given daily for three days.
- Then reduce to 5–7.5% daily.
- Increase this amount if there are ongoing fluid losses (e.g. diarrhoea, polyuria).
- Divide total daily requirement into two or three doses.

HYPOTHERMIC SHOCK
Clinical presentation
Feathers are fluffed to trap body heat and the bird is lethargic and sleeping a lot to conserve energy. It may be unable to remain on the perch, and often found on the floor of the cage.

Management
Exogenous heat should be provided by placing the bird in a heated cage (**97**) or by placing a reading light

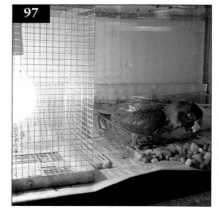

97 This simple hospital cage, a modified aquarium, meets many of the requirements of a hospital cage (i.e. heat, humidity, security and ease of cleaning and disinfection).

(with incandescent bulb, not Fluorescent tube) beside the cage, preferably next to a perch. Ideally, birds should be hospitalized in a heated room. The ambient temperature around the bird should be raised to 30–32°C. The bird should be monitored for signs of heat stress: panting, wings held away from the body.

Covering a cage with a towel or blanket does not help to keep a bird warm.

CATABOLISM
Clinical presentation
Food may be untouched in dishes and droppings reduced in size and quantity; faeces are often dark (or even black) and urates are small and sometimes yellow. There is wasting of the pectoral muscles and weight loss (all patients should be weighed on every visit so that a record of their normal weight is maintained in their records).

Management
Placing food and water bowls in easily accessible places and offering favourite foods can encourage an ill patient to start eating. Placing food in a dish on the floor of a cage for a patient that is perching (and reluctant to leave the perch) will not encourage appetite. The food bowls may need to be placed adjacent to the perch where the bird is easily able to reach them.

If the patient is not eating, but not vomiting or moribund, crop gavage with a hand-rearing formula or other appropriate food can be instituted. Oesophagostomy feeding tubes, placed into the proventriculus, can be used to bypass the patient's head and used in cases such as head trauma where eating or passing a stomach tube is not feasible. Duodenal catheters have been used with a degree of success by some clinicians. This is a reasonably complex surgical procedure.

Total parenteral nutrition via an intravenous catheter is not routinely practised in avian medicine at this time.

RESPIRATORY COMPROMISE
Clinical presentation
Signs include open-mouth breathing, increased respiratory effort (seen as tail bobbing and inspiratory sternal lift), audible respiratory noise and collapse.

Management
If the dyspnoea is of an acute nature, the clinician must consider the possibility of tracheal obstruction. If this is the case, an air sac catheter placed in the left caudal thoracic air sac can be life-saving (see Chapter 3, Clinical Techniques, p. 63) (**98**).

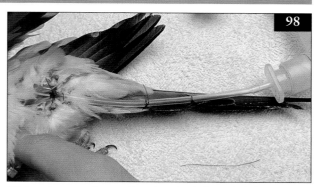

98 An air sac catheter placed in the left caudal thoracic air sac.

Oxygen therapy supplied either through a face mask or in an oxygen chamber can help patients with respiratory compromise. Clinicians must be aware that prolonged exposure to 100% oxygen can cause perivascular oedema and increase the degree of respiratory compromise.

ANALGESIA
Clinical signs of pain
Birds, unlike domestic mammals, indicate pain in a less obvious manner than many clinicians are accustomed to. They will respond to painful stimuli in one of two ways:
- 'Fight-or-flight' responses:
  - Excessive vocalization.
  - Wing flapping.
  - Decreased head movement.
- Conservation–withdrawal responses:
  - Immobility.
  - Closure of eyes.
  - Inappetence.
  - Fluffing of feathers.

It is thought that the 'fight-or-flight' response is more common with acute pain from which the bird attempts to escape. In contrast, with chronic or overwhelming pain, from which perhaps the bird feels it cannot escape, the bird may adopt the 'conservation–withdrawal' responses, perhaps in an attempt to minimize the further pain that struggling would induce. Care must be taken not to misinterpret lack of movement or vocalization as an indication that the bird is not in pain.

It is wise, therefore, to make the assumption that what would be painful to another species would be painful to humans, and adequate analgesia should therefore be provided.

Management

- Butorphanol appears to be more effective in many birds than buprenorphine. Dose: 1–4 mg/kg q6h IM, orally.
- Meloxicam 0.2–0.5 mg/kg q12h IM, orally.
- Carprofen 2–4 mg/kg q24h IM, orally.

The combination of an opioid (e.g. butorphanol) and a nonsteroidal anti-inflammatory drug (NSAID) (e.g. meloxicam) may achieve better analgesia than either alone. Other analgesic protocols can be found in the formulary (Chapter 27).

BLOOD LOSS

Birds are able to withstand comparatively greater blood loss than mammals. This is thought to be the result of:

- An increased capillary surface area within skeletal muscle allowing for rapid extravascular fluid resorption to maintain vascular volume.
- The ability to mobilize large numbers of immature erythrocytes.
- The absence of the autonomic response to haemorrhage that contributes to haemorrhagic shock.

Clinical presentation

There may be a history or physical evidence of recent blood loss. Mucous membranes are pale and the respiratory rate and effort are increased. The bird may be weak and lethargic. The PCV is usually less than 0.2 1/l.

Management

Many cases of blood loss do not require a transfusion. In mild cases, or when a blood donor is not available, intravenous or intraosseous colloids or crystalloids, alone or in combination, may be sufficient. When given together, crystalloids are administered at doses of 30–40 ml/kg while the colloid is administered at 5 ml/kg. With the bird's ability to mobilize immature erythrocytes, it is not uncommon for the PCV to return to normal within seven days with this therapy alone.

In more severe cases or where a significant blood loss is anticipated (e.g. surgery), a blood transfusion may be necessary (**99**). Homologous transfusions are ideal, preferably between the same species, but the same genus will give similar results. The half-life of a homologous transfusion is believed to be 6–11 days. Heterologous transfusions, on the other hand, have a half-life of three days or less. Transfusion reactions can occur with repeated transfusions, particularly heterologous transfusions.

Blood may be collected into syringes containing an anticoagulant such as sodium citrate (0.1 ml/0.9 ml blood), heparin (0.25 ml/10 ml blood), acid citrate dextrose (0.1 ml/0.9 ml blood) or citrate phosphate dextrose (0.1 ml/0.9 ml blood). Up to 10% of the donor's blood volume (1% of its bodyweight) can be collected. Once collected the blood is used within 12–24 hours. Nucleated avian erythrocytes are very metabolically active, metabolizing fat and protein and consuming 7–10 times more oxygen than mammalian erythrocytes. Consequently, they do not store well.

Transfusions can be given via an indwelling intravenous catheter (**100**) or intraosseous catheter. They can be administered as a constant rate infusion over 1–2 hours, or a slow bolus over 1–5 minutes. If using a bolus approach, care must be taken to avoid fluid overload.

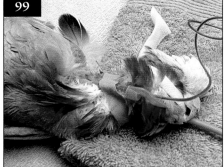

99 This galah is receiving a blood transfusion prior to a surgical procedure where blood loss is anticipated.

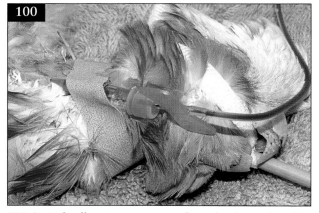

100 An indwelling intravenous catheter has been placed in the right jugular vein and sutured to the skin. Freshly collected blood is being administered via a luer plug and extension set.

HOSPITAL CARE

Hospital care for companion birds requires a veterinary clinic to make accommodation for their differing requirements, often far removed from those needed by dogs and cats.

SECURITY

Most companion birds are 'prey' species, and they do not feel safe or secure when housed near predators (i.e. dogs, cats, birds of prey and reptiles). Loud noises and constant movement around a cage can be stressful to a sick bird.

WARMTH

Although it is obvious that a hypothermic bird (see page 92) needs a focal heat source, most companion birds, sick or healthy, are more comfortable in warmer temperatures. Air conditioning, for example, adds to a bird's energy requirements to maintain its body temperature.

Care must be taken when heating a room that humidity levels do not decrease excessively, predisposing a bird to dehydration.

BIOSECURITY

Many of the diseases for which birds require hospitalization are infectious. All hospitalized birds are stressed to some degree, and therefore likely to be immunocompromised. Attention must therefore be taken to prevent aerosol or mechanical transmission of disease within an avian hospital facility.

FEEDING

Most companion birds cannot withstand long periods of food deprivation. Therefore, every effort must be made to ensure that hospitalized birds are eating. No attempt should be made to convert a seriously ill bird to a new diet until it is stable. Eating an unhealthy diet is still better than not eating anything at all. Favourite foods should be offered in a way that the bird is likely to show interest in:

- Place food and water bowls in easily accessible places (e.g. the food bowls may need to be placed adjacent to the perch where the bird is easily able to reach them).
- Scattering a small amount of food on the floor of the cage often encourages a bird to browse and begin eating.

If the patient is not eating, but not vomiting or moribund, crop gavage with a hand-rearing formula or other appropriate food can be instituted.

PSYCHOLOGICAL CARE

Many companion birds are closely bonded to their owner. In these cases, hospitalization can result in separation anxiety evidenced by anorexia, lethargy or hyperexcitability. In some cases feather picking may develop. In these cases consideration must be given to discharging a patient to home care, on the proviso that the bird is returned to hospital if it fails to improve when back in familiar surroundings.

FURTHER READING

De Matos R, Morrisey JK (2005) Emergency and critical care of small psittacines and passerines. In: *Seminars in Avian and Exotic Pet Medicine: Emergency and Critical Care*. TN Tully, MA Mitchell, JJ Heatley (eds). **14(2)**:90–105.

Graham JE (2004) Approach to the dyspneic avian patient. In: *Seminars in Avian and Exotic Pet Medicine: Emergency Medicine*. AM Fudge, MS Johnston (eds). **13(3)**:154–159.

Harrison GJ, Lightfoot TL, Flinchum GB (2006) Emergency and critical care. In: *Clinical Avian Medicine, Vol 1*. GJ Harrison, TL Lightfoot (eds). Spix Publishing Inc, Palm Beach, pp. 213–232.

Jaensch SM, Cullen L, Raidal SR (2001) The pathology of normobaric oxygen toxicity in budgerigars (*Melopsittacus undulatus*). *Avian Pathology* **30(2)**:135–142.

Jenkins JR (1997) Hospital techniques and supportive care. In: *Avian Medicine and Surgery*. RB Altman, *et al.* (eds). WB Saunders, Philadelphia, pp. 232–252.

Jenkins JR (1997) Avian critical care and emergency medicine. In: *Avian Medicine and Surgery*. RB Altman, *et al.* (eds). WB Saunders, Philadelphia, pp. 839–863.

Lichtenberger M (2004) Principles of shock and fluid therapy in special species. *Seminars in Avian Exotic Pet Medicine* **13(3)**:142–153.

Lichtenberger M (2005) Determination of indirect blood pressure in the companion bird. *Seminars in Avian Exotic Pet Medicine* **14(2)**:149–152.

Lichtenberger M (2006) Emergency case approach to hypotension, hypertension and acute respiratory distress. In: *Proceedings of the Annual Conference of the Association of Avian Veterinarians*, pp. 281–290.

Lichtenberger M, Chavez W, Thamm DH, *et al.* (2007) Use of hetastarch and crystalloids for resuscitation of acute blood loss shock. In: *Proceedings of the Annual Conference of the Association of Avian Veterinarians*, pp. 103–106.

Paul-Murphy J (2006) Pain management. In: *Clinical Avian Medicine, Vol 1*. GJ Harrison, TL Lightfoot (eds). Spix Publishing Inc, Palm Beach, pp. 233–240.

CHAPTER 6
DIFFERENTIAL DIAGNOSES

Listed below, by clinical signs, are the differential diagnoses that the clinician should be considering when examining a patient. Although every effort has been made to make this list as exhaustive as possible, it would be difficult, if not impossible, to guarantee that every possible differential diagnosis was included in this list.

In many cases the list goes only as far as describing the organs likely to be involved. Clinicians are referred to the chapters dealing with those organs for a more comprehensive discussion of diseases that could affect them.

CHANGE IN DROPPINGS
DIARRHOEA (101)
- Bacterial, fungal or viral enteritis.
- Intestinal parasites.

101 Diarrhoea.

- Proventricular dilatation disease.
- Chlamydiosis.
- Megabacteria (*Macrorhabdus*).
- Liver disease.
- Zinc and lead poisoning.

CHANGE IN COLOUR OF THE FAECAL PORTION
- Black: anorexia, melena (40).
- Pale: exocrine pancreatic insufficiency, maldigestion due to *Macrorhabdus* or other gastrointestinal diseases.
- Brown: pelleted diet.
- Dietary change (e.g. purple with berries).

ENLARGED FAECAL PORTION (39)
- Egg laying.
- Space-occupying lesion in abdomen.
- Exocrine pancreatic insufficiency.
- Formulated diets.
- Malabsorptive diseases.

FRANK BLOOD IN THE DROPPINGS
- Oviductal disease:
  - Egg binding.
  - Salpingitis.
  - Metritis.
  - Neoplasia.
- Cloacal disease:
  - Internal papilloma disease.
  - Cloacoliths.
  - Cloacitis.
  - Cloacal neoplasia.

WHOLE SEED IN THE DROPPINGS
- Increased intestinal motility.
- Any condition affecting proventricular and ventricular function:
  - Proventricular dilatation disease (**102**).
  - Candidiasis.
  - *Acuaria* (gizzard worm) infection.
  - Megabacteria (*Macrorhabdus*).

POLYURIA
- Stress or fear, especially on initial presentation ('stress polyuria').
- Renal disease.
- Diabetes mellitus.
- Diabetes insipidus.
- Hepatic disease.
- Pancreatic disease.
- Hyperadrenocorticism.
- Heavy metal toxicosis.
- 'Phosphate flush' due to an all-seed diet.
- Psychogenic polydypsia, usually seen in juvenile birds.
- Pituitary adenoma in budgerigars.
- Normal in lories and lorikeets.
- Birds being hand fed or crop fed.

CHANGE IN COLOUR OF THE URATES
- Green: hepatic disease.
- Pink/crimson: renal disease, lead poisoning.
- Yellow: anorexia, early or resolving hepatic disease.
- Orange: vitamin B injection.

MALODOROUS DROPPINGS
- Clostridial overgrowth.
- Cloacoliths.

APPETITE AND THIRST
INCREASED APPETITE
- Diabetes mellitus.
- Disorders of digestion, including megabacteria (*Macrorhabdus*) and endoparasitism.
- Jaw injuries (the bird is actually not eating, but rather is attempting to do so).
- Exocrine pancreatic insufficiency.
- Starvation (check there is food, and not just husks, in the food dish).

DECREASED APPETITE
- Nonspecific sign of illness.
- Mouth or jaw injuries.

POLYDYPSIA
- See above for causes of polyuria.
- Formulated diets may cause a moderate increase in thirst in some birds.

DECREASED THIRST
- Nonspecific sign of illness.
- Sufficient water in green foods and vegetables.

WEIGHT LOSS
- Nonspecific sign of illness.
- Response to controlled diet.
- Increasing fitness due to increasing exercise.
- Normal weaning response (if less than 10% weight loss).

102 Undigested seed in droppings from a bird with proventricular dilatation disease.

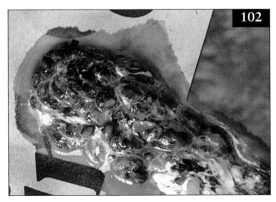

POSTURE

FLUFFED, IMMOBILE, EYES CLOSED, BOTH LEGS ON PERCH

- Nonspecific sign of illness. (Note: Some sick birds will make an effort to appear normal when being examined, but can rarely maintain this for more than a minute or two before reverting to the 'sick bird look') (103).

FLUFFED, IMMOBILE, EYES CLOSED, HEAD TUCKED UNDER ONE WING, ONLY ONE LEG ON PERCH

- Sleeping.

TAIL POINTING DOWN, PERPENDICULAR TO CAGE FLOOR, WHILE WINGS REMAIN AT A NORMAL ANGLE

- May be increased respiratory effort as evidenced by tail bobbing.
- Spinal kyphosis (104).
- Egg binding.

TAIL BOBBING UP AND DOWN IN AN EXAGGERATED MOVEMENT

- Respiratory disease: tracheal obstruction, pulmonary disease, severe air sac disease.
- External pressure on air sacs: internal organ enlargement, egg binding, kyphosis compressing abdominal space.

HEAD HELD DOWN BUT BIRD IS LOOKING UP, WINGS SPREAD OUT, TAIL SPREAD

- Reproductively active hen: courting posture.
- Heat stress.
- Egg binding.

WING DROOP

- Bilateral: generalized weakness, heat stress.
- Unilateral: wing injury. As a general rule, the lower the droop, the more distal the injury.

SITTING ON THE FLOOR OF THE CAGE, BODY UPRIGHT, PERHAPS PANTING

- Leg injuries.
- Egg binding.

NEUROLOGICAL SIGNS (ATAXIA, FITTING, PARALYSIS/PARESIS, TREMOR)

- Weakness due to illness.
- Agonal signs.
- Lead poisoning.
- Head trauma.
- Hypocalcaemia.
- Hypoglycaemia.
- CNS lesions (e.g. proventricular dilatation disease (217), encephalitis, neoplasia).
- Cardiovascular disease.

BILATERAL LEG PARESIS/PARALYSIS

- Spinal disease: trauma, neoplasia.
- 'Obturator' paralysis in hens that are egg-bound or have recently laid eggs.
- Hypocalcaemia.
- Barraband paralysis syndrome.
- Lorikeet paralysis syndrome.
- Bilateral leg trauma.

UNILATERAL LEG PARESIS/PARALYSIS

- Fractured leg.
- Soft tissue trauma.

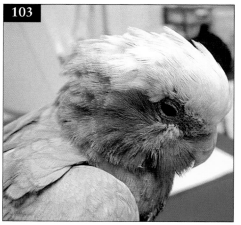

103 Sick bird look. The feathers are fluffed and the eyes are sunken.

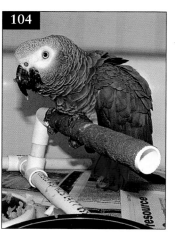

104 Kyphosis in an African grey parrot.

- Renal enlargement (e.g. neoplasia) pressing on the sciatic nerve, predominantly seen in budgerigars (**219**).
- Neoplasia.

ONE WING HELD OUT TO THE SIDE, RESTING ON THE FLOOR OR PERCH
- Check for broken/dislocated leg on that side.

FEATHERS AND SKIN
GENERALIZED FEATHER LOSS
- PBFD.
- Polyomavirus.
- Feather damaging behaviour. (Note: If this is self-inflicted, the head will appear normal).
- Extreme age.
- Obesity.
- Normal lack of feathers along apterylae.
- Excessive mutual grooming by cage mate (**105**).
- Bald patch on crown of head, behind crest, is normal in lutino cockatiels.

FEATHERING GRADUALLY DARKENING OR BECOMING 'GREASY-LOOKING' (115)
- Liver disease.
- Malnutrition.
- Hypothyroidism?
- Age.

BROKEN PRIMARY FEATHERS ON WINGS AND/OR TAIL
- Heavy falls, often associated with poorly done wing clips.
- Small caging combined with wing flapping or inability to perch steadily.

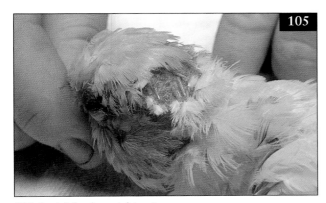

105 Social feather picking in a sun conure.

- Cage mate aggression.
- Malnutrition.

'STRESS LINES' (HORIZONTAL BREAKS IN THE FEATHER VANE)
- Physiological stress or illness at the time the feather was emerging through the skin. If severe, it could indicate generalized disease in the bird.
- Fenbendazole if administered while feathers were growing.

LONG STRAW-LIKE FEATHERS OVER THE THIGHS OR OTHER FEATHERS STILL ENCASED IN KERATIN SHEATHS
- 'Straw feathers' in canaries, a lethal genetic disorder.
- Inability to groom properly:
  - Illness.
  - Obesity.
  - Spinal abnormalities.
  - Elizabethan collar to prevent feather picking.
  - Beak malformations.

ABNORMALLY COLOURED FEATHERS
- Red feathers on African grey parrots:
  - PBFD.
  - Chronic feather plucking.
  - Malnutrition.
  - Liver disease.
  - Normal genetic variation.
- Abnormally coloured eclectus parrots:
  - PBFD.
  - Polyomavirus.
  - Nutritional issues, especially with hand-rearing formulae.
  - Liver disease.
  - Thyroxine medication.
- Green feathers turning black: saprophytic fungal growth resulting in grossly visible opaque black discoloration. This fungal growth is usually due to the oils from human hands left on the feathers after petting or holding the bird. This is not seen in birds with powder down (e.g. cockatoos and African greys) because the powder keeps the feathers clean.
- Lutino cockatiels becoming a deep 'buttercup' yellow; feathers have a 'greasy' appearance:
  - Chronic liver disease.
  - Hypothyroidism?
- Green feathers turning yellow, blue feathers turning white (**112**)
  - PBFD.
  - Malnutrition.
- Young white cockatoos with dirty feathering: PBFD

RAGGED LOOKING PLUMAGE WITHOUT PRURITUS
- Delayed moult:
  - Malnutrition.
  - Endocrine disorders.
  - Abnormal diurnal rhythm.
  - Excessive egg production.
- Incompatibility of cage mates (e.g. aggressive plucking is common in zebra finches, red-eared waxbills, golden-breasted waxbills and orange-cheeked waxbills).
- Improper housing.
- Dermatophytosis.

CONTINUED GROWTH OF FLIGHT, TAIL AND CONTOUR FEATHERS IN BUDGERIGARS UNABLE TO FLY
- 'Feather–duster':
  - Associated with a lethal recessive gene.
  - Some reports of association with a herpesvirus.

PRURITIS (134)
- Lice and mites.
- Malnutrition.
- Dermatitis.
- Polyfolliculosis.
- Feather inclusion cysts.
- Allergic dermatitis.

FEATHERS MISSING ON THE HEAD (133)
- Cage mate aggression.
- Dermatitis.
- Folliculitis.
- Cutaneous neoplasia.
- Dermatophytosis.
- Cutaneous candidiasis.
- Trauma.

GREENISH DISCOLORATION OF SKIN
- Bruising (253).

FLAKY, DRY SKIN (113)
- Malnutrition.
- Lack of bathing opportunities.
- Dermatophytosis.
- Cutaneous candidiasis.

FEATHER CYSTS (117)
- Retained feathers: often pruritic. Usually seen on wings or over sternum:
  - Traumatic, often associated with incorrect housing.
  - Incomplete removal of a broken 'blood feather'.
  - Overpreening by bird.
  - Secondary to folliculitis.
- Benign follicular tumours, commonly seen in canaries, but can be seen in other species. Usually not pruritic and can occur anywhere on the body.
- Mycobacterial granulomas in the skin can be confused with feather cysts.

POLYFOLLICULOSIS
- Chronic condition most commonly seen in budgerigars and lovebirds.
- Newly emerging feathers have short, stout quills with retained sheaths.
- Usually intensely pruritic.
- Unclear whether it is a primary problem or secondary to folliculitis.

ENLARGED UROPYGIAL (PREEN) GLAND
- Hyperplasia.
- Neoplasia.
- Blockage with keratin plug (sometimes associated with hypovitaminosis A).
- Infection.

YELLOW SUBCUTANEOUS DEPOSITS
- Fat.
- Lipoma.
- Xanthoma.

SELF-MUTILATION OF AFRICAN LOVEBIRDS (*AGAPORNIS* SPP.)
- Seen on the shoulder region and prepatagial membrane or, less commonly, on the inguinal region, chest, back, base of tail and around the cloaca.
- Can be unilateral or bilateral.
- Intensely pruritic.
- Cause still undetermined.

FEATHER PICKING
- Physical problems:
  - Dermatitis/folliculitis.
  - Underlying painful lesions (e.g. arthritis, neoplasia, internal organ disease or enlargement [if painful or uncomfortable]).

- Malnutrition.
- Nicotine sensitivity.
- Reproductive-associated feather picking.
- Giardiasis in cockatiels.
- Psychological causes:
  - Fear.
  - Boredom.
  - Insecurity.
  - Anxiety.
  - Attention-seeking behaviour.
  - Sexual frustration.

WINGS

BLOOD ON FEATHERS
- Wing tip trauma, often associated with excessively severe wing trimming and improper housing (**106, 36**).
- Broken 'blood feather'.
- Trauma to bone, muscle or skin.

WING DROOPING
- Broken bones.
- Muscle damage.
- Weakness.
- Respiratory disease.

SWELLINGS
- Neoplasia.
- Healing/healed broken bone.
- Soft tissue trauma.
- Feather cyst.
- Granuloma.

WINGS HELD AWAY FROM THE BODY
- Heat stress.
- Behavioural:
  - Courtship.
  - Fear.
  - Aggression.

GREEN DISCOLORATION
- Bruising.

FEET AND LEGS
LIMPING
- Injury to bone, muscle or joints.
- Pododermatitis (bumble foot).
- Hypocalcaemia.
- Pre-existing deformity (e.g. developmental varus/valgus deformity).

SWOLLEN JOINTS
- Articular gout.
- Arthritis:
  - Degenerative.
  - Infectious.
- Neoplasia.
- Trauma.

MISSING NAILS OR TOES
- Aggressive cage mates.
- Unsafe caging or cage furniture.
- Ergotism (**107**).
- Toe constriction due to fibrous band formation (constricted toe syndrome) or foreign bodies (e.g. cotton thread).
- Frost damage.

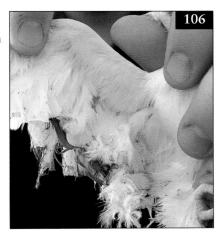

106 Feather damage due to an excessive wing trim.

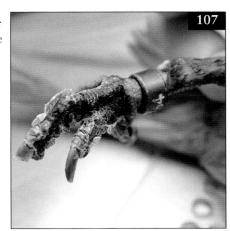

107 Avascular necrosis of the digits.

ABNORMAL SHAPE OR DIRECTION OF THE LEGS
- Coxofemoral subluxation: splay leg.
- Nutritional secondary hyperparathyroidism.
- Incorrectly aligned healed fractures or joint luxations.
- Slipped tendon (the gastrocnemius tendon 'slips' out of the groove on the back of the hock). Associated with trauma, poor diet, poor conformation and perhaps a genetic influence.

HYPERKERATOSIS OF THE SCALED PART OF THE LEG
- *Cnemidocoptes*.
- Nutritional deficiency, especially zinc and/or biotin.
- Dermatophytosis.

SELF-MUTILATION OF FOOT AND TOES
- Osteomyelitis.
- Myositis/tendonitis.
- Pododermatitis.
- Neuralgia.
- Necrosis of the extremities (see above: Missing nails or toes).

BEAK
OVERGROWN BEAK
Sometimes with bruising present in the keratin of the beak (**146**):
- Liver disease.
- *Cnemidocoptes*.
- Lack of occlusal wear.

BEAK TWISTED TO THE LEFT OR RIGHT
- Scissor beak (**137**):
  - Congenital.
  - Acquired.

UPPER BEAK INSIDE THE LOWER BEAK
- Prognathism (**139**).

INABILITY TO CLOSE BEAK PROPERLY
- Subluxation of the palatine bone due to hyperextension of the maxilla in macaws.
- Hyperextension of the mandible.
- Fractured jaw.

FLAKES OF KERATIN ON THE BEAK
- Malnutrition.
- Lack of an abrasive surface in the cage to groom beak on.

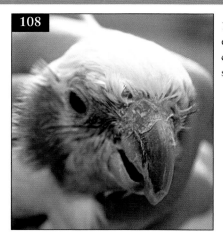

108 Nasal exudate in a cockatiel with sinusitis.

WHITE, CRUSTY, HONEYCOMBED LESIONS ON THE BEAK
Sometimes also on feet and vent:
- Scaly face mite (**148**).

NARES UNEQUAL IN SIZE
- Chronic respiratory disease (**154**).

THICKENING AND HYPERTROPHY OF CERE OF BUDGERIGAR HENS
- Cere hypertrophy associated with hyper-oestrogenism (**153**).

NARES BLOCKED OR STAINING/MATTING OF FEATHERS ABOVE NARES (108)
- Chronic respiratory disease.
- Choanal atresia (African grey parrots).

EYES
FEATHER LOSS AROUND EYES (109)
- Rubbing of the face against a perch or sides of cage
  - Conjunctivitis.
  - Sinusitis.
  - Ocular and periocular pain due to other causes (e.g. neoplasia, avian poxvirus).
- Overgrooming by companion bird.

EYELID ABNORMALITIES
- Congenital:
  - Cryptophthalmos (failure of eyelid formation, resulting in fusion of the eyelid margins) is occasionally seen in cockatiels. (**159**)

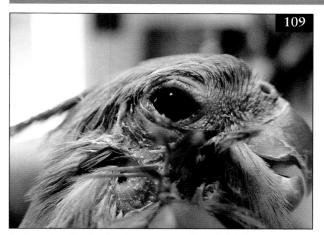

109 Periocular feather loss and conjunctivitis in a cockatiel.

- Blepharophimosis (narrowing of the palpebral fissures without fusion of the eyelid margins) is occasionally seen in all species.
- Acquired:
  - Symblepharon (adhesion of the eyelid(s) to the globe) can be seen as a sequela to severe conjunctivitis.
  - Acquired blepharophimosis is occasionally seen after conjunctivitis or other ocular inflammatory conditions.
  - Scarring and deformity is occasionally seen after avian poxvirus infections.

THICKENING AND HYPERAEMIA OF THE CONJUNCTIVA
Often associated with epiphora or ocular discharge:
- Conjunctivitis:
  - Chlamydiosis.
  - Mycoplasma.
  - Mycobacteria.
  - Parasites ('eye' worms): *Oxyspirura mansoni*, *Ceratospira* spp. and *Thelazia* spp.
  - Other chronic infections.
  - Allergic, especially secondary to nicotine.
- Sinusitis.
- Avian poxvirus.
- Neoplasia.

EXOPHTHALMOS
- Sinusitis.
- In chicks it is often associated with stunting or nutritional secondary hyperparathyroidism.

- Retrobulbar neoplasia, especially lymphoma.
- Pituitary adenomas in budgerigars.

ENOPHTHALMOS
- Dehydration.
- Sinusitis in macaws.

CORNEAL CHANGES
- Usually multifocal, white, glistening, raised, noninflammatory corneal lesions: lipid or cholesterol deposits associated with high-fat diets and obesity.
- Keratitis or corneal ulceration:
  - Primary: bacterial, fungal or viral (avian poxvirus).
  - Secondary: trauma or exposure due to eyelid deformity or malformation.
- Mass on cornea:
  - Dermoid.
  - Staphyloma: uveal herniation into a weakened, distorted area of the cornea.
  - Descemetocoele.

HYPHEMA
- Trauma.
- Warfarin toxicosis.
- Neoplasia.

CATARACTS
Similar aetiology to mammals; can be inherited or acquired.

FACE
SWELLINGS ON THE FACE
- Sinusitis.
- Neoplasia.
- Insect bite.
- Trauma.

MATTING/STAINING OF FEATHERS BELOW AND CAUDAL TO EYE
- Otitis externa.

MATTING OF THE FEATHERS OVER FACE AND HEAD
- Vomiting (46).

SMALL NODULES ON THE FACIAL SKIN OF MACAWS
- Macaw acne: ingrown feather follicles that produce a reactive nodule.

BODY
PROMINENT KEEL BONE ('GOING LIGHT')
- Chronic illness, resulting in catabolism of the muscle.
- Inability to fly, causing the muscles to atrophy due to disuse. (Note: This degree of muscle wastage is usually not as severe as seen with illness.)

TWISTED KEEL BONE
- Nutritional secondary hyperparathyroidism.
- Genetic abnormality.

SPLIT KEEL BONE (NONTRAUMATIC)
- Genetic abnormality where the two halves of the sternum have failed to fuse correctly.

ULCERATIVE LESION ON THE CRANIAL END OF THE KEEL
- Chronic self-mutilation and trauma resulting from falling heavily to the ground. Most commonly seen in birds with overly severe wing trims (**110**).
- Ulcerating lipoma or 'fat abscesses'.

OVERABUNDANCE OF PECTORAL MUSCLE MASS (I.E. 'CLEAVAGE') ALONG KEEL
- Obesity.

ENLARGED ABDOMEN
Increased space between the sternum and the pubic bones (**224**).

- Solid enlargement:
  - Obesity.
  - Hepatomegaly.
  - Internal neoplasia (e.g. renal, gonadal).
  - Egg binding.
  - Oviductal enlargement in breeding season.
  - Normal in young birds still being fed.
  - Intestinal parasitism (severe).
- Fluid enlargement:
  - Yolk-related peritonitis.
  - Ovarian cyst.
  - Neoplastic cyst.
  - Ascites associated with heart and/or liver disease.
- Hernia.

SUBCUTANEOUS EMPHYSEMA (204)
- Trauma.
- Postendoscopy air leakage.
- Rupture of cervicocephalic air sac due to trauma or air sacculitis.

SPLIT IN SKIN BETWEEN VENT AND TAIL
- Heavy landing associated with overly severe wing trim (**114**).

SUBCUTANEOUS MASSES
- Lipomas (**111**).
- Xanthomas.
- Fat deposits.
- Hernias.
- Abscesses.

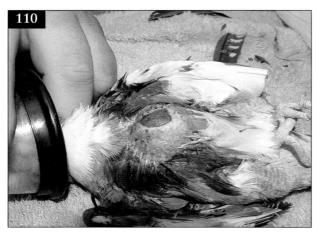

110 Sternal trauma associated with heavy falls due to excessive wing trim.

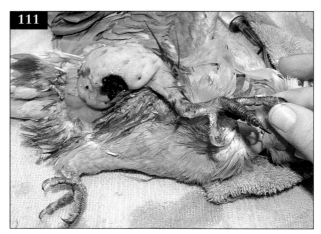

111 Lipoma in a galah.

PAEDIATRICS

CROP NOT EMPTYING OR SLOW TO EMPTY
- Generalized illness with ileus.
- Bacterial or yeast ingluvitis.
- Hand-rearing formula mixed incorrectly: incorrect temperature or consistency.
- Foreign body obstruction.

CERVICAL EMPHYSEMA
- Ruptured cervicocephalic air sac, often due to rough handling while being fed.
- Gulping air while feeding (in this case the air is in the crop, not under the skin).

ERYTHEMATOUS SKIN
- Dehydration.
- Heat stress.
- Generalized illness.

PALLOR
- Cold stress.
- Illness.

OVERLY LARGE HEAD
- Stunting: reduced rate of growth due to any cause (250).

BRUISING ON THE SKIN
- Severe bacterial or viral infection, especially polyomavirus.
- Injections (e.g. enrofloxacin).
- Trauma from parents or siblings.

FEATHERS NOT GROWING NORMALLY
- Stunting: reduced rate of growth due to any cause.
- Polyomavirus.

SWOLLEN TOES
- Constricted toe syndrome (164).
- Bedding or thread wrapped around toe, acting as a tourniquet.

THIN TOES
- Stunting: reduced rate of growth due to any cause.

VOMITING
- Ingluvitis.
- Generalized illness.
- Foreign body obstruction (e.g. from chewing on substrate).
- Weaning, particularly South American species.

REFUSING TO EAT
- Weaning.
- Nonspecific sign of illness.

REDDENED SKIN OR SCAB OVER THE CROP
- Crop burn.
- Trauma from crop needle.

FURTHER READING

Doneley B, Harrison GJ, Lightfoot TL. (2006) Maximizing information from the physical examination. In: *Clinical Avian Medicine, Vol 1.* GJ Harrison, TL Lightfoot (eds). Spix Publishing Inc, Palm Beach, pp. 153–212.

CHAPTER 7
DISORDERS OF THE SKIN AND FEATHERS

CONGENITAL DISORDERS
'FEATHER DUSTER' OR 'CHRYSANTHEMUM' SYNDROME IN BUDGERIGARS
Definition/overview
Juvenile birds exhibit continued growth of flight, tail and contour feathers.

Aetiology
This is believed to be a lethal recessive genetic disorder. There is thought to be an association with budgerigar herpesvirus, but a 'cause and effect' has not been established.

Clinical presentation
Affected birds are unable to fly and make a barely audible noise. Most die within the first few years of life.

'STRAW FEATHER' IN CANARIES
Definition/overview
Feathers fail to emerge from the feather sheath, giving them a straw-like appearance.

Aetiology
This is a lethal disorder, believed to be hereditary in canaries.

Differential diagnosis
It must be differentiated from any condition that prevents the bird from grooming properly.

FEATHER CYSTS IN CANARIES
Definition/overview
These appear as in-grown feathers forming hard, yellow nodules on the skin of canaries with complex feathering such as the Norwich, Border and Gloucester strains.

Aetiology
They may actually be benign neoplasms of the feather follicle. Several dermal papillae form in each follicle, resulting in a tangle of feathers that fail to erupt from the skin. It is believed to be an hereditary condition.

Clinical presentation
The dorsal thoracic area is a frequent site of multiple cysts, but they can occur anywhere on the body and wings. They often occur in several sites along a feather tract.

Management
Treatment of individual cysts can be conservative, simply lancing and expressing the contents of the cyst. Recurrence is common, but surgical excision of the affected follicle is generally curative. When multiple cysts are present, surgical excision of the affected tract may be required. Cysts on the wings may not be amenable to surgery without partial wing amputation. Therefore, conservative therapy may be warranted, so long as the owner is aware of the probability of an ongoing problem.

'PORCUPINE FEATHERS' IN HOMER AND FANTAIL PIGEONS
A similar condition to 'straw feather' in canaries.

BALDNESS IN LUTINO COCKATIELS
A bald patch is present behind the crest feathers on the crown of the head in lutino cockatiels. No treatment is required or available.

NUTRITIONAL DISORDERS
Malnutrition may affect the skin and feathers in several ways.

FEATHER QUALITY
- Brittle feathers.
- Abnormal moulting resulting in frayed or damaged feathers.
- Inability to preen, resulting in retained feather sheaths.
- Stress bars. Breaks in the feather vane due to brief episodes of dysfunction of epidermal collar associated with release of corticosteroid hormones during some stress. It can be associated with periods of malnutrition, especially during the weaning process.

FEATHER COLOUR
Colour in birds is the result of a combination of feather structure (affecting the passage or reflection of light), melanin pigments (black, grey and brown) and carotenoid pigments (yellow and red). Nutrition will affect both the feather structure and the amount and type of carotenoids in the feather. Malnutrition can therefore produce some of the following effects on feather colour:
- Fading and dullness of plumage (**112**).
- Red feathering in African grey parrots.
- Abnormal colours in eclectus parrots.
- Colour changes in other parrots (e.g. green feathers turning yellow, blue feathers turning white).

It must be remembered that other agents can also affect feather colour, notably genetics and viral diseases such as PBFD.

SKIN CHANGES
- Increased scaliness of the skin (**113**).
- Subcutaneous fat deposits giving the skin a yellowish hue.
- Increased skin fragility such that the skin tears easily. A common example of this is 'tail split' injuries in cockatiels with badly done wing clips. The combination of a heavy fall and fragile skin leads to a split in the skin between the vent and the tail (**114**).

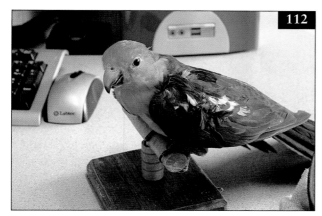

112 A king parrot fed an all-seed diet for many years. Note the general dullness of the plumage, the red feathers turning orange and the green feathers turning yellow.

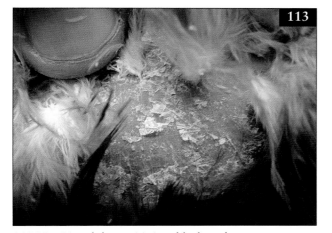

113 Nutritional dermatitis in a black cockatoo.

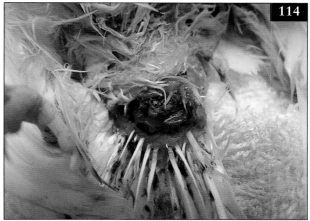

114 'Tail split' injury associated with a heavy fall in a cockatiel.

Management

A dietary assessment to identify and correct nutritional deficiencies is an essential component of the evaluation of any dermatological problem in birds.

ENDOCRINE DISORDERS
HYPOTHYROIDISM
Clinical presentation

Poultry with thyroiditis demonstrate changes in feather quality and colour. Black, brown and yellow feathers become red, longer and more pointed and have fewer pennaceous barbules than normal. A similar syndrome has been seen by the author in galahs with suspected hypothyroidism. These birds develop long, narrow primary flight feathers and develop a pink–red discoloration of the grey plumage. At the same time, the normally pink feathers deepen in colour intensity.

An obese scarlet macaw with confirmed hypothyroidism had nonpruritic feather loss, mild nonregenerative anaemia, mild leucocytosis, heterophilia, hypercholesterolaemia and sparse feathers, and it had not moulted in over a year. It responded well to thyroxine therapy.

Lutino cockatiels with suspected hypothyroidism may show deepening colour intensity and a loss of barbs and barbules in the feathers, giving the bird a 'greasy' deep yellow colour (**115**). Results of liver function tests in these birds are often normal.

Diagnosis

Hypothyroidism is much overdiagnosed. Diagnosis is difficult because normal resting T_4 levels in birds are much lower than in mammals and are often below the detectable limits of many laboratory techniques and equipment. Diagnosis requires demonstration of a failure to respond to TSH administration, but avian TSH is not commercially available.

Management

Despite the lack of laboratory confirmation, some obese birds that demonstrate a lack of weight loss following a rigid diet, accompanied by poor quality feathers and infrequent moults, respond favourably to thyroxine therapy.

DELAYED MOULTING
Aetiology

Delayed moult is usually caused by a combination of malnutrition, abnormal diurnal rhythm, especially for companion birds kept indoors, concurrent illness and endocrine disorders (e.g. hypothyroidism). Excessive egg production may cause abnormal or delayed moulting due to endocrinal effects on feather growth.

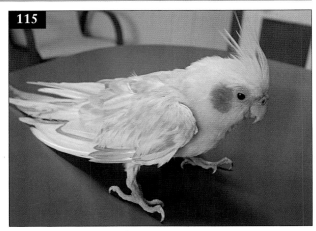

115 Darkening of the feathers and a 'greasy' appearance in a cockatiel with suspected hypothyroidism.

Clinical presentation

Birds present with untidy plumage, bald spots and damaged, brittle feathers. The ends of the feathers often become frayed and lose their colour. Other (non-dermatological) signs may include decreased vocalization in male canaries, excessive or decreased egg production and general lethargy.

Management

Normal diurnal rhythms should be re-established by ensuring the bird gets at least 12–14 hours of 'sleep time' in a darkened, quiet environment. Simply covering a cage in a busy family area is insufficient to meet the sleep requirements for most birds. Nutritional problems must be corrected.

Egg production should be controlled through nutritional, environmental, social and hormonal manipulation (see Chapter 20, Disorders affecting the reproductive tract).

BACTERIAL INFECTIONS
Definition/overview

Staphylococcus spp. are suspected of being the most common bacterial skin pathogens. They may result in generalized skin infections, which may appear as a folliculitis or a dermatitis (**116**). Localized or multifocal swellings may be abscesses from infected wounds, damaged feather follicles or foreign bodies (**117**), or *Mycobacterium* infection.

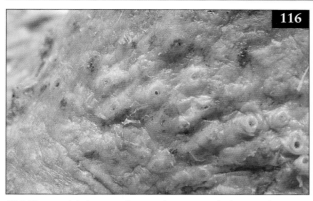

116 Dermatitis in a cockatoo due to staphylococcal infection following a dog 'mouthing' the bird.

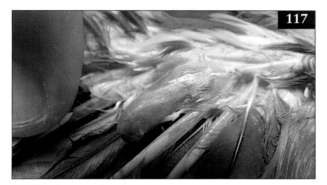

117 Feather cyst in a sun conure.

Clinical presentation

In generalized *Staphylococcus* infections the skin is usually very pruritic, and often erythematous.

Mycobacterium infection causes localized or multifocal lesions that may be wart-like, dry flaky swellings of the skin, granulomatous skin lesions or raised ulcers.

Diagnosis

Diagnosis requires skin biopsy (including follicles) and culture. MRSA is becoming a more recognized entity in these cases.

Management

Systemic antibiotic therapy is given as indicated by culture. Washing the bird two to three times weekly with benzyl peroxide or chlorhexidine shampoos can be beneficial by removing a lot of the scale and debris on the skin and reducing the bacterial load. Surgical excision of localized lesions may be curative.

The zoonotic potential of *Mycobacterium* and MRSA must be discussed with the owner before attempting treatment (see Chapter 13, Disorders of the gastrointestinal tract, p. 167).

FUNGAL INFECTIONS
Aetiology

Candida albicans, *Malassezia pachydermatis*, dermatophytes (*Microsporum gallinae*, *M. gypseum*, *Trichophyton verrucosum*, other *Trichophyton* spp.), *Cryptococcus bacillisporus* (formerly *C. neoformans* var. *gattii*) and *C. neoformans* var. *grubii* (formerly *C. neoformans* var. *neoformans* serotype A), *Aspergillus* spp.

Clinical presentation

Candida causes lesions around the commissures of the mouth and nares and occasionally around feather follicles on the head, back and ventral abdomen.

Malassezia results in generalized pruritus, sometimes with crusting and folliculitis.

Dermatophytes are a slow-spreading infection causing scabs, crusts and alopecia on the body and thin-skinned areas of head and upper beak, and a rough, porous appearance of the podotheca. In gallinaceous birds the characteristic scaly, crusty lesions of the wattle, comb and legs are known as 'favus'.

Cryptococcus has been reported to cause subcutaneous nodules on the head and body and raised nodular lesions on the face and beak.

Cutaneous aspergillosis has been associated with focal ulcerative pruritic lesions.

Diagnosis

Cytology can be used with caution: feather dust stains similarly to yeast organisms and can be nearly impossible to distinguish from yeast bodies. Biopsy and fungal culture can be used.

Management

Systemic antifungals (itraconazole, fluconazole, ketoconazole, terbinafine) are given for 1–3 months. Topical treatment may be carried out using enilconazole wash, clotrimazole wash or cream, or miconazole shampoos.

VIRAL INFECTIONS

Viral infections can cause dystrophic feathers (PBFD virus, polyomavirus, adenovirus and parvovirus [waterfowl]) or skin lesions (poxvirus, papillomavirus and herpesvirus).

PSITTACINE BEAK AND FEATHER DISEASE
Aetiology
PBFD virus, a circovirus, is a nonenveloped single-strand DNA virus measuring 14–17 nm.

Pathogenesis
The virus has a minimum incubation period of 21–25 days, but it could be as long as several years. The virus is shed in faeces, crop secretions and feather dust. Vertical transmission is suspected but not confirmed.

Clinical presentation
There are two forms of PBFD: acute and chronic. All psittacines are susceptible, but New World psittacines and cockatiels appear to be rarely affected. PBFD is more common in juveniles than in adults, but naïve adults are susceptible.

Acute PBFD is seen in juveniles, around weaning age. They are lethargic, fluffed and anorexic.

Haematology may show a pancytopenia and nonregenerative anaemia. Affected birds may die with severe hepatic necrosis before feather abnormalities develop. Feather lesions have been noted in fledgling birds at 28–32 days old.

Chronic PBFD causes progressive replacement of normal feathers with dystrophic feathers (retained sheaths and blood supply, clubbed appearance, stress lines, constrictions and abnormal shapes). The degree and location of the feather loss may depend on the state of moult when the bird was initially infected. Typically lesions develop in order of powder down, contour, primaries, secondaries, tail and then the crest. Poicephalus species and lories may only lose tail feathers and primary flight feathers (**118**, **119**). These feathers may then regrow. Neophemas may develop untidy plumage and lose feathers easily when handled. Many parrots develop feather colour changes: blue feathers become white, green feathers become yellow. Beak lesions including palatine necrosis, ulceration, elongation and easily fractured beaks (**120**) are seen in cockatoos. Immunosuppression is common in all species.

Diagnosis
Histopathology
Basophilic intracytoplasmic inclusion bodies found in feather follicles and the cloacal bursa are considered diagnostic (**121**). Care must be taken not to confuse them with herpesvirus or adenovirus. Feathers and skin show multifocal necrosis of epidermal cells, epidermal hyperplasia and epidermal hyperkeratosis. Diffuse necrosis of epidermal cells is seen throughout the epidermal collar and in basal and intermediate layers of developing feathers. Beak histopathology shows hyperkeratosis and separation of the cornified outer layer from underlying tissues and bones. Atrophy and focal aggregation of necrotic cells are seen in the thymus and bursa.

Serology
Haemagglutination inhibition is a sensitive method for measuring antibody responses to PBFD. When combined with haemagglutination it allows a review of the bird's PBFD status.

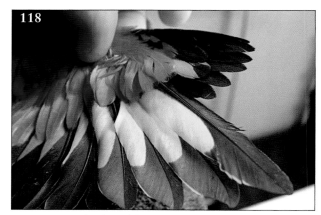

118 Psittacine beak and feather disease in a lorikeet, showing loss of distal primary feathers.

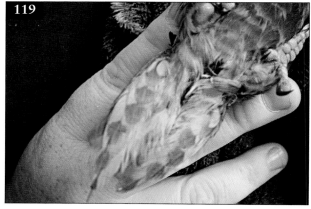

119 Psittacine beak and feather disease in a lorikeet, showing loss of primary feathers and colour changes.

PCR
Viral-specific PCR probes are the most sensitive test, but they give no indication of whether the bird is infected or transiently viraemic.

Management
Avian interferon may be of value if given before the bird shows clinical signs. Otherwise, supportive care (e.g. treating secondary infections and providing a good diet) is all that can be done at this time.

Prognosis
Some birds (e.g. lorikeets) may be able to mount an effective immune response and apparently recover. It is unclear at the time of writing if these birds become inapparent carriers. Some birds, despite showing

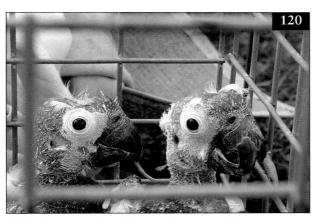

120 Psittacine beak and feather disease in wild cockatoos.

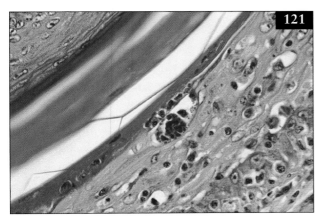

121 Botryoid inclusion follicle from a case of psittacine beak and feather disease. (400×)

clinical signs, may live for 10–30 years, but most infected birds die within two years of secondary diseases related to immunosuppression.

POLYOMAVIRUS
Aetiology
Polyomavirus is a nonenveloped virus that is relatively environmentally stable. All parrots can be affected, but it is most common in macaws, conures, eclectus parrots and caiques. It is rare in African grey parrots, cockatoos and cockatiels. Passerines, including grass finches, canaries, goldfinches and greenfinches can also be infected. It is unknown if the virus in passerines is antigenically related to the virus in psittacines, or if it can be transmitted between psittacines and passerines.

Infection does not always result in disease. Disease determinants include species of the bird, age at which it is infected and concurrent immunosuppression (e.g. PBFD). The age of peak susceptibility varies between species:
- Budgerigars: 10–25 days old.
- Conures: <6 weeks old.
- Macaws and eclectus: <14 weeks old.
- Lovebirds: up to 1 year (concurrent PBFD may be a factor).
- Older birds usually do not show clinical signs unless secondarily immunosuppressed (e.g. PBFD).

Adult birds can be infected, but they rarely show signs of disease.

Pathophysiology
Infected birds of any age that do not develop disease will still have viral replication and shed the virus. The length of time the virus is shed is determined by the age at which the bird is infected (the older the bird, the shorter the shedding period) and the species of bird:
- Budgerigars shed for up to six months, stopping at sexual maturity or the first breeding cycle.
- Conures shed for 4–8 weeks, rarely up to 16 weeks.
- Macaws shed for 6–14 weeks.
- Cockatoos shed for 8–10 weeks.

The virus is passed horizontally in urine, faeces and respiratory and skin secretions. Vertical transmission is suspected, but not yet adequately proven. Infected non-budgerigar parrots shed the virus 2–7 days after being experimentally inoculated.

In larger parrots the time between exposure and death is usually 10–14 days.

Clinical presentation

Polyomavirus infection causes acute death in most parrots, especially those <15 days old. In larger parrots, death may occur between 20 and 140 days old.

In budgerigars (the primary reservoir of polyomavirus) signs include decreased hatchability and embryonic death, abdominal distension, subcutaneous haemorrhages and feather dysplasia that may resolve after several months (primary and secondary feathers on the wings and tail are lost or fail to erupt — in the budgerigar fancy these birds are known as runners and the condition is known as French Moult) (**122, 123**). There may be neurological signs if the cerebellum is affected.

In other parrots the virus causes sudden death or crop stasis, weakness, yellow urates, pallor, bleeding from feather follicles and subcutaneous bruising.

In estrilid finches (grass finches) the virus causes acute mortality in two- to three-day-old fledglings, young adults and mature finches. Survivors may demonstrate poor feather development and misshapen lower beaks.

Infection is rare in fringillidae finches (canaries, goldfinches, greenfinches), where three types of lesions have been described: pulmonary (firm lungs with pale areas amongst congestion); hepatic/splenic (hepatosplenomegaly, focal haemorrhages in the liver); and cutaneous (warts have been described on the beaks of canaries). Other concurrent infections are common (e.g. *Atoxoplasma*, poxvirus).

Diagnosis

Antemortem diagnosis can be achieved using PCR probes. After initial infection there is a viraemia that can be detected by blood PCR. After a short period, the virus can be detected in the cloaca by PCR. When the bird is about to stop shedding, the blood PCR becomes negative. After 6–8 weeks the cloacal shedding stops. Therefore:

- Blood positive, cloaca negative: early stages of infection, or intermittent shedding.
- Blood and cloaca positive: bird actively infected and shedding.
- Blood negative, cloaca positive: bird is about to stop shedding.
- Blood and cloaca negative: bird has cleared infection, no longer shedding.

Blood should be tested first. If it is negative, the bird should be quarantined for eight weeks and can then be considered clear. If it is positive, the bird should be retested in 2–3 months.

Gross pathology findings include hydropericardium, cardiomegaly, hepatomegaly, splenomegaly, generalized pallor (muscles may appear an orange colour) and petechial haemorrhages.

Histopathological findings include:

- In larger parrots, clear to basophilic intranuclear inclusions can be found in the spleen, in mesangial cells in the kidneys and in Kupffer cells.
- In budgerigars inclusions can be found in most organs including the cerebellum, renal tubules, splenocytes and hepatocytes. The most prominent are often found in the feather follicles and growing feathers.
- Massive hepatocellular necrosis.
- Immune-mediated glomerulonephropathy.

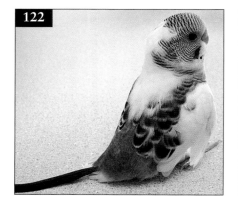

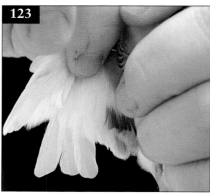

122, 123 Shortened tail and wing feathers in a budgerigar with polyomavirus infection. In the budgerigar fancy this disease is known as 'French moult' and the birds are known as 'runners' or 'creepers' because of their inability to fly.

Management
Non-budgerigar aviaries
By the time the first case is recognized, most other birds will already be infected. Therefore vaccination or testing may not be of any benefit. Hand rearing should stop and chicks allowed to be parent reared, as there is less incidence of disease in parent-reared birds (except in budgerigars). All birds to be sold should be tested by blood PCR and held for two weeks after a negative result before selling.

Budgerigar aviaries
Nestlings and young birds are the reservoir of infection, therefore breeding should be stopped for four months (until all birds are at least six months old). All young birds should be removed and the adults moved to a clean environment. Disinfection is carried out with phenolics, sodium hypochlorite or stabilized chlorine dioxide.

Prevention
Non-budgerigar aviaries
It is best not to keep budgerigars, cockatiels or lovebirds without testing them. Other people's birds should not be brought into the nursery. A closed aviary should be maintained (i.e. no movement in without testing first). PBFD is tested for at the same time. If birds do have to be moved out, and then back in, they must be at least 18 weeks old and, if vaccinations are being used, they should be given four and two weeks prior to movement. Traffic control is used to prevent movement from adults to chicks.

Budgerigar aviaries
A random number of birds should be tested to determine if disease is present. Only PCR-negative birds should be brought in, including own birds returning from shows.

AVIAN POXVIRUS
Aetiology
Avian poxvirus is a large (up to 400 nm) enveloped DNA virus. All avipoxviruses are morphologically similar, but they have differing host specificity.

Pathophysiology
The virus is environmentally stable and can survive for years in dried organic debris. The virus must enter the body through mucous membranes or abraded skin. It is unable to penetrate intact epithelium. It can be transmitted directly through fighting, feather damaging behaviour or preening, or

it can be indirectly transmitted by blood-sucking insects (e.g. mosquitoes). The virus will either remain at the point of entry, causing localized infection, or spread haematogenously to the liver and bone marrow, producing a systemic infection. The incubation period is 7–9 days in pigeons and four days to three weeks in canaries.

Clinical presentation
There are four different syndromes:
- Dry pox: discrete scabby lesions on unfeathered parts of the body (e.g. combs, wattles, beaks, eyelids).
- Wet pox: fibronecrotic diphtheritic lesions in the oropharynx.
- Septicaemic form in canaries.
- Viral-induced neoplastic lesions in the skin and lungs.

The presenting syndrome is determined by the strain of the virus, the mode of transmission and the age, species and health of the infected bird. Lesions may become infected and painful, and may interfere with eating, respiration and vision.

Diagnosis
Intracytoplasmic inclusion bodies, known as Bollinger bodies, are considered pathognomonic. Virus isolation and PCR can be utilized.

Management
Most localized lesions are self-limiting, healing in 3–4 weeks (although diphtheritic lesions may persist for several months) and producing immunity for 6–12 months or longer. If lesions are infected, antibiotics and gentle cleansing are indicated. Forceful removal of scabs may result in scarring and deformity.

Control revolves around isolation of affected birds, minimizing fighting and preventing access of biting insects. Sodium hypochlorite is an effective disinfectant. Attenuated live vaccines are available for pigeons and poultry. The fowl pox vaccine is effective in ostriches. There is also a canary pox vaccine available.

PAPILLOMAVIRUS
Aetiology
Papillomavirus is a double-stranded nonenveloped DNA virus.

Clinical presentation
Cutaneous papillomas (small fleshy pedunculated masses originating primarily from featherless areas

such as the feet and face) are seen in African grey parrots, canaries and finches. Their effects are usually simply mechanical, and so the clinical signs are determined by their location.

This is a different disease syndrome from Internal Papilloma Disease seen in macaws, conures and hawk-headed and Amazon parrots (see Chapter 13, Disorders of the gastrointestinal tract, p. 170).

Diagnosis
Koilocytosis (large dense cytoplasmic perinuclear space with irregular edge) is the hallmark of papillomaviruses. Virus isolation is the gold standard, but papillomavirus viral particles may be rare or absent. Western blot immunoassay and immunohistology are ideal along with standard histology.

Management
Radiosurgery, cryosurgery and laser surgery have all been used to remove the papillomas and, possibly, stimulate an immune response to delay or prevent recurrence.

PARASITIC INFECTIONS
MITES
Mites are the most important and commonly encountered external parasite of birds. Adult mites have eight legs; the larval stage has six legs.

Cnemidocoptes pilae
See Chapter 8, Disorders of the beak and cere, p. 129 (**124**).

Dermanyssus gallinae (red or roost mites)
This mite lives in the environment, where it can survive long periods without feeding. It takes blood meals at night and leaves the bird in the day. It causes skin irritation, scaliness and anaemia (especially in juveniles or small birds). Heavy infestations may kill chicks in the nest box.

Ornithonyssus spp. (fowl mite)
These host-dependent blood-sucking mites remain on the bird, where they congregate at the eyelids and vent. They may cause anaemia, pruritis and damaged plumage. They may also transmit *Borrelia* and *Lankesterella*.

Epidermoptic mites
This group includes *Myialges* spp., *Epidermotes* spp. and *Microlichus* spp. They may be carried mechanically by the hippoboscid fly. They cause depluming dermatitis with scale formation in passerines.

Quill mites
This group includes *Syringophilus* spp., *Dermoglyphus* spp., *Pterolichus* spp., *Analges* spp. and *Harporhynchus* spp. (**125**). Their entire lifecycle is spent on the host. They can be found by examining the pulp material within a developing or damaged feather. They cause partial or complete loss of the feather.

LICE
Definition/overview
Lice are six-legged, wingless, crawling external parasites with chewing mouthparts. Sucking lice do

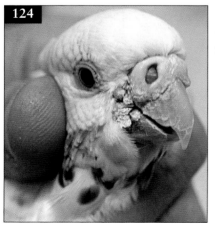

124 *Cnemidocoptes* infestation.

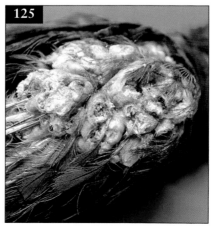

125 *Harporynchus*, a mite, causes these lesions in lorikeets and other species.

not infect birds. They are species specific. They may serve as a vector for some contagious diseases (e.g. eastern equine encephalitis).

Species

There are many hundreds of species of lice found on birds. Just a few examples include:
- Biting lice of psittacines include *Neopsitta-conirmus*, *Psittaconirmus*, *Eomenopon* and *Pacifimenopon*.
- Biting lice of pigeons include the Philopteridae and Menoponidae families.
- Biting lice of raptors include *Mallophaga* spp.

Life cycle

Lice usually live on just the one host. Eggs are glued to feather shafts and hatch in 4–7 days. Nymphs go through three moults before maturing.

Clinical presentation

Lice feed on skin scales, feather debris and hair, causing pruritus and poor feather quality.

FLEAS

The stickfast flea, *Echidnophaga gallinacea*, is a bloodsucking ectoparasite. It occasionally attaches to the skin of the head of nonpoultry birds and causes irritation and blood loss, resulting in depression, anaemia and pruritis on the skin of the head.

FLIES

Flies that cause problems with aviary and companion birds include *Pseudolynchia canariensis* (the pigeon fly) and the hippoboscid fly (louse fly, parrot fly). Blood-sucking flies are found on many species of birds. They seldom leave the host, but are not host specific. They lay their eggs off the host, in a secluded spot. They also act as vectors of *Haemoproteus*.

TICKS

Argas persicus, the fowl tick, is a soft-bodied tick that feeds for 3–7 days on the bird before dropping off. It normally lives in the environment.

Ixodes cornuatus, a hard-bodied tick, causes ascending paralysis.

MANAGEMENT

Sprays and washes can be effective. Natural and synthetic pyrethrins are effective and generally safe. Organophosphate washes are not recommended because of the high incidence of adverse effects. Ivermectin and moxidectin are effective against blood-sucking and keratin-feeding parasites.

NEOPLASTIC AND PSEUDONEOPLASTIC CONDITIONS
LIPOMAS
Incidence

Lipomas can be seen in any bird, but are most common in Amazons, budgerigars and galahs. They usually occur in older birds; there does not appear to be a sex predilection. They are associated with an exclusively, or at least predominantly, all-seed diet, combined with a sedentary life style.

Clinical presentation

Masses are usually located along the main fat deposits on the body (around the crop, the ventral abdomen, thighs and down the legs). They are occasionally found around the cloaca. They are rarely seen on the back or the wings. They are firm masses, often embedded in subcutaneous fat, with the overlying skin often yellow in colour (126). The masses may be mobile. Birds are occasionally presented for bleeding due to the lipoma ulcerating.

Diagnosis

Diagnosis is based on the history and clinical appearance. Lipomas must be distinguished from hernias and xanthomas. Radiography can be useful for differentiating lipomas and hernias.

Management

Lipomas are often an indication of extensive underlying disease processes including cardiovascular disease, hepatic lipidosis, hypothyroidism and, occasionally, diabetes mellitus. Before starting any treatment it is important that this information is communicated to the owner and the patient's health (as a whole) is determined.

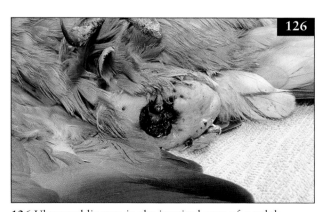

126 Ulcerated lipoma in the inguinal area of a galah.

Surgical excision, while curative, is often not the first treatment of choice. The author's preference is to only excise ulcerating lipomas or those that are mechanically interfering with the bird's lifestyle (e.g. interfering with the normal range of motion of the leg). If surgery is decided upon, great care must be taken to monitor for coagulopathies, often not apparent until the postoperative period. In the case of ulcerating lipomas, where surgery is required urgently, fresh whole blood transfusions may be required during and after the procedure (see Chapter 5, Supportive therapy, p. 94).

If the lipoma is not ulcerating, the bird should be converted to a formulated diet and its weight monitored. In many cases the lipoma will shrink to a size where it is either no longer clinically significant (and therefore no further treatment is required) or, if surgery is indicated, it becomes a more simple procedure with fewer postoperative complications.

Some clinicians report that treatment with L-levothyroxine is beneficial in shrinking lipomas. If the decision is made to use this therapy, care must be taken to monitor for adverse side-effects.

NEOPLASIA OF THE UROPYGIAL GLAND
Incidence
These tumours are seen in those parrots that possess an uropygial gland (see Chapter 1). They are most commonly seen in budgerigars.

Clinical presentation
There is abnormal swelling of the uropygial gland. It will occasionally present as an ulcerated mass with bleeding from the dorsal tail area.

Diagnosis
Tumours must be distinguished from adenitis, hypovitaminosis A with glandular metaplasia and hyperkeratosis, abscessation and impactions. Biopsy is the best means of achieving a diagnosis.

Management
Surgical excision can be achieved in the early stages, but these masses are often very vascular and extensive by the time they are noticed by the owner. Chemotherapy appears to have little success in treating this condition. Irradiation with Strontium-90 has shown promise as an effective therapy. Surgical debulking may be necessary in some cases. Response time after therapy is directly related to the mitotic activity of the neoplasm (the higher the mitotic rate, the faster the response time).

OTHER NEOPLASMS
Fibromas/fibrosarcomas can occur anywhere on the body. They may be subcutaneous or proliferative with a nodular, red appearance. They tend to be locally invasive and recurrent (**127**). Surgical excision has been followed by both radiation and chemotherapy with some success.

Squamous cell carcinomas also may occur anywhere on the body, being most prevalent at mucocutaneous junctions of the head, on the distal wing and on the phalanges. They also tend to be locally invasive, and radiation therapy has been attempted with some success.

Soft tissue sarcomas, including haemangiomas and haemangiosarcomas, have been reported in several locations in birds.

Lymphoma and lymphosarcoma (**128**) will occasionally present as hyperkeratotic, alopecic areas of skin, often on the head. Chemotherapy has been used successfully in some cases.

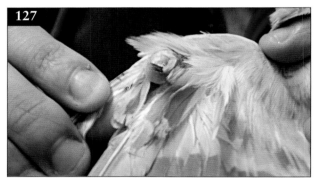

127 Fibroma/fibrosarcoma on the wing of a budgerigar.

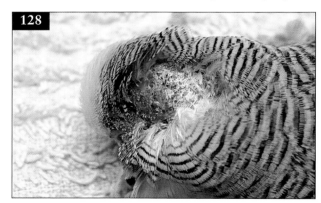

128 Epitheliotropic lymphosarcoma on the crown of the head of a budgerigar.

XANTHOMAS
Incidence
Xanthomas can be seen in any bird at any age. They are considered by some authors to be a metabolic problem (hypercholesterolaemia) combined with an inflammatory response following localized trauma. Xanthomas are thought to be the result of haemorrhage into soft tissue (due to trauma), with the resultant deposition of cholesterol triggering an inflammatory response.

Clinical presentation
Xanthomas are generally friable, yellow-coloured, fatty-appearing masses that may be located anywhere on the body, but are often seen on the distal wing, on the ventral abdomen and on the sternum. Occasionally they will bleed due to repeated trauma.

Diagnosis
Cytology or histopathology shows macrophages laden with cholesterol crystals accompanied by inflammatory cells.

Management
Surgical excision is often difficult or not feasible due to the widespread nature of the lesion, the friability of the tissue and overlying skin and the vascularity of the lesion, which requires good haemostasis. Severe painful xanthomatosis on the distal wings may require amputation.

Medical therapy involves treating the underlying causes of the hypercholesterolaemia (e.g. diet, hepatopathy), NSAIDs (e.g. meloxicam) to control the inflammatory response and prevention of further trauma to the area.

TOXIC CONDITIONS
Fenbendazole can damage feathers if given during new feather growth. The feathers that develop during this period appear dysplastic and brittle, breaking easily.

Silver sulphadiazine, used as a topical antibacterial cream, has been reported to cause agyria (e.g. silver poisoning) after excessively prolonged application. It causes a bluish discoloration of the skin, feathers and mucous membranes.

CONDITIONS AFFECTING THE UROPYGIAL GLAND
IMPACTION
This is associated with hypovitaminosis A, infection, neoplasia or trauma. The gland becomes distended with a caseous-like secretion.

Hot compresses and gentle expression of the gland can temporarily relieve the impaction, but underlying causes need to be addressed.

INFECTION AND ABSCESSES
Untreated impactions can become infected and go on to form abscesses. These usually are painful and erythematous. Surgical ablation of the gland may be required if the abscess fails to respond to debridement, flushing, antibiotics and NSAIDs.

NEOPLASIA
See above under Neoplastic and pseudoneoplastic conditions.

IATROGENIC TRAUMA
The most common iatrogenic trauma seen in companion birds is that resulting from an excessive wing trim. One-winged trims and/or trimming secondary and tertiary flight feathers reduce the bird's ability to slow while in flight and control its descent. The result is a heavy fall. Repeated (or even single) heavy falls can result in broken 'blood feathers' (newly erupted feathers with a rich blood supply in the shaft) (129), bruising to the cranial sternum that leads the bird to mutilate the area, often resulting in an ulceration in the skin

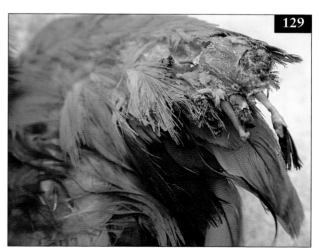

129 Severely traumatized wing tip associated with heavy falls to the ground.

and muscle, sometimes with an underlying osteomyelitis (**130**), and tail splits (splits in the skin between the vent and the tail [**114**]).

Treatment must be aimed at treating the existing trauma while preventing further trauma. Badly broken feathers may need to be removed. (If more than one feather needs to be removed, general anaesthesia and analgesia are appropriate.) If the feather(s) are not badly broken, it may be possible to leave them *in situ* if the haemorrhage has stopped. Sternal trauma, if mild, may respond to antibiotic and analgesic therapy while preventing the bird from further damaging the area (Elizabethan collar +/– a neck brace). If osteomyelitis is present or the ulceration is deep, surgical debridement may be necessary. Tail splits can be debrided and sutured.

Further trauma can be reduced by restoring flight. This can be achieved by 'imping' new primary feathers onto the stumps of those that have been trimmed and/or removing the stumps of trimmed feathers (under anaesthesia) to encourage the regrowth of new feathers. The bird should be confined in a large cage and not allowed free flight until it is able to fly safely. The perches in the cage should be lowered and the floor padded with soft towels to prevent heavy falls and hard landings within the cage.

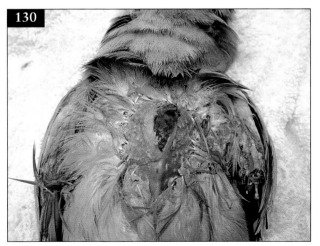

130 Sternal and wing tip trauma resulting from heavy falls to the ground.

FEATHER DAMAGING BEHAVIOUR AND OTHER SELF-MUTILATING CONDITIONS
POLYFOLLICULOSIS
Definition/overview
This is a chronic pruritic condition that can cause multiple small feather cysts in budgerigars and lovebirds.

Aetiology
Histologically there is the appearance of multiple feather shafts from the same follicle, with a thin layer of epidermis separating the shafts. Chronic inflammation occurs beneath the pulp cap and the feather sheath is thickened. There is some discussion as to whether this condition is the cause of the bird's intense pruritis or is the result of damage done by the bird in response to the pruritis.

Clinical presentation
Newly emerging feathers have short, stout quills with retained sheaths. There appear to be several feathers emerging from a single, enlarged follicle.

Management
Surgical excision of affected follicles or feather tracts may be of benefit. NSAIDs such as Meloxicam may be of benefit.

SELF-MUTILATION IN *AGAPORNIS* SPECIES
Clinical presentation
This is an intensely pruritic self-mutilation problem affecting the shoulder region and prepatagial membrane. Less commonly it can involve the inguinal region, chest, back, base of tail and around the cloaca. It can be unilateral or bilateral. Polyfolliculosis is found in some cases.

Long-term scarring of the prepatagial membrane often restricts the bird's ability to fly, and often the affected area cracks and bleeds when the bird stretches its wings.

Management
Treatment is often unrewarding. Placing an Elizabethan collar until the skin wounds have healed can be of benefit, but recurrence once the collar is removed is common. Antibiotics and anti-inflammatory therapies should be given.

COCKATIEL FEATHER MUTILATION SYNDROME
Definition/overview
This is associated with intestinal giardiasis and has been reported in cockatiels only. It appears to be less common now than ten years ago.

Aetiology

It is postulated that giardiasis causes an intestinal malabsorption syndrome, leading to a vitamin E/selenium deficiency which in turn leads to dry, flaky skin that can progress to episodes of feather pulling, alopecia and pruritis.

Clinical presentation

Dry, flaky skin that can progress to episodes of feather pulling, alopecia and pruritis. Other clinical signs include weight loss, depression, ruffled feathers, chronic diarrhoea, neonatal mortality, cachexia and weakness.

Diagnosis

Eosinophilia and hypoproteinaemia are commonly reported; the eosinophilia is most likely to be due to the tissue damage associated with feather damaging behaviour. Detection of the trophozoites (on very fresh faecal smears suspended in normal saline) and cysts (using centrifuged zinc sulphate flotation) is very suggestive that this syndrome is present.

Management

Treatment with nitroimidazoles is usually effective, with a rapid response usually noted.

QUAKER MUTILATION SYNDROME

Aetiology

The aetiology is unclear. There is no histopathological evidence of a pathogen. Insufficient cases have been fully worked up to determine a pattern.

Clinical presentation

There is acute onset of severe self-induced skin trauma, often directed at the neck and sternum and usually unrelated to prior episodes of feather-damaging behaviour (**131**).

Management

Treatment is directed at preventing further trauma through the use of neck braces and/or Elizabethan collars. Analgesia is given through the use of NSAIDs and antibiotic coverage is provided. Euthanasia is often requested because of the severity and recurrence of the trauma.

FEATHER DAMAGING BEHAVIOUR DIRECTED TOWARDS OTHER BIRDS

Towards nestlings

Some parents will start to pluck feathers from their nestlings while they are still in the nest box. Mild cases involve removal of feathers, usually from the back, dorsal wings and head (**132**). Severe cases will see the parent(s) remove wing tips or toes, or even kill the nestling.

Two theories exist as to why this behaviour occurs:
- A learnt behaviour: feather pluckers were often feather plucked themselves as chicks
- A desire to remove the nestlings so as to prepare the nest box for another clutch of eggs.

Affected chicks are best removed for hand rearing. They should not be used for breeding if possible.

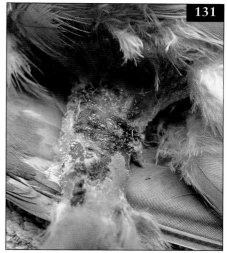

131 Quaker self-mutilation. Note the severe self-inflicted trauma to the inguinal region.

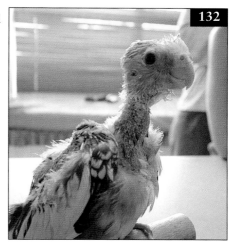

132 Cockatiel chick feather picked by parents.

Towards a bonded mate

Some individuals will pluck feathers from their mate, often at the beginning of the feather season. Both hens and cocks may do the plucking. Usually it is the feathers on the head and face that are plucked (133). It is unusual to see this plucking extend to traumatic mutilation. Many of these pairs will breed successfully. They should be separated if mutilation is likely to result in injury.

Towards cage mates

In overcrowded or otherwise stressful living conditions some birds (particularly finches, budgerigars, *Agapornis* spp., *Neophema* spp. and gallinaceous birds) will pluck the head and back of their cage mates. Occasionally this behaviour can lead to cannibalism and death. Some birds will also chew and pluck flight and tail feathers of cage mates, even in good living conditions.

Affected birds and, if possible, the offending bird(s) should be removed. Stocking density and stress factors need to be addressed and corrected. Foraging activities and toys should be provided for birds that appear to be indulging in this behaviour due to a lack of environmental enrichment.

FEATHER DAMAGING BEHAVIOUR DIRECTED TOWARDS THE BIRD ITSELF
Definition/overview
This is one of the most common and most frustrating conditions that veterinarians can be presented with.

The causes for this condition are often multifactorial and cascading in their effects. By the time the bird is presented to the clinician the original inciting cause may have disappeared or been obscured by other complicating or reinforcing factors.

It must be stressed to the bird's owner that a successful outcome may simply be a reduction, rather than elimination, of the activity. In other words, a feather picker will nearly always remain a feather picker, but may pick less.

Aetiology
Feather damaging behaviour may be due to either physical or psychological problems. It is simplistic and inaccurate to diagnose 'boredom' or 'fear/anxiety' without a thorough investigation to rule out physical problems first (134, 135). It is also simplistic to feel that a single aetiology exists for each individual case. In many cases several factors, both physical and psychological, have combined to produce the clinical sign of feather damaging behaviour.

Physical causes of feather damaging behaviour
- Dermatitis: infectious (bacterial, fungal, viral), chemical (e.g. nicotine absorbed from the owner's fingers) or allergic (still unproven, but strong evidence exists for allergic dermatitis to be a factor in some feather-pickers). Allergies are suspected to occur in birds, but a reliable diagnostic test has yet to be developed.
- Folliculitis: bacterial, fungal, viral.

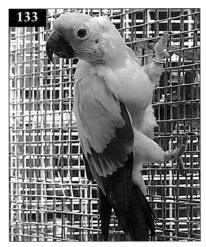

133 Not all feather picking is self-inflicted. This sun conure has been feather picked by her mate.

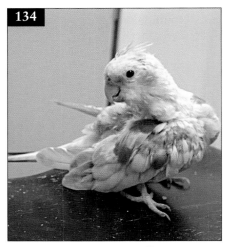

134 Pruritis needs to be differentiated from psychological feather damaging behaviour.

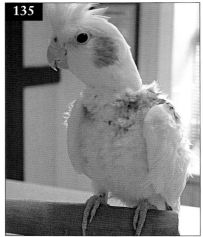

135 Feather picking cockatiel. Note the untouched head and neck feathers, evidence that the feather picking on the torso is self-inflicted.

- Malnutrition: an all-seed diet often results in dry, flaky skin that is predisposed to superficial infections, with resultant pruritis.
- Environmental conditions: extremes of humidity, aerosol contamination and cigarette smoke have been associated with feather damaging behaviour.
- Heavy metal toxicoses are often implicated as a cause of feather damaging behaviour. However, all reported cases are anecdotal and there is no reliable evidence that heavy metal toxicosis causes feather damaging behaviour.
- Underlying painful lesions: hepatopathy (e.g. chlamydiosis), osteomyelitis, pancreatic disease, renal disease, neoplasia, underlying abscesses.
- Reproductive activity, perhaps through ovarian and oviductal enlargement and liver changes (vitellogenesis), is believed to cause abdominal discomfort that may be seen as feather damaging behaviour of the thighs and ventral abdomen of some reproductively active hens.
- Parasites — external (mites, lice) and internal (*Giardia*) — are often overdiagnosed as a cause of feather damaging behaviour (**136**). Pet shop employees, in particular, often advise bird owners to treat feather damaging behaviour birds for lice. *Giardia* has only been associated with feather damaging behaviour in cockatiels, yet many case studies report *Giardia* testing in non-cockatiel species.

136 Feather lice are an exaggerated cause of feather damaging behaviour.

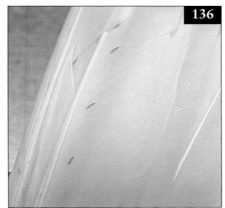

Psychological causes of feather damaging behaviour
- Attention seeking behaviour: this occurs when the bird uses feather damaging behaviour to obtain attention from an owner when that owner is not engaged in an activity with the bird.
- Anxiety: a state of apprehension, uncertainty and fear resulting from the anticipation of a realistic or fantasized threatening event or situation, often impairing physical and psychological functioning. Anxiety disorders may have biological and/or environmental causes: improper socialization that many companion parrots receive during the hand-rearing process may be reflected in an inability to cope with otherwise normal situations; fear, real or imagined, of a person or situation that the bird is exposed to; and 'lack of self-confidence' due to a history of undermining events. An example of this is severe wing clips in juvenile birds that are learning to fly. The resultant heavy falls to the ground may trigger feather damaging behaviour. Anxiety disorders include separation anxiety and obsessive compulsive disorders. Separation anxiety is the presence of behavioural signs of distress (screaming, feather disruptive behaviour) that occurs when the bird is left alone, as a distress response to separation from the person or persons to whom it is attached. This form of anxiety often results from inadequate social skills due to a failure to teach the bird coping behaviours while being hand reared or weaned. Obsessive compulsive disorders are characterized by repetitive, stereotypic motor, locomotor, grooming, ingestive or hallucinogenic behaviours that occur out of context to their normal occurrence or in a frequency or duration that is in excess of that required to achieve a goal. They interfere with the bird's ability otherwise to function normally in its social environment. An example of this is compulsive grooming (i.e. grooming in excess of that which is normally required for grooming and which interferes with normal behaviour). It cannot be interrupted. (This must be distinguished from excessive grooming, which is unrelated to hygienic or maintenance requirements and is more frequent or intensive than previously exhibited. However, unlike compulsive grooming, it can be interrupted.)
- Boredom: parrots are intelligent animals who need to be kept occupied. As a general rule, wild birds spend up to 80% of daylight hours foraging for, and consuming, food. The other 20% of the

day is spent socializing and grooming, and occasionally sleeping. For captive birds, with food provided in a dish every day, this situation can be reversed (i.e. only 20% of the day is spent foraging and eating food, the other 80% is spent socializing and grooming). When socializing opportunities are limited (e.g. the lone bird in a household where everyone is at work during the day), overgrooming may occur and feather damaging behaviour results.

Diagnosis

A thorough history of both the bird and the problem is required. In particular, this history needs to focus heavily on the bird's interaction with its environment and the people (and other animals) around it. A detailed physical examination should be performed and a minimum database on the bird's health status gathered (haematology and clinical biochemistries, whole body radiographs). Based on this physical examination and clinical database, the following additional diagnostic tests may be warranted:

- Skin biopsy.
- Pathogen detection through culture or PCR.
- Endoscopy.

If a physical cause is unable to be determined and the patient's history supports it, a diagnosis of psychological feather damaging behaviour can then be made (*Table 3*). At this stage every effort should be made to incorporate the services of a veterinary behaviourist or a suitably qualified parrot behaviour consultant.

Management

Elizabethan collars are rarely indicated unless self-mutilation and/or physical trauma is occurring. In many cases Elizabethan collars and other restraints may worsen the patient's anxiety state and aggravate the original problem.

Psychotropic drugs may be of benefit as a short-term therapy to break a feather damaging behaviour 'cycle', but are rarely, if ever, warranted as a long-term solution. They can be used to suppress, modify or change unwanted behaviour, but should be used in conjunction with behavioural modification. Most exert their effect by enhancing or inhibiting the effects of excitatory or inhibitory neurotransmitters. Examples of drugs that may have a role in short-term therapy include:

Table 3 Diagnosis of feather damaging behaviour.

Timing and nature of feather damaging behaviour	Differential diagnoses	Reinforcing factors
Occurs when owner is not present	Separation anxiety; boredom	Habit; lack of environmental enrichment/foraging activities
Occurs when owner is present but not paying attention to the bird	Attention seeking behaviour	Owner's behaviour (drama, attention); habit
Bird interrupts other behaviour to damage feathers	Obsessive/compulsive disorder; true pruritus	Owner's behaviour (drama, attention); habit
As well as the feather damaging behaviour, the bird exhibits signs of unwarranted fear, anxiety or stress	Generalized anxiety disorders	Owner's behaviour (avoidance); habit; major changes in household
Problem starts at an extremely young age; handfed bird	Improper preening; poor early socialization	Owner's behaviour (drama, attention); habit
Involves primarily remiges and retrices. The feathers are frayed and splintered	Anxiety disorders. Iatrogenic: improper wing trim, feather trauma due to small cage	Owner's behaviour (drama, attention); habit
Overly bonded, sexually mature bird that displays sexual behaviours out of context	Reproductively related	Owner's behaviour (drama, attention); habit

- Benzodiazepines (e.g. diazepam) inhibit dopamine and potentiate gamma-amino butyric acid (GABA). They are also muscle relaxants, and can interfere with learning.
- Phenothiazines (e.g. acepromazine) are dopamine antagonists. They are rarely used in birds.
- Butyrophenones (e.g. haloperidol) inhibit dopamine and are used for self-mutilation and feather damaging behaviour.
- Antihistamines (e.g. diphenhydramine) inhibit histamine receptors, producing sedation.
- Progestins (e.g. medroxyprogesterone acetate) potentiate GABA; they have a calming and an anti-inflammatory effect. However, they have multiple side-effects including obesity, hepatopathy and diabetes mellitus.
- Tricyclic antidepressants (e.g. clomipramine, doxepin and amitriptyline) potentiate serotonin, producing sedation and anticholinergic activity. They can be used to alleviate anxiety and depression. They must be used with care because of side-effects including constipation and arrhythmias.
- Serotonin specific re-uptake inhibitors (e.g. fluoxetine) have serotonergic effects.
- Narcotic antagonists and agonist/antagonists (e.g. naltrexone) act at the opiate centres in the brain, blocking endorphin response to self-injurious behaviour. This may be useful in some birds.

As mentioned earlier, psychotropic drugs, if used at all, should be employed as a short-term solution. Psychological feather damaging behaviour is a behavioural problem and the real solutions lie in behavioural modification. It must be ensured that stability and security are present in the bird's lifestyle at home. Anxiety disorders arising from, for example, fear of human interaction or fear of falling due to an inappropriate wing trim can lead to feather damaging behaviours. These types of factors should be identified and eliminated if present. Triggering events that may have had a role in the development of feather damaging behaviour, such as changes in the household or a perceived lack of attention, should be identified. Techniques can be used to teach the bird to accept these triggering environmental events if, indeed, it is appropriate for the bird to accept them.

Basic training is implemented and strengthened using a system of positive reinforcement. Once this has been achieved, training can be extended to guide more normal behaviours. The '80–20 rule' is important: 80% of the bird's day should be spent foraging for food, the remaining 20% on grooming and socializing activities. In practical terms, for a companion parrot, this can be done by:

- Providing foraging activities both with and without the owner being present. The bird may need to be taught how to participate in these activities, as at first it might be afraid of new objects or activities.
- Enhancing 'normal' feather care through gentle misting with water and by providing other items that can be groomed in addition to the bird's feathers.
- Developing more normal social interactions between the bird and its owners. The aim is to provide social interaction that is engaging, stimulating and changing for the bird. If there is a 'one-person bond' present between the bird and an owner this must be modified into a more normal flock and social interaction. It must be remembered, though, that it is essential to replace unwanted behaviours with more desirable behaviours; at no time should a behavioural void develop through removing an activity or interaction without replacing it with others.

The goal is to decrease the feather damaging behaviour; it is unlikely that a permanent cure will be achieved. Regular communication and follow-up evaluations are essential to monitor changes in the bird's behaviour and environment. If the result is a healthy, well socialized bird that actively engages its environment and its human companions, the state of its plumage becomes less significant.

FURTHER READING

Briscoe JA, Reisner IR, Rosenthal KL (2004) Incorporating the veterinary behaviourist: a new model for the diagnosis and treatment of a feather damaging pet parrot. In: *Proceedings of the Annual Conference of the Association of Avian Veterinarians*, pp. 293–296.

Chitty J (2005) Feather pulpitis in plucking parrots. In: *Proceedings of the Annual Conference of the Association of Avian Veterinarians*, pp. 259–265.

Clubb SL (2006) Clinical management of feather damaging behaviour associated with inflammatory skin disease in parrots. In: *Proceedings of the Annual Conference of the Association of Avian Veterinarians*, pp. 73–78.

Clubb SL, Buerkle M, Crosta L, Ciembor PG, Latima KS, Garner MM, Ritchie BW (2004) Feather damaging behaviour in Lories and its association with psittacine circovirus. In: *Proceedings of the Annual Conference of the Association of Avian Veterinarians*, pp. 319–320.

Clubb SL, Elmo N, Buerkle M, Crosta L, Enders F (2004) Incidence and characterisation of feather damaging behaviour in a large parrot collection. In: *Proceedings of the Annual Conference of the Association of Avian Veterinarians*, pp. 321–332.

Clubb SL, Garner MM, Cray C, Goodman M (2004) Diagnostic assessment of feather picking behaviour in African Grey Parrots (*Psittacus erithacus*). In: *Proceedings of the Annual Conference of the Association of Avian Veterinarians*, pp. 313–318.

Ferrell ST (2002) Avian integumentary surgery. *Seminars in Avian and Exotic Pet Medicine* 11(3):125–135.

Garner MM (2006) Inflammatory skin disease in feather picking birds: histopathology and species predispositions. In: *Proceedings of the Annual Conference of the Association of Avian Veterinarians*, pp. 17–20.

Gartrell BD, Rogers L, Alley MR (2005) Eosinophilic dermatitis associated with *Trichophyton asahii* in a cockatiel (*Nymphicus hollandicus*). *Journal of Avian Medicine and Surgery* 19(1):25–29.

Gill JH (2002) Avian skin diseases. *Veterinary Clinics of North America: Exotic Animal Practice* 4(2):463–492.

Greenacre CB (2005) Viral diseases of companion birds. *Veterinary Clinics of North America: Exotic Animal Practice* 8(1):85–106.

Hochleithner M, Hochleithner C (1996) Surgical treatment of ulcerative lesions caused by automutilation of the sternum in psittacine birds. *Journal of Avian Medicine and Surgery* 10(2):84–88.

Johnston MS, Preziosi DE, Morris DO, Rosenthal KL, Rankin S (2004) The role of *Malassezia* in feather destructive behaviour in psittacines. In: *Proceedings of the Annual Conference of the Association of Avian Veterinarians*, pp. 89–90.

Koski MA (2001) Dermatological diseases in psittacine birds: an investigational approach. *Seminars in Avian and Exotic Pet Medicine* 11(3):104–125.

Lightfoot TL, Nacewiz CL (2006) Psittacine behaviour. In: *Exotic Pet Behaviour*. TB Bays, TL Lightfoot, J Mayer (eds). Saunders Elsevier, St Louis, pp. 51–102.

Martin KM (2004) Behavioural approach to psittacine feather-picking. In: *Proceedings of the Annual Conference of the Association of Avian Veterinarians*, pp. 307–312.

Merryman JI, Buckles EL (1998) The avian thyroid gland. Part One: a review of the anatomy and physiology. *Journal of Avian Medicine and Surgery* 12(4):234–237.

Merryman JI, Buckles EL (1998) The avian thyroid gland. Part Two: a review of function and

pathophysiology. *Journal of Avian Medicine and Surgery* 12(4):238–242.

Nemetz LP (2004) Strontium-90 therapy for uropygial neoplasia. In: *Proceedings of the Annual Conference of the Association of Avian Veterinarians*, pp. 15–20.

Phalen DN (2006) Implications of viruses in clinical disorders. In: *Clinical Avian Medicine, Vol 2*. GH Harrison, TL Lightfoot (eds). Spix Publishing Inc, Palm Beach, pp. 721–746.

Powers LV, Van Sant F (2006) Axillary and patagial dermatitis in African Grey Parrots (*Psittacus erithicus*). In: *Proceedings of the Annual Conference of the Association of Avian Veterinarians*, pp. 101–105.

Raidal SR (1995) Viral skin diseases of birds. *Seminars in Avian and Exotic Pet Medicine* (4):77–82.

Ritchie BW (1995) Circoviridae. In: *Avian Viruses: Function and Control*. BW Ritchie (ed). Wingers Publishing, Lake Worth, pp. 223–252.

Ritchie BW (1995) Papoviridae. In: *Avian Viruses: Function and Control*. BW Ritchie (ed). Wingers Publishing, Lake Worth, pp. 127–170.

Ritchie BW (1995) Poxviridae. In: *Avian Viruses: Function and Control*. BW Ritchie (ed). Wingers Publishing, Lake Worth, pp. 285–312.

Rosenthal KL, Morris DO, Mauldin ES, Ivey ES, Peikes H (2004) Cytologic, histologic and microbiologic characterization of the feather pulp and follicles of feather-picking psittacine birds. *Journal of Avian Medicine and Surgery* 18(3):137–143.

Schmidt RE (2002) Avian thyroid metabolism and diseases. *Seminars in Avian and Exotic Pet Medicine* 11(2):80–83.

Schmidt RE, Lightfoot TL (2006) Integument. In: *Clinical Avian Medicine, Vol 2*. GH Harrison, TL Lightfoot (eds). Spix Publishing Inc, Palm Beach, pp. 395–410.

Schmidt RE, Reavill DR, Phalen DN (2003) Integument. In: *Pathology of Pet and Aviary Birds*. RE Schmidt, DR Reavill, DN Phalen (eds). Iowa State Press, Ames, pp. 177–196.

Seibert LM (2006) Feather-picking disorder in pet birds. In: *Manual of Parrot Behaviour*. AU Luescher (ed). Blackwell Publishing, Oxford, pp. 255–266.

Tully TN, Foil CS, Nett-Mettler C, Columbini-Osborn S, Heatley JJ, Hosgood G (2006) Status of intradermal skin testing in avian species. In: *Proceedings of the Annual Conference of the Association of Avian Veterinarians*, pp. 33–37.

Welle K (2005) Clinical approach to feather picking disorders in pet birds. In: *Proceedings of the Annual Conference of the Association of Avian Veterinarians Australian Committee*, pp. 83–87.

CHAPTER 8
DISORDERS OF THE BEAK AND CERE

MALFORMATION
Definition/overview
Malformation of the beak may be congenital or acquired. Congenital conditions include lateral deviations of the maxilla (wry/scissor beak) (137) and mandibular prognathism (138, 139). Acquired conditions include lateral deviations of the maxilla (wry/scissor beak), compression deformities of the mandible or maxilla (140) and other malformations, often associated with a 'softening' of the beak due to malnutrition.

Aetiology
Congenital malformations are thought to be associated with incorrect incubation parameters (temperature, humidity, ventilation or turning of the egg) or parental nutrition. Acquired malformations are thought to be due to damage to all, or part of, the germinal epithelium of the beak or to the poorly calcified beaks of neonates.

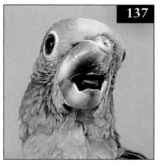
137 Congenital scissor beak in a juvenile Amazon parrot.

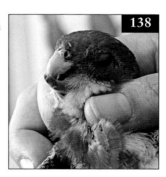
138 Congenital prognathism in an eastern rosella.

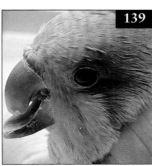
139 Acquired prognathism in an adult quaker.

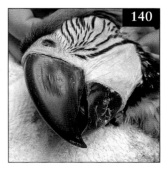
140 Lateral beak compression in a juvenile macaw, due to excessive holding pressure while hand feeding.

Clinical presentation

In lateral deviations of the maxilla (wry/scissor beak), the maxillary beak is deviated laterally from the level of the cere or beak tip. The side of the mandible no longer in wear and the maxilla often overgrows. This condition is most common in macaws up to two months of age, but acquired scissor beak can occur in any species at any age.

Mandibular prognathism is most common in cockatoos aged 1–2 weeks. The maxilla sits inside the mandible.

Compression deformities of the mandible are most commonly seen in macaws up to five weeks of age. Other malformations are often associated with *Cnemidocoptes* infection, trauma and PBFD.

Management

Conservative treatment may be effective in very young chicks. Applying gentle digital pressure for ten minutes two to three times daily may straighten a deviated maxilla or lift the maxilla up and forward in prognathic chicks. Cases that do not respond to this treatment, or older birds with calcified beaks, will need more aggressive therapy.

Deviated maxilla

Beak trimming, involving grinding the overgrown gnathotheca on the side contralateral to the maxillary deviation and the overgrown tomia on the maxilla, allows the maxilla to move back into a normal position. At the same time the occlusal ledge inside the maxilla has to be reshaped so that it is perpendicular to the lateral walls of the rhinotheca. The bird should then be encouraged to chew hard objects (e.g. branches) frequently and the beak reshaped every two weeks until normal.

Acrylic ramps or prostheses can be used to augment the trimming described above. An acrylic ramp is built up on the gnathotheca on the same side as the maxillary deviation, forcing the maxilla into a normal position. The ramp needs to be high enough so that the bird cannot open its mouth wide enough to get its maxilla over the top of the ramp. This technique frequently fails due to damage to the gnathotheca during the attachment of the ramp.

Trans-sinus pinning is an 'orthodontic' procedure, designed to provide constant lateral tension on the deviated maxilla to guide it into a more anatomically normal position. A K-wire or small Steinmann pin is placed perpendicular to the skull, through the frontal sinuses just caudal to the craniofacial hinge joint on a line between the lateral canthus of the eye and the cere. Care must be taken not to position this pin too caudally or too low. In macaws, a small bony protuberance marks the point where the pin is introduced on one side and exits on the other. On the side of beak contralateral to the direction of the deviation, the pin is bent 90° as it leaves the skin. The pin should run the length of the maxilla, and the end (level with the beak tip) is curled over on itself. The other end of the pin is trimmed and curled over on itself so that it is flush against the skin and cannot be pulled through the skull.

The tip of the beak is then placed under tension by means of a rubber band around the beak and the distal end of the wire. In older birds this rubber band is replaced by a piece of wire running through a hole in the distal rhinotheca. The tension is maintained until the beak has straightened. In young birds this can be as soon as 10–14 days; older birds may require 10–14 months. The tension can be adjusted by loosening or tightening the wire/rubber band as required.

Once the beak has straightened the wire/rubber band should be removed. If, after several days, the beak has remained in a normal position, the pin can be removed.

Prognathism

An acrylic prosthesis can be placed over the rhinotheca. One or two small pins can be placed through the rhinotheca to provide 'anchor points' to prevent the prosthesis falling off. The goal is to force hyperextension of the craniofacial hinge joint into a more normal range of motion, allowing for a 'firming' up of the joint so that the upper mandible cannot be overflexed to the point of mandibular prognathism. There is no correction of 'growth' of the beak, but rather guidance and reduction of the abnormal range of motion of the craniofacial hinge joint. The prosthesis must be long enough to prevent the bird opening its mouth wide enough to place the prosthesis inside the gnathotheca.

A trans-sinus pinning technique can be used in older birds. It requires a pin placed through the frontal sinuses as described above. The ends of the pin are then bent forwards to meet just rostral to the beak tip and are linked to form a triangle. A second pin is placed through the rhinotheca midway along its length, with the triangular trans-sinus pin resting on it. Cerclage wire is then used to link the tip of the beak with the apex of the triangle. This arrangement also extends the craniofacial hinge joint into a more normal position.

Prognosis

Many birds with untreated malformations will adapt to the deformity and learn to eat well. However, they will usually do better if the malformation can be corrected. With appropriate techniques, follow-up and care, the prognosis for most beak malformations is good.

TRAUMA

Definition/overview

Common injuries include puncture wounds of the rhinotheca or gnathotheca (**141**), avulsion of the rhinotheca or gnathotheca or both (**142**, **143**), mandibular or maxillary fracture and mandibular symphyseal fracture (**144**).

Aetiology

Causes include bite wounds from other birds and occasionally from other animals, entrapment in wire or metal objects, particularly in cages, and blunt force trauma resulting from striking objects while in flight (e.g. ceiling fans, walls, windows).

Management

Initial treatment should be aimed at relieving pain, stopping bleeding and controlling infection. Once this initial assessment and treatment are finished, attention needs to be given to providing nutritional and fluid support to the patient. Tube feeding or placing an oesophagostomy tube may be required until the patient is able to eat for itself.

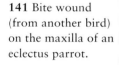

141 Bite wound (from another bird) on the maxilla of an eclectus parrot.

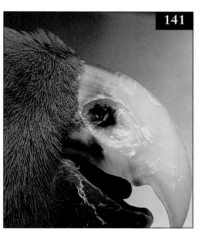

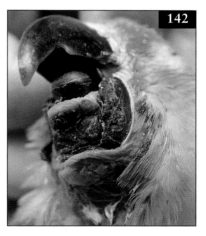

142 Traumatic avulsion of the mandible in a sun conure.

143 Despite the loss of the entire lower beak, this sun conure (same bird as **142**) is still able to eat normally.

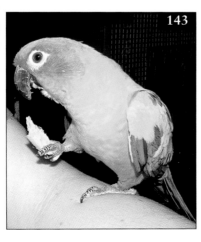

144 Traumatic split in the gnathotheca of a sulphur-crested cockatoo. This is a common injury in breeding pairs that sometimes fight.

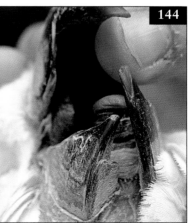

Once the patient is stable, consideration must be given to how to repair the injury, if indeed repair is feasible.

Puncture wounds, if superficial, can be treated conservatively by keeping them clean and giving antibiotics and analgesics as appropriate. Deeper wounds that may affect the structural integrity of the beak should be carefully debrided, dried and then 'plugged' with dental acrylic. As granulation tissue fills in the wound, the acrylic plug will be forced out. This may be a matter of days or perhaps weeks. The plug can be replaced until the clinician is assured the beak's integrity is no longer at risk.

Avulsion of all or part of the mandible or maxilla is a common injury. As a general rule, avulsions of less than the rostral third of the maxilla will usually result in regrowth of the avulsed portion. Loss of more than this amount will usually result in permanent deformity. Surprisingly, many birds will adapt to this deformity and do well, so long as infection and pain are controlled and the bird is nutritionally supported until the wounds have healed. Overgrowth of the opposing rhinotheca or gnathotheca is common, requiring regular trimming. Beak prostheses rarely work in birds, as the kinetic forces transmitted into the prosthesis by normal beak actions (e.g. eating, gripping objects) rapidly lead to implant failure.

Fractures of the mandible or maxilla are more difficult to handle. With fresh injuries, repair with cerclage wire may be effective in some cases. Splinting the fractured area by taping the beak shut may also be of benefit. Nutritional support via an oesophagostomy tube is obviously essential.

Mandibular symphyseal fractures, if fresh, can be treated by wiring with cerclage wire and sealing the fracture line with tissue glue. Care must be taken not to allow the tissue glue to seep into the fracture line. If nonunion results, or if the injury is already several days old when first presented, many of these birds will adapt and be able to eat well. Again, nutritional support may be required via tube feeding or an oesophagostomy tube until the bird is able to eat by itself.

Prognosis
Most beak injuries have a good prognosis. Despite severe injuries, many birds will adapt and survive quite well.

HYPEREXTENSION OF THE MAXILLA
Definition/overview
This is predominantly a problem in macaws. The maxilla is hyperextended, leaving the beak slightly open. Simple reduction, even under anaesthetic, is usually unsuccessful.

Aetiology
Trauma, particularly biting hard on to a solid object and forcefully hyperextending the maxilla, leads to a dorsal subluxation of the palatine bone. This then engages the infraorbital septum, locking the maxilla into a hyperextended position.

Management
Under anaesthesia a Steinmann pin or closed artery forceps is introduced through a lateral approach through the infraorbital sinus just caudal to the beak commissure. It is inserted to a depth half the width of the skull. This can be done blindly or with the guidance of an endoscope. Several large blood vessels are in this area.

The beak is hyperextended further to 'disengage' the palatine bone from the septum. With the beak still hyperextended, the pin or forceps are used to lever the palatine bone ventrally, disengaging it from the septum and allowing the beak to close. The bird is treated with analgesics for 5–7 days and prevented from climbing or biting hard foods for two weeks.

Prognosis
The prognosis is usually good.

OVERGROWN MAXILLA
Aetiology
An overgrown maxilla is associated with chronic liver disease, although the exact pathogenesis is unclear (**145**). Other factors include damage to the germinal epithelial layer, malnutrition, lack of wear or opportunity to wear (**146**), *Cnemidocoptes* and neoplasia. See also **147**.

Diagnosis
A thorough review of the patient's history, including diet and history of head trauma, is required.

CBC and biochemistries are carried out to determine health status, with a particular emphasis on the liver. Radiography of the head may be necessary.

Treatment
The diet should be corrected and appropriate treatment given for liver disease if present. Corrective

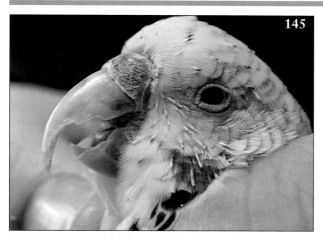

145 An overgrown beak, probably due to chronic hepatopathy in a budgerigar after ten years on an all-seed diet.

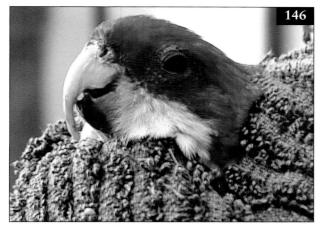

146 Overgrown rhinotheca in an eastern rosella. The cause was not determined, but may have been due to the lack of opportunity to chew on branches, etc.

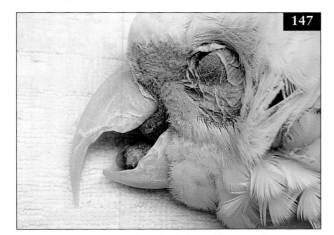

147 Normal beak in a long-billed corella – not be confused with an abnormality!

trimming is carried out as required and the opportunity for increased chewing behaviour should be provided.

CNEMIDOCOPTES
Aetiology
The species of mite are *Cnemidocoptes pilae* (psittacines and passerines) and *Cnemidocoptes mutans* (poultry). It appears that the mite spends its entire life cycle on its host, although it may be transmitted between birds via dead skin and scales. It is probable that immunosuppression and genetic factors play a role in the development of clinical signs.

Clinical presentation
There is slight variation between affected species:
• Budgerigars, kakarikis, neophemas and *Polytelis* spp. develop proliferative crusty, exuberant growths the beak, cere, face, legs, the margin of the vent and on the wing tips. A characteristic 'honey-combed' appearance is due to the mite tunnelling through the keratin (**148**). With severe infection, marked beak deformities can occur through damage to the germinal epithelium. These include thickening of the beak, overgrowth of all of the beak or overgrowth of part of the beak. Weakening of the keratin can cause part of the beak to crumble and break off.

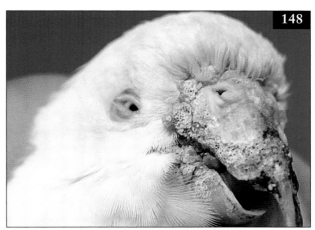

148 Cnemidocoptic mange in a budgerigar, showing advanced beak lesions.

- Lorikeets can develop proliferative hyperkeratotic 'lice nests' all over the body, which may appear neoplastic.
- Canaries develop 'tassel foot', keratin tags arising from the caudal edge of the podotheca along the tarsometatarsus, giving the appearance of 'tassels'. The scales on the podotheca may also become hyperkeratotic.
- Poultry also develop hyperkeratosis on their legs, which can become swollen and painful, causing the bird to limp.
- Owls are rarely affected. They may develop bilateral, proliferative papillary hyperkeratosis on the feet and legs.

Diagnosis
The classical 'honeycomb' appearance is typical. Skin scrapes are usually rewarding. The mite can be identified by its dorsal shield and scapular setae.

Management
Ivermectin or moxidectin is used at 0.2 mg/kg topically, orally or parenterally, repeated every two weeks until the crusts disappear (usually three treatments are required). Topical creams and liquids are often not effective, as the whole bird must be treated.

Prognosis
The prognosis is good, although beak deformities may become permanent if treatment is left too late.

INFECTION
BACTERIAL AND FUNGAL INFECTIONS
Aetiology
Bacterial and fungal infections may result from extension of nasal and sinus infections into the bone and keratin of the beak, or they may be the result of trauma (see above). Causative organisms include *Candida*, *Aspergillus*, *Cryptococcus*, *Mycobacterium* and *Pseudomonas* spp. Other bacteria can also be isolated.

Clinical presentation
The beak and nares become distorted. Underrunning of the keratin occurs, which could lead (in severe cases) to sloughing of all, or part of, the rhamphotheca (**149**).

Diagnosis
Diagnosis is based on cinical signs, transillumination of the beak to determine the depth and extent of the lesion, and biopsy and culture.

Management
Surgical debridement is carried out as required and antimicrobial therapy administered as indicated by culture.

VIRAL INFECTION
Aetiology
Viruses affecting the beak include PBFD in cockatoo species (**150**), avipox virus in all species and polyomavirus in finches.

Clinical presentation, diagnosis, management
See Chapter 7, Disorders of the skin and feathers, p. 110.

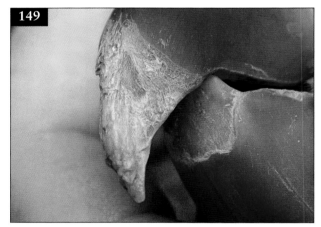

149 Keratin loss on the rhinotheca (upper beak) of an alexandrine parrot. The inciting cause was determined to have been a fungal infection.

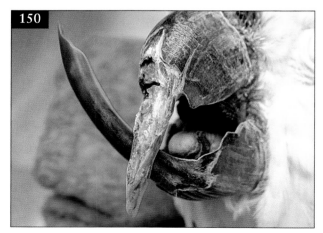

150 PBFD affecting the beak of a sulphur-crested cockatoo.

NEOLPLASIA

Definition/overview

Tumour types involved in the beak include fibrosarcoma (**151**), squamous cell carcinoma, liposarcoma and keratoacanthoma (**152**).

Diagnosis

Diagnosis is by biopsy.

Management

The use of chemotherapy and radiation in the treatment of avian neoplasia continues to be explored.

Prognosis

The prognosis is guarded, although newer treatment protocols, including radiation, offer more hope.

DISORDERS OF THE CERE

The cere is the naked skin situated at the base of the maxilla found in parrots, pigeons and owls. The nares are located within the cere.

HYPERTROPHY

This may be caused by *Cnemidocoptes* (see above). Cere hypertrophy due to hyperoestrogenism in female budgerigars presents as a smooth hypertrophic growth on the cere (**153**). It is easily peeled off with a fingernail, with no underlying haemorrhage. Malnutrition, especially hypovitaminosis A, may result in cere hypertrophy.

COLOUR CHANGE

Increasing brown coloration of the cere in female budgerigars is indicative of oestrogenic activity associated with the onset of the breeding season.

Sertoli cell tumours in male budgerigars may present as a blue cere turning brown. Treatment with radiation or surgery may be successful in selected cases.

Pallor of the cere is often seen in budgerigars with chronic illness of any type.

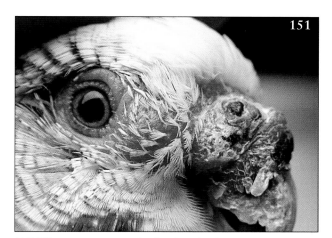

151 Fibrosarcoma on a budgerigar beak.

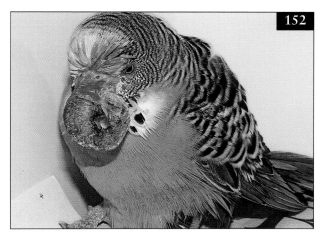

152 Keratoacanthoma in a budgerigar.

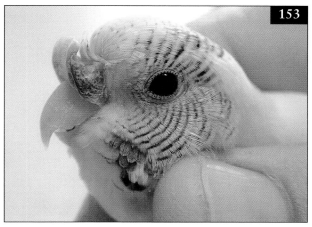

153 Cere hypertrophy in a budgerigar.

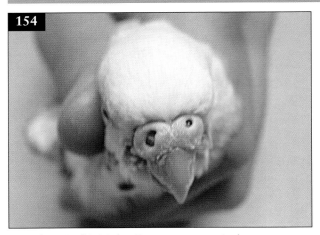

154 Chronic rhinitis leading to asymmetrical nares.

DISTORTION

Chronic respiratory infections may present as 'cere abscesses', swelling and distortion of the cere due to an underlying accumulation of caseated pus in the frontal sinus and nasal cavity. Rhinoliths, large plugs of caseated debris in the nasal cavity under the nares, are commonly seen in African greys, but can be seen in any species. Affected birds commonly present for sneezing, swelling of the cere and occlusion of the nare (usually unilateral). Rhinoliths must be differentiated from tumours and fungal granulomas. Many can be gently debrided under general anaesthesia, with the area thoroughly flushed after completion. In some cases surgical debridement may be necessary. Samples must be submitted for histopathology and culture to identify the underlying cause.

Asymmetry of the size and shape of the nares often results after cere abscesses or untreated chronic infections erode the supporting bone and soft tissues (**154**).

FURTHER READING

Altman B (1997) Beak repair, acrylics. In: *Avian Medicine and Surgery*. RB Altman, SL Clubb, GM Dorrestein, K Quesenberry (eds). WB Saunders, Philadephia, pp. 787–799.

Clipsham R (1997) Beak repair, rhamphorthotics. In: *Avian Medicine and Surgery*. RB Altman, SL Clubb, GM Dorrestein, K Quesenberry (eds). WB Saunders, Philadephia, pp. 773–786.

Gelis S (2006) Evaluating and treating the gastrointestinal system. In: *Clinical Avian Medicine, Vol 1*. GJ Harrison, TL Lightfoot (eds). Spix Publishing Inc, Palm Beach, pp. 411–440.

Olsen GH (2003) Oral biology and beak disorders of birds. *Veterinary Clinics of North America: Exotic Animal Practice* 6(3):505–521.

Schmidt RE, Lightfoot TL (2006) Integument. In: *Clinical Avian Medicine, Vol 1*. GJ Harrison, TL Lightfoot (eds). Spix Publishing Inc, Palm Beach, pp. 395–410.

Speer BL (2002) Trans-sinus pinning to address scissor-beak deformities in psittacine species. In: *Proceedings of the Annual Conference of the Association of Avian Veterinarians Australian Committee*, pp. 283–290.

CHAPTER 9
DISORDERS OF THE EYE

ASSESSING THE EYE
DISTANT EXAMINATION
Initially the bird should be watched at a distance (flying, moving around the cage or room). If there are eye problems, the bird may have difficulty finding food or show reluctance to fly or move around. There may be abnormal head posture; many birds with unilateral blindness will tilt their head so that the 'good' eye is uppermost. The bird may have an exaggerated startle reaction.

PHYSICAL EXAMINATION
Symmetry, position and mobility of globes should be assessed. The eyes of a normal bird are clear, symmetrical and centred in the socket. The normal conjunctiva is pale pink and moist.

Hydration can be evaluated by tenting the skin over the eyelids.

The periorbital area is assessed for swelling, discoloration, pustules, scars, scabs or abnormal growths. Conjunctivitis, sunken eyes and ocular discharges are abnormal. Pale or white coloration of the conjunctiva can indicate anaemia.

The iris colour should be noted. The colour is an indication of age or sex in many species of birds. Young Amazon parrots have brown irises that become red–orange as they age. Young African grey parrots have brown irises that change to grey, then white, by 15 months of age (155, 156). Young macaws have brown irises that change to grey within the first year, and then between one and three years of age the colour changes from grey to yellow. Young cockatoos have brown irises. In some species the adult female cockatoo has red–brown irises (157) and adult males have dark brown to black irises. (Note that not all hens have red–brown irises.)

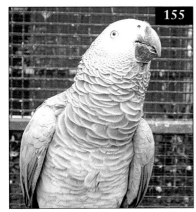

155 The pale iris of an adult African grey parrot.

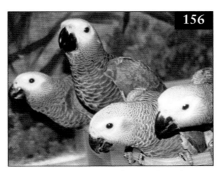

156 The dark irises of juvenile African grey parrots.

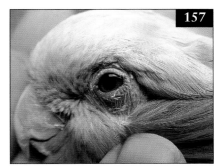

157 Mature galah hens often (but not always) have a reddish iris.

The cornea and anterior chamber should be examined with focal illumination and transillumination.

Fundic examination can be difficult, as the striated muscle in the iris makes pupillary dilation difficult. Atropine and tropicamide are ineffectual. Techniques that have been used include:

- Intracameral injection of d-tubocurarine (do not use a commercial preparation, as it has an irritant preservative). Topical d-tubocurarine (3 mg/ml) does not work well, as it does not penetrate the cornea sufficiently.
- Topical vecuronium bromide (4 mg/ml). Vecuronium is a synthetic curariform nondepolarizing neuromuscular blocking agent. It competes for nicotinic acetylcholine receptors at the motor end plate. It does not work topically in South African black-footed penguins, but has worked in citron-crested and sulphur-crested cockatoos and African grey and blue-fronted Amazon parrots with minimal systemic effects.
- General anaesthesia, especially with ketamine or air sac perfusion. Note that while air sac perfusion has been reported to be successful in inducing mydriasis in pigeons, it does not appear to work in cockatoos.

Responses and reflexes

- Menace reflex (assesses cranial nerves II and VII). Eye-blink, pulling away of the head or aggressive action of the beak can be provoked by bringing the hand towards each eye.
- Pupillary light response (assesses cranial nerves II and III). The avian pupil's movements are poor in response to light, but rapid in response to accommodation or voluntary control. Although there is no consensual pupillary light response (as there is complete decussation of the optic nerves at the chiasm), the orbital bone is so thin that a response can often be detected in one eye after a light is shone in the other.
- Corneal reflex. A symmetrical eye-blink normally occurs when the cornea is gently touched with a moist cotton swab. Failure to do so indicates a lesion in cranial nerves V and VII.
- Palpebral reflex and facial sensation. A symmetrical eye-blink should be elicited by touching each side of face or the lateral canthus of the eye. Failure to do so suggests a lesion in cranial nerves V and VII.
- There should be symmetrical deviations of the eyes when the head is moved in different positions, with the eyes always returning to the centre. Failure to do so suggests either a bilateral lesion in cranial nerve VIII or a brainstem lesion (especially in the pons and midbrain).

Ancillary testing

- Cytology and culture of the conjunctival flora.
- Schirmer tear test — normal result is 3–12 mm in clinically normal birds. There is a wide variation between species. Local anaesthesia in the cornea significantly reduces tear movement along the strip.
- The Phenol Red Thread Test (Zone-Quick, San Mateo) is a new test available in the evaluation of tear production in animals. It is a yellow cotton thread, 75 mm long, impregnated with the pH indicator phenol red (phenolsulphonephthalein). One end of the thread is folded to a length of 3 mm and, at the time of use, opened to an appropriate angle and placed within the ventral conjunctival fornix. The thread remains in this position for 15 seconds. The colour of the thread changes to red when wet and, once the thread is removed, the length of this change is measured in millimetres similar to the Schirmer tear test. The Phenol Red Thread Test is faster and causes less reflexive tearing than the Schirmer tear test due to the significantly less irritating contact with the cornea in species where it has been evaluated. Normal results appear to lie in the range of 8–23 mm, with no effect from local anaesthesia discerned.
- Fluorescent staining of the cornea can detect small ulcerations and lacerations.
- Intraocular pressures are between 9.2 and 22 mmHg in normal bird eyes. The Tonopen® is ideal for birds, as it can be used with a minimal corneal diameter of 9 mm. Readings of eyes with corneal diameters of 5 mm or less (budgerigar range) are not reliable.
- Ultrasonography allows detection of retinal detachment or sequestration of the pecten bridge.
- More advanced tests include:
  - Electroretinography. Recording of electrical potentials after light stimulation. It gives no information about vision, but does assess retinal function.
  - Fluorescein angiography. Observation of the distribution of fluorescein within ocular blood vessels following intravenous injection. This enables diagnosis of subtle haemorrhages of the pecten and choroid, atrophy of vessels and retinal disease.

DISORDERS OF THE EYE
LIDS AND PERIORBITAL REGION

Poxvirus (in mild cases) may cause a unilateral blepharitis with eyelid oedema, starting about 10–14 days after infection. It may also cause keratitis and, less commonly, anterior uveitis. Prophylactic vitamin A injections and antibiotic therapy may decrease the severity of the infection. Most cases are self-limiting and resolve over a few weeks. In severe cases there may be distortion and scarring of the eyelids.

Chlamydial infections and other causes of sinusitis may lead to blepharitis, thickening of the eyelids and matting or loss of periorbital feathering (due to lacrimation and rubbing).

Proliferative lesions on the eyelids and periorbital region may be due to *Cnemidocoptes pilae*, papillomas or vitamin A deficiencies.

Feather loss around the eye without any evidence of inflammation or conjunctivitis can be due to excessive grooming by a cage mate. This is often seen in finches when they are overcrowded, or in parrots during the breeding season.

Eyelid abnormalities include:
- Cryptophthalmos (failure of eyelid formation, resulting in fusion of the eyelid margins) is occasionally seen in cockatiels (**158, 159**). Surgical correction is usually unrewarding, but affected birds appear to have some degree of vision through their eyelids.
- Blepharophimosis (narrowing of the palpebral fissures without fusion of the eyelid margins) is occasionally seen in all species. Again, surgical correction is usually unrewarding.
- Symblepharon (adhesion of the eyelid to the globe) can be seen as a sequela to severe conjunctivitis. Surgical correction is possible in some cases.
- Scarring and deformity is occasionally seen after avian poxvirus infections.

CONJUNCTIVA
Definition/overview

Thickening and hyperaemia of the conjunctiva, often associated with epiphora or ocular discharge, may be seen with conjunctivitis, sinusitis (see Chapter 16, Disorders affecting the respiratory system) or neoplasia.

Aetiology

Conjunctivitis may be due to:
- Bacterial infections.
- Chlamydiosis.
- *Mycoplasma*.
- Mycobacteria.
- Viral infections (e.g. adenovirus, poxvirus, cytomegalovirus [in gouldian finches]).
- Fungal infections (*Aspergillus*, *Candida*, *Cryptococcus*).
- Parasites: 'eye' worms (*Oxyspirura mansoni*, *Ceratospira* spp. and *Thelazia* spp.); cryptosporidial infections; *Plasmodium* spp. can cause eyelid swelling in canaries and domestic poultry; microsporidiosis has been reported to cause conjunctivitis.
- Foreign bodies and physical irritants such as smoke or chemical fumes.
- Allergies, especially secondary to nicotine.

Neoplasia involving the eyelids includes conjunctival papillomas, squamous cell carcinomas and melanomas (**160**).

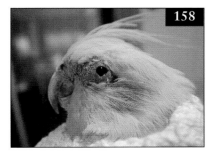

158 Acquired cryptophthalmos in a cockatiel following severe chlamydial infection.

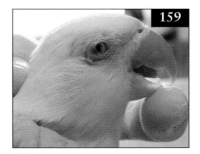

159 Congenital cryptophthalmos in an Indian ring-neck.

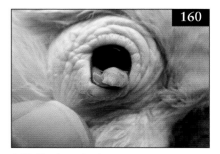

160 Conjunctival tumour (haemangioma) in a cockatoo.

Diagnosis

Diagnosis involves cytology and culture of the conjunctiva. Conjunctival biopsy or PCR of a conjunctival swab may be required.

Management

This is determined by the aetiological agent. Topical therapy, if indicated, should be in drop form. Eye ointments should be avoided, or at least used very sparingly, because of the likelihood that grooming will see the ointment spread throughout the feathering. Ointments containing cortisone should not be used at all, as systemic absorption and subsequent immuno-suppression and hepatopathies can be significant.

In many cases, especially chlamydiosis, systemic as well as topical therapy is indicated.

CORNEA
Definition/overview

Xerophathalmia, a lack of tear production, is a classical sign of vitamin A deficiency. A long-term deficiency may result in an irreversible kerato-conjunctivitis sicca.

Cholesterol deposits are seen frequently in parrots, especially Amazons, usually on a high-fat diet or with other metabolic issues. They appear as painless, multifocal, white, noninflammatory corneal lesions. Even with resolution of the dietary problems, these corneal precipitates do not resolve, but rarely seem to cause a problem.

Infectious keratitis may be bacterial or fungal or be caused by microsporidia. Noninfectious keratitis may be caused by trauma or a foreign body.

Management

Antimicrobial therapy, topically and/or systemically, is given as indicated. Flubiprofen topically or meloxicam systemically may be used for analgesia and anti-inflammatory therapy.

The cornea can be protected by a temporary tarsorrhaphy. Third eyelid flaps have been used, but they are difficult to perform and experience in other species indicates they are not as useful as originally thought.

In severe cases, enucleation may be required. If possible, a specialist opinion should be sought before taking this step.

UVEA
Acute uveitis
Aetiology

Acute uveitis may be caused by trauma, infection (e.g. reovirus), lens rupture or toxoplasmosis.

Clinical presentation

Signs include photophobia, blepharospasm, corneal oedema, aqueous flare, hyphaema, hypopyon, miosis, dyscoria, iris thickening or discoloration, and anterior/posterior synechiae.

Management

Anti-inflammatory therapy is required using topical (e.g. flubiprofen) and systemic (e.g. meloxicam) NSAIDs.

Chronic uveitis
Aetiology

This is a sequela to acute uveitis.

Clinical presentation

Signs include diffuse corneal oedema, posterior synechiae causing pupillary seclusion and iris bombé, anterior synechiae, secondary glaucoma, cataract, retinal atrophy and chronic detachment, and blindness.

Management

Anti-inflammatory therapy is given as for acute uveitis: topical (e.g. flubiprofen) and systemic (e.g. meloxicam) NSAIDs.

LENS
Cataracts (161)
Aetiology

Familial cataracts are reported in Yorkshire and Norwich canaries. A fully penetrant autosomal recessive gene is responsible.

Acquired cataracts can be due to uveitis (see above), toxins or ageing. Idiopathic cataracts have been noted in a number of species.

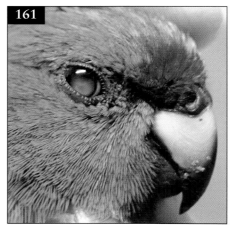

161 Cataracts in a mature kakariki hen.

Treatment

In many cases no treatment is required or feasible, due to other disease processes in the eye affecting vision. Phaecoemulsification has been used successfully in many species and may be used if the retina is believed to be intact.

Luxation

This may occur secondary to trauma or uveitis. Lens luxation also leads to further uveitis. If this lens-induced uveitis does not respond to NSAID therapy, phaecoemulsification is necessary to remove the lens.

RETINA

Retinitis may occur due to infectious agents (e.g. *Toxoplasma*), trauma or diseases of the CNS. Retinal detachment may occur following trauma or retinitis. Retinal dysplasia has been noted sporadically. Retinal degeneration may be due to malnutrition, toxins or hypoxia, but no specific cause has yet been identified.

THE EYE AS A WHOLE
Panophthalmitis
Aetiology

Panophthalmitis may be caused by infection or trauma.

Clinical presentation

Early clinical signs are referable to extension of the inflammatory process throughout the eye, and include pain, blepharospasm, hypopyon, corneal oedema and ulceration, and secondary glaucoma. Chronically the eye may develop phthisis bulbi, a shrunken, fibrotic globe.

Diagnosis

Diagnosis is based on the clinical appearance.

Management

Aggressive antimicrobial therapy, NSAIDs and temporary tarsorrhaphy may help in early cases. Enucleation is often the preferred treatment.

Glaucoma
Aetiology

Glaucoma may be primary, or secondary to trauma.

Clinical presentation

The globe is enlarged and painful. Glaucoma must be differentiated from exophthalmos (see below).

Diagnosis

Diagnosis is based on the clinical signs and intraocular pressure, as measured by a Tonopen® (see p. 134 for normal values).

Management

Topical dorzolamide is given three times daily initially, then titrated to effect.

Exophthalmus
Aetiology

Exophthalmus may be caused by orbital rim malformation associated with stunting in neonatal chicks, retrobulbar caseated sinusitis or neoplasia, or pituitary adenoma.

Clinical presentation

Unilateral or bilateral exophthalmos.

Diagnosis

Diagnosis is based on the clinical appearance. Exophthalmus must be differentiated from glaucoma. CT scanning may assist in evaluating the retrobulbar area.

Management

Retrobulbar sinusitis is difficult and frustrating to treat because of the caseous nature of the exudate and the lack of surgical access to the sinus. Surgical trephination of the sinus followed by flushing and mechanical debridement may assist in some cases.

The appearance of stunted chicks often improves as the cause of the stunting is identified and remedied.

FURTHER READING

Gancz AY, Malka S, Sandmeyer L, Cannon M, Smith DA, Taylor M. (2005) Horner's syndrome in a red-bellied parrot (*Poicephalus rufiventris*). *Journal of Avian Medicine and Surgery* **19(1)**:30–34.

Kern TJ (1997) Disorders of the special senses. In: *Avian Medicine and Surgery*. RB Altman, SL Clubb, GM Dorrestein, K Quesenberry (eds). WB Saunders, Philadelphia, pp. 563–589.

Korbel RT (2000) Avian ophthalmology: a clinically oriented approach. In: *Proceedings of the Annual Conference of the Association of Avian Veterinarians*, pp. 439–456.

Korbel RT (2007) Avian ophthalmology: principles and application. In: *Proceedings of the Annual Conference of the Association of Avian Veterinarians*, pp. 191–200.

CHAPTER 10
DISORDERS OF THE EAR

OTITIS EXTERNA
Aetiology
Otitis externa is an uncommon disorder. It may result from infection with bacteria (*Escherichia coli, Staphylococcus aureus, Pasteurella multocida, Proteus mirabilis, Pseudomonas aeruginosa, Klebsiella oxytoca, Enterococcus* spp.), fungi (*Candida* spp., *Microsporum gallinae*) or mycobacteria, or infestation with arthropod parasites (*Cnemidocoptes*). It may occur as an extension of generalized skin disease or may be due to neoplasia or trauma.

Clinical presentation
Affected birds have an aural exudate (serous, purulent or haemorrhagic). There may be caseated material in the ear canal. Swelling and erythema, auricular feather loss and self-inflicted excoriation are seen. There may be hyperkeratosis.

Diagnosis
Diagnosis is based on clinical signs, cytology and culture. The narrow ear canal makes visualization with anything larger than a 1.9 mm endoscope difficult, if not impossible.

In cases that fail to respond to therapy, judicious biopsy may be required.

Management
Systemic and topical antibiotics are given as indicated by culture. Meloxicam or another NSAID can be given if the ear appears to be particularly painful or swollen. Careful flushing with saline may assist in the removal of exudate. Careful debridement with a loop curette may be required if caseous exudate cannot be flushed out.

OTITIS MEDIA AND OTITIS INTERNA
Aetiology
Otitis media and otitis interna are uncommon, although more common than otitis externa. They can occur as a result of developmental abnormalities seen in some canaries. Other causes include an extension of otitis externa or sinusitis; PMV-3 infection, especially in Australian *Neophema* spp., canaries and finches; poxvirus; iatrogenic damage following treatment with aminoglycoside antibiotics (e.g. gentamicin); and neoplasia.

Clinical presentation
Signs include head tilt, 'star gazing', torticollis and vestibular disorders (loss of proprioception).

Diagnosis
Diagnosis is based on clinical signs, PMV-3 serology or virus isolation (from tissue samples), if appropriate. In larger birds CT or MRI may be of value in confirming a diagnosis.

Management
Antimicrobial and anti-inflammatory therapy may be of some value. The prognosis is guarded.

FURTHER READING
Kern TJ (1997) Disorders of the special senses. In: *Avian Medicine and Surgery*. RB Altman, *et al.* (eds). WB Saunders, Philadelphia, pp. 563–589.

Schmidt RE, Reavill DR, Phalen DN (2003) Special sense organs. In: *Pathology of Pet and Aviary Birds*. RE Schmidt, *et al.* (eds). Iowa State Press, Ames, pp. 197–212.

Shivaprasad HL (2007) The avian ear: anatomy and diseases. In: *Proceedings of the Annual Conference of the Association of Avian Veterinarians*, pp. 127–133.

DISORDERS OF THE LEGS, FEET AND TOES

MALFORMATIONS

It can be difficult to distinguish between congenital and acquired malformations, especially in neonates and juveniles.

Factors that can have an effect on normal skeletal conformation include:

- The bird's parents:
  - Genetics: hereditary malformations have been identified in some birds.
  - Health: in particular, subclinical heavy metal toxicosis has been associated with congenital limb malformation in the offspring of affected birds.
  - Diet: poor quality diets fed to parent birds are often reflected in the health and conformation of the offspring. In particular, calcium–phosphorus imbalances in the parental diet will often result in chicks with limb malformations.
- Incubation procedures and parameters. Artificial incubation is more likely to produce chicks with limb malformations than natural incubation. Incorrect incubator temperature, humidity, ventilation and rate and degree of egg turning can have deleterious results on the development of the embryo and result in malformations.
- The nesting environment. Nest box design can have an effect of neonates in several ways: slippery floors are believed to contribute to coxofemoral subluxation ('splay leg') in budgerigars; inexperienced parents who can enter the nest box quickly and land heavily on the chicks can cause injuries resulting in malformations.
- Birds that are hand reared in a brightly lit, roomy container are often encouraged to move around more than they would in a dark and relatively cramped nest box. This can lead to excessive weight bearing on the legs, with subsequent bowing and malformations.

Nutritional secondary hyperparathyroidism and rickets (collectively referred to as metabolic bone disease) are underlying factors behind many of these problems. Rickets is a metabolic bone disease in growing animals caused by a vitamin D3 deficiency. (This can be due to inadequate nutrition, lack of exposure to sunlight, defective vitamin D activation, defective vitamin D receptors, hypoparathyroidism, renal failure, renal phosphate loss or gastrointestinal malabsorption.) The result is impaired mineralization of osteoid tissue or epiphyseal cartilage, leading to thinning and weakening of the bones and excessive growth of cartilaginous structures. This, in turn, causes deformity at the ends of the bones, particularly in the proximal tibiotarsus, the beak (rubber beak), the head of the ribs and, sometimes, the costochondral junction (rachitic rosary). Radiographically there may be widening and distortion of the growth plates.

Nutritional secondary hyperparathyroidism is commonly seen in adult birds fed a diet that is either calcium deficient or has an excess of phosphorus (or both). For example, seed-only diets may have a calcium:phosphorus ratio as low as 1:10. Fruits, nuts and most vegetables are also calcium deficient. When these diets are fed to birds, especially parents rearing chicks or to recently fledged juveniles, the parathyroid gland releases parathyroid hormone which, amongst other effects, withdraws calcium from the bone to maintain normal serum calcium levels. The result is thin bones which bend or break easily, leading to malformations.

COXOFEMORAL SUBLUXATION (SPLAY LEG)
Aetiology

Splay leg may be the result of a lack of nonslip substrate in the nest box. This allows the legs to splay out laterally away from the body, subluxating the coxofemoral joint and leading to laxity or damage of the medial collateral ligaments of the stifle, angular limb deformities of the femur, tibiotarsus and tarsometatarsus, or slipped tendons. Sometimes, if the chicks have metabolic bone disease as well, folding fractures of the tibiotarsus will result in secondary 'splay' deformities.

Management
Early recognition and correction are important; once skeletal ossification occurs conservative techniques such as splinting or hobbling are unlikely to be effective. Very young birds can have their legs hobbled into a normal position in order to guide the leg into a normal position during growth. Various techniques have been used to achieve this goal, including tying the feet together with bandages or placing the chick's legs into a foam block. However, if the chick is not presented until after ossification is complete, surgical derotational osteotomies may be required.

ANGULAR LIMB DEFORMITIES
Aetiology
Angular limb deformities (ALDs) occur when more weight is borne on one side of the growth plate than the other (**162, 163**). On this side of the physis, growth is inhibited, while on the other side, growth continues normally. Common causes include incubation problems, nutritional imbalances and trauma. In precocious chicks (e.g. ratites), ALDs may occur for a range of reasons including insufficient exercise, high-energy diets, trauma and heated flooring.

Clinical presentation
The result of an ALD is a deviation of the growth of the limb from the midline: if the growth is directed laterally, it is termed a valgus deformity; if medial to the midline, it is termed a varus deformity. The deformity may be a bowing or rotation of the affected bone. This then has a cascading effect on the muscles, tendons and joints of the affected leg.

Management
Corrective surgery, in the form of derotational osteotomies, is the treatment of choice, but it must be done sooner rather than later. Timing is essential when addressing affected joints; waiting until the bird has finished growing may result in irreversible tendon and joint contracture.

PATHOLOGICAL FRACTURES
Aetiology
Pathological fractures commonly occur in chicks with nutritional secondary hyperparathyroidism or rickets. The fractures most commonly occur in the long bones — the humerus, the radius and ulna, the femur and the tibiotarsus.

Management
Some of these fractures will heal with minimal intervention, but this invariably results in some degree of bone deformity. Attempts to repair these fractures surgically can be frustrated when the contralateral leg is required to support the bird's weight and lacks the cortical strength to do so, resulting in another fracture or bowing of that leg. Slinging the chick to minimize this problem can cause other problems such as compression of the sternum and ribs. These factors need to be considered before undertaking such a procedure.

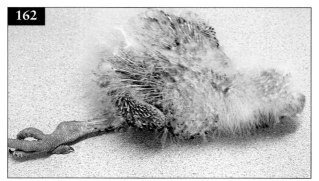

162 Femoral and tibiotarsal rotation in a black cockatoo chick. Although this chick was artificially incubated and hand reared, its parents were on a calcium-deficient, all-seed diet.

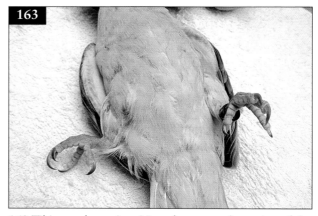

163 Tibiotarsal rotation. Note the outward rotation of the right leg compared with the left.

TOE MALPOSITIONS

Definition/overview

Anteroflexion of P4 is a developmental issue in psittacine paediatrics, more often encountered where there has been subclinical stunting or substrate mismanagement. Once the first phalangeal bone has ossified normally, it is fused to the tarsometatarsus and becomes less flexible. If the anteroflexion has not been corrected (by splinting) by that time, the anteroflexion may be permanent.

Management

The affected digit can be splinted out into a normal position, but the abnormal angulation of P1 means that once the splint has been removed, the digit will return to an abnormal position.

SLIPPED TENDON

Definition/overview

The gastrocnemius tendon 'slips' medially or laterally out of the intercondylar groove on the back of the hock, causing a valgus or varus deformity of the lower leg. This is associated with trauma, poor diet, poor conformation and perhaps a genetic influence. It is most commonly seen in ratites and gallinaceous birds, but can be seen in any species.

Management

Simple surgical repair of the tendon sheath is usually unrewarding, and a rotational osteotomy or arthrodesis may be required.

SWOLLEN JOINTS

Swollen joints, often associated with pain and lameness, is a common presentation at any age.

ARTICULAR GOUT

Definition/overview

The metabolism of aspartate, glutamine and glycine produces purines, which are then metabolized in the liver (and to a small extent in the kidney) to form uric acid. Ninety percent of this uric acid is secreted by the proximal convoluted tubule; the remainder is filtered by the glomerulus. The thick sludge formed by this uric acid in the ureters is flushed down to the cloaca by hypotonic urine, which is then retrograded into the caudal rectum for resorption.

Renal disease, and possibly dehydration, leads to hyperuricaemia. The levels of uric acid can spike in cases of water deprivation and then return to normal, so persistent hyperuricaemia is not always present.

Uric acid in plasma is soluble and relatively inert until it reaches a saturation threshold that is temperature dependent and also is different for each species. It is thought that the lower temperature of the extremities, compared with the rest of the body, allows plasma uric acid to precipitate out of solution at a lower concentration. Consequently, chronic renal insufficiency, with a gradual elevation of plasma uric acid levels, results in the deposition of uric acid crystals in the synovial capsules and tendon sheaths of the joints. Conversely, acute renal failure with a rapid rise in plasma uric acid leads to the precipitation of uric acid crystals onto the serosa of internal organs (visceral gout).

Aetiology

Uric acid crystals, when deposited in and around joints, provoke an inflammatory response that causes the swelling and pain associated with articular gout.

Clinical presentation

Gross lesions typically consist of soft painful swellings on the feet at the metatarsophalangeal and interphalangeal joints.

Diagnosis

Fine needle aspiration can be used to confirm the presence of uric acid crystals, but the procedure may be painful to the patient and haemorrhage can be difficult to control. Radiographically, urate tophi can be identified if dystrophic calcification is occurring.

Management

Reducing the hyperuricaemia can be achieved by treating the underlying renal disease (see Chapter 21, Disorders of the urinary system, p. 223). The use of allopurinol (a xanthine oxidase inhibitor) to reduce the production of uric acid and/or probenecid (a uricosuric drug) to increase the secretion of uric acid by the kidney is beneficial in some patients.

Colchicine reduces the inflammatory changes seen around uric acid tophi. NSAIDs can be used to relieve pain only if renal function is adequate. Butorphanol given orally can assist with the comfort of some patients. Surgical excision of prominent tophi can be undertaken, but haemorrhage may be significant.

Prognosis

Prognosis is usually guarded, although some patients can be given a good quality of life for an extended period.

LUXATION OF THE JOINT

See Chapter 12, Disorders of the musculoskeletal system, p. 152.

ARTHRITIS
Aetiology
Swollen painful joints (arthritis) can be due to traumatic injuries, septic inflammation (*Streptococcus* spp., *Pseudomonas* spp., *Chlamydophila psittaci*, *Mycoplasma* spp., *Reovirus*), microfilaria, especially in wild-caught Indonesian cockatoo species, articular gout (see above), degenerative changes or neoplasia.

Diagnosis
Diagnosis is based on the patient's history, physical examination, haematology and biochemistries, radiography and fine needle aspirate with cytology and culture where appropriate.

Management
The cause should be identified and removed if possible (e.g. weight reduction in obese birds); septic joints may need to be opened and lavaged; caseated debris should be removed if possible. Long-term antibiotic therapy (as dictated by culture and sensitivity testing) will be required in cases of bacterial infection.

Pain relief may be achieved with NSAIDs or oral butorphanol.

Attempts have been made to improve the joint physiology using pentosan polysulphate and glucosamine. These are unproven therapies in birds at this time. Anecdotal reports are encouraging and no adverse effects have been recorded, so these therapies may be worth trialling.

Husbandry should be adapted to cater for disabilities. Arthritic birds may have mobility problems and may have difficulties grasping small diameter perches. Wide flat perches and providing easier access to food and water may be beneficial.

PODODERMATITIS
Definition/overview
Pododermatitis is also known as bumblefoot. It refers to an inflamed and often infected lesion on the plantar surface of the foot. It is most commonly seen in raptors, but can be seen in other species as well, especially gallinaceous birds, passerines and small parrots. It is a disease of captivity, being rare or nonexistent in wild birds.

Aetiology
The plantar surface of the foot is protected by a thick layer of stratified squamous epithelium, which in turn is covered by a layer of keratin. Over the surface of this keratin is a layer of papillae, which are thought to spread evenly the weight-bearing requirement of the foot.

When this barrier is eroded or breached, an inflammatory response is often provoked and infection can be introduced. These infections are usually associated with *Staphylococcus aureus*, but other bacteria including *E. coli*, *Pasteurella* spp., *Klebsiella* spp., *Clostridium* spp., *Corynebacterium* spp., *Bacillus* spp., *Diplococcus* spp., *Nocardia* spp., *Actinobacillus* spp., *Actinomyces* spp., *Aeromonas* spp., *Proteus* spp. and *Pseudomonas* spp. have been implicated. *Candida* spp. and *Aspergillus* spp. may also be involved in some cases.

The inflammation and/or infection may extend into the joints, tendons and bones of the foot.

Contributing factors to the erosion or breaching of the keratin barrier include trauma, hypovitaminosis A, obesity, perches (smooth, regular surfaces or fine sandpaper-covered perches), long periods of inactivity leading to excessive weight bearing without relief, and excessive weight bearing on one leg due to a problem with the other leg (e.g. a unilateral lameness may lead to pododermatitis in the contralateral leg). In many cases, pododermatitis in one foot will lead to some degree of pododermatitis in the other foot.

Clinical presentation
Raptor veterinarians have developed a classification scheme for pododermatitis that provides clinicians with a treatment plan and guide to prognosis. This classification scheme can be extended to other species with good results.

Class I
There is early devitalization of a prominent plantar area without disruption of the epithelial barrier. It is subdivided into:
- Hyperaemia (bruise) or early ischaemia (a blanched area with compromised capillary perfusion) (**164**).
- Hyperkeratotic reaction (an early callus) (**165**).

Class II
There is localized inflammation/infection of underlying tissues in direct contact with devitalized area, with no gross swelling. It is subdivided into:
- Puncture wound.
- Ischaemic necrosis of epithelium (a penetrating callus or scab).

Class III
More generalized infection; gross inflammatory swelling of underlying tissues is present. The origin may be puncture wounds or ischaemic necrosis; however, by this stage the initial cause is of minor

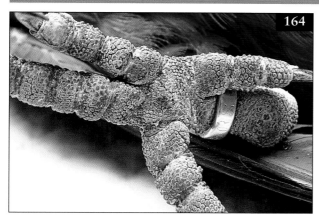

164 Early pododermatitis in a scarlet macaw; note bruising on the plantar surface of the foot.

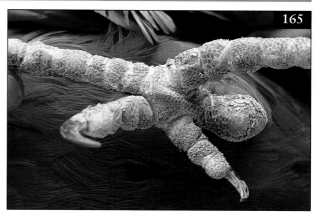

165 The opposite foot on the same bird as shown for comparison; note the early callus on the ventral hock.

significance in comparison with the ongoing pathology. It is subdivided into:

- Serous (acute): oedema and hyperaemia of the tissues.
- Fibrotic (chronic): attempt at encapsulation and confinement.
- Caseous: accumulation of necrotic debris.

Class IV

There is established infection with gross swelling and involvement of deeper vital structures. Radiology and surgical exploration will often be required to differentiate class III from class IV. Class IV is a chronic condition causing tenosynovitis and occasionally arthritis and osteomyelitis.

Class V

This is an extension of class IV, characterized by crippling deformities.

Diagnosis

A thorough history is taken to investigate the bird's husbandry, diet and previous medical problems. A thorough physical examination is carried out to classify the pododermatitis and identify any concurrent or predisposing problems (e.g. leg or spinal injuries). Ancillary diagnostic steps include culture and sensitivity testing of infected lesions and radiography of any case worse than class II.

Management

This is usually determined by the classification of the condition, as outlined above:

- Class I carries a favourable prognosis, as there is no evidence of infection. The changes generally respond to conservative husbandry changes including changing perching surfaces and application of topical emollients.
- Class II carries a good prognosis, as infection is localized. Such lesions respond well to surgery, as the total affected area is easily resected and epidermal defects are characteristically small, hence the architecture of the weight-bearing structures of the plantar aspect are maintained intact. This class will generally not respond to conservative treatment.
- Class III traditionally carries a good to guarded prognosis, as infection is well established and structural changes have affected the foot. Some can be treated as for class II; however, the majority should be treated by complete surgical removal of all affected tissue, followed by first-intention healing.
- Class IV carries a guarded to poor prognosis, as infection is harboured in and affects deeper vital structures, making surgical debridement difficult or impossible. In view of the chronicity, pockets of encapsulated infective tissues are often present, which if not cleared will result in later recurrence.
- Class V carries a poor to hopeless prognosis and may require euthanasia.

Treatment regimes include improving the bird's health and nutritional status, usually by conversion to a formulated diet, and improving the bird's husbandry by supplying natural branches for perches. Some cases of pododermatitis may benefit from padded perches until the condition has resolved.

If surgery is contemplated, culture and sensitivity testing should be performed in advance so that the results are available at the time of surgery. This allows an appropriate antibiotic to be used at the time of surgery rather than several days later when postsurgical fibrotic encapsulation of pathogenic bacteria is underway. While waiting for the results, broad-spectrum antibiotic coverage and analgesia can be commenced.

Surgery is aimed at debulking the infection, removing all caseous debris and infected and fibrotic tissue, and closing the site so that primary-intention healing can occur. Placing antibiotic-impregnated methylmethacrylate beads into the area before closure can assist with long-term delivery of antibiotics into the affected area.

After surgery it is important that pressure is relieved from the surgery site. This is achieved by padded bandages or gauze/rubber 'doughnuts' to distribute pressure evenly while keeping the surgery site clean and away from potentially contaminated surfaces.

Close attention must be given to the contralateral foot to ensure it does not develop pododermatitis as well.

CONSTRICTED TOE SYNDROME

Definition/overview

This is a circumferential constriction caused by foreign material or fibrous bands, which may result in avascular necrosis of the digit distal to the constriction (**166**).

Aetiology

Two forms are seen:
- The formation of constricting fibrous bands on the toes of neonatal chicks, possibly due to low humidity in the nest box, incubation issues or ergot-like intoxication.
- Entanglement of the toes with artificial or natural fibres in birds of any age.

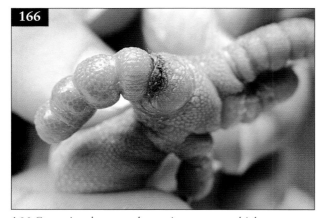

166 Constricted toe syndrome in a macaw chick.

Clinical presentation

In the early stages the toe distal to the constriction may appear swollen and oedematous. If the bird is perching, lameness may be noted. As the condition progresses, circulation to the toe is lost. Cyanosis of the toe is followed by a desiccated appearance; finally, the affected area drops off, sometimes leaving a nub of necrotic bone protruding.

Management

Early recognition and prompt treatment increase the chances of a successful outcome. After 24 hours the prognosis for saving the toe becomes poor. If the patient is presented after circulation loss is severe and necrosis is apparent, amputation is usually required.

Artificial or natural fibres need to be carefully removed. The use of general anaesthesia and magnification is strongly recommended.

Mild or early neonatal cases may respond to increasing the humidity around the toe (by using moisturising creams) and massage.

More advanced or severe cases will require surgery. Two techniques have been advocated:
- A deep longitudinal incision on either side of the toe to sever the band and relieve the constriction.
- Complete excision of the band followed by a circumferential skin anastomosis using only two or three sutures to establish skin apposition without tension. Following the anastomosis a release incision should be made on the medial and lateral aspects of the digit longitudinally across the anastomosis to allow swelling to occur without compromising circulation.

After surgery a hydroactive dressing should be used to keep the area moist and prevent scar formation while the incisions heal. The toe must be monitored during healing for any reformation of the constricting band.

PARESIS OR PARALYSIS

BILATERAL

Spinal trauma or neoplasia

Definition/overview

If trauma or neoplasia severs or compresses the spinal cord, it can result in paresis or paralysis. Depending on the level and extent of the injury or neoplasm, cloacal and vent tone may also be lost. Most spinal trauma will occur at the lumbar–synsacral junction, where there is some spinal flexibility.

Management

Conservative or surgical therapy is rarely successful.

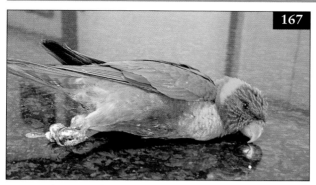

167 Lorikeet paralysis syndrome in a Swainson's (rainbow) lorikeet.

Obturator paralysis
Definition/overview
An 'obturator paralysis' syndrome is sometimes seen in hens that are egg-bound or have had difficulty passing an egg. Calcium deficiencies, pelvic fractures and bruising of the sciatic and other nerves, acting in concert or individually, can lead to leg paresis.

Clinical presentation
Affected birds are otherwise bright and alert. Cloacal and vent tone may be affected.

Management
Supportive care, NSAIDs and calcium supplementation are indicated. Prognosis is fair to good, with most birds recovering within a week.

Lorikeet paralysis syndrome
Clinical presentation
Lorikeet paralysis syndrome (clenched foot syndrome) (167) is seen in both wild and captive lorikeets. Affected birds, which can be of any age and either sex, are presented throughout the year with leg paralysis and clenched feet. They are otherwise bright and alert and usually have a good appetite. Occasional individuals will become progressively more extensively paralysed.

Diagnosis
Histopathology of the cerebellum, brain stem, spinal cord and brain shows nonsuppurative leptomeningitis, perhaps consistent with a viral encephalomyelitis. However, no virus has yet been identified.

Management
There is no specific therapy, but some birds that are given supportive care may recover over a period of weeks or months.

Barraband (or *Polytelis*) paralysis syndrome
Barraband (or *Polytelis*) paralysis syndrome, seen most commonly in the barraband or superb parrot (*Polytelis swainsonii*), is a now uncommon condition similar to lorikeet paralysis syndrome. No known cause has been identified. With supportive care some birds will recover, but recurrence is seen occasionally.

Bilateral leg trauma
Definition/overview
Fledgling parrots with nutritional secondary hyperparathyroidism (see p. 139, Malformations) may present with bilateral pathological fractures of the legs.

Management
Surgical therapy is warranted, but the prognosis is guarded.

Lead toxicosis
This may present as a bilateral paresis.

UNILATERAL
Unilateral trauma
Unilateral trauma, either skeletal or soft tissue, may result in a unilateral paresis.

Sciatic nerve compression
Definition/overview
Sciatic nerve compression by a renal tumour (nephroblastoma or adenocarcinoma) is seen occasionally in budgerigars, but rarely in other species (219). The sciatic nerve, as it passes between the middle and caudal divisions of the kidney, is compressed by the tumour.

Clinical presentation
Affected birds show unilateral paresis and may also have polyuria, polydypsia, a distended abdomen and hyperuricaemia, depending on the extent of renal involvement.

Management
An anecdotal report of treatment with carboplatin indicated a short-term response only. Radiation therapy has yet to be evaluated for efficacy with this disease. At the moment, the prognosis remains poor for patients diagnosed with this disease.

Spinal neoplasia

Spinal neoplasia may produce a unilateral paresis/paralysis, although bilateral effects are more common.

HYPERKERATOSIS

Definition/overview

This is seen in most species, but canaries and poultry are the most commonly reported.

Aetiology

Usually associated with *Cnemidocoptes* infection (see Chapter 8, Disorders affecting the beak and cere), but there is some suspicion that a nutritional deficiency (possibly zinc and/or biotin) associated with all-seed diets may be involved in some cases. Secondary bacterial and fungal infections may contribute to the pain sometimes seen with this condition.

Clinical presentation

The scales and skin on the podotheca become hyperkeratotic and may be painful.

Management

Treatment with ivermectin or moxidectin, combined with correction of nutritional deficiencies, is usually curative. In refractory cases, biopsies and/or culture may be needed to identify secondary pathogens.

SELF-MUTILATION OF THE FEET AND TOES

Definition/overview

This is a complex problem, with no simple answers or solutions. Affected birds will bite and chew at their feet and toes, sometimes to the point of amputating their own toes.

Aetiology

Suggested/proven causes include: dermatitis; allergic dermatitis; underlying pain due to conditions such as osteomyelitis, healing fractures, soft tissue infection or inflammation, tendonitis, arthritis; chemical irritants (e.g. nicotine); vasculitis (e.g. immune-mediated, frost bite); obsessive — compulsive disorders.

Neuritis is the inflammation of a nerve or group of nerves characterized by pain, loss of reflexes and atrophy of the affected muscles. It may be viral (e.g. PDD), traumatic (e.g. entrapment of the superficial nerves by a fracture or external skeletal fixator) or toxic (e.g. lead).

Neuralgia is pain that follows the path of a specific nerve. In humans the causes of neuralgia are varied and can include chemical irritation, inflammation, trauma (including surgery), compression of nerves by nearby structures (e.g. tumours) and infections. In many cases, however, the cause is unknown. Neuralgia is suspected, but not yet proven, in some birds that self-mutilate their feet and toes.

Management

Wherever possible, causative agents and secondary infections should be identified and eliminated. The bird should be prevented from mutilating the area through the use of bandages or Elizabethan collars. NSAIDs can be given to reduce inflammation and provide analgesia.

Gabapentin has been used to treat neuralgia in humans and small mammals. Limited use in birds suggests that it may be a useful medication for self-mutilation disorders.

TOE TAPPING IN ECLECTUS PARROTS

Definition/overview

Toe tapping is the bilaterally symmetrical rhythmic extension and contraction of the digits of both feet, manifested when the bird is at full rest. Wing tip 'flipping' may also be seen in some individuals. When stimulated, these 'toe tappers' are able to stop the behaviour. Self-inflicted trauma is not a feature of this condition.

Aetiology

Numerous aetiologies have been suggested including post-polyomavirus neuritis, nutritional deficiencies and lead toxicosis. Oversupplementation with vitamins appears to be emerging as the 'favourite' aetiology. A dietary history usually reveals the excessive use of vitamin supplements, often in conjunction with a formulated diet.

Management

Discontinuing the supplementation often resolves the problem. In some cases, reducing the amount of formulated diet or simply changing brands is also required. As more research is done into this condition, it is likely that more appropriate therapies will be developed.

LEG BAND CONSTRICTION

Definition/overview

Swelling and vascular necrosis of the distal foot occurs due to the tourniquet effect of a constricted leg band (**168**).

168 Leg band constriction in a sun conure. In this case a plastic band had slipped up on to the tibiotarsus.

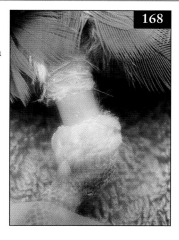

169 Constricted split aluminium leg band.

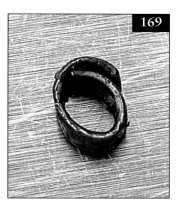

Aetiology
This constriction develops as the result of applying too small a band to a growing bird; applying a soft 'split band' (usually made of aluminium) that is chewed on by the bird, causing it to overlap and constrict (**169**); accumulation of scale and debris under the band (this is sometimes seen in budgerigars with *Cnemidocoptes* infection); or trauma and resultant swelling of the leg, with the (once loose) band becoming too tight (**47**).

Clinical presentation
Initially there is pain (shifting lameness, chewing at foot), followed by swelling and more pain. Eventually the foot may necrose and 'fall off'.

Management
Treatment in the early stages requires removal of the band and NSAIDs (e.g. meloxicam). However, owners need to be advised that constriction of the periosteum

of the tarsometatarsus often leads to avascular necrosis of the bone below the band. In these cases, and where there is significant superficial necrosis, amputation of the leg may be required. In some cases the ring is all that is holding the foot on to the leg; removing the band results in the foot coming away with it.

MISSING NAILS AND TOES
Aetiology
It can be due to aggressive cage mates; unsafe caging or cage furniture; ergotism; toe constriction due to fibrous band formation (constricted toe syndrome) or foreign bodies (e.g. cotton thread); or frost damage.

Management
This is usually diagnosed after the event and treatment is rarely required. Birds that are missing toes or nails rarely appear to be handicapped.

FURTHER READING
Echols MS (2007) Avian kidney disease, Part I: types of renal disease. In: *Proceedings of the Annual Conference of the Association of Avian Veterinarians Australian Committee*, pp. 101–116.

Echols MS (2007) Avian kidney disease, Part II: diagnosis of renal disease. In: *Proceedings of the Annual Conference of the Association of Avian Veterinarians Australian Committee*, pp. 117–128.

Echols MS (2007) Avian kidney disease, Part III: treatment of renal disease. In: *Proceedings of the Annual Conference of the Association of Avian Veterinarians Australian Committee*, pp. 129–137.

Quesenbery K (1997) Disorders of the musculoskeletal system. In: *Avian Medicine and Surgery*. RB Altman et al. (eds). WB Saunders, Philadelphia, pp. 523–539.

Remple JD, Forbes NA (2000) Antibiotic-impregnated polymethyl methacrylate beads in the treatment of bumblefoot in raptors. In: *Raptor Biomedicine III*. JT Lumeij, et al. (eds). Zoological Education Network, Lake Worth, pp. 255–266.

Stanford M (2006) Calcium metabolism. In: *Clinical Avian Medicine, Vol 1*. GJ Harrison, TL Lightfoot (eds). Spix Publishing Inc, Palm Beach, pp. 141–151.

148

CHAPTER 12

DISORDERS OF THE MUSCULOSKELETAL SYSTEM

SKELETAL
HEREDITARY, CONGENITAL AND DEVELOPMENTAL

These may be caused by genetics; teratogens (e.g. organophosphates); malnutrition, either parental or of the juveniles; malpositioning within the egg; or artificial incubation (problems with temperature, humidity, ventilation, and turning frequency).

Spinal bifida

Incomplete closure of the embryonic neural tube results in an incompletely formed spinal cord. In addition, the vertebrae overlying the open portion of the spinal cord do not fully form and remain unfused and open. This allows the abnormal portion of the spinal cord to protrude through the opening in the bones. There may or may not be a fluid-filled sac surrounding the open spinal cord.

Spinal bifida occurs sporadically in pet birds.

Kyphosis (104)

Flexion of the spine occurs due to collapse or malformation of a vertebra, usually a thoracolumbar vertebra. The condition can be congenital or acquired (as a result of metabolic bone disease or osteomyelitis). The result is a 'hunchback'; the spine is bent in a dorsal direction such that the tail points perpendicular to the floor. There may be dyspnoea evident due to compression of the abdominal and thoracic air sacs.

Scoliosis

Lateral deviation and curvature of the spine occurs due to apical malformations of vertebrae.

In poultry it has been associated with genetics, melatonin deficiency through pinealectomy or continuous light exposure. The indication is that there is a threshold level of serum melatonin below which scoliosis may develop, probably in conjunction with other factors that have yet to be identified. Deficiencies of copper, manganese or vitamin B6 have been shown to aggravate the condition.

How this correlates with the occasional scoliosis seen in companion birds remains unclear, but it raises issues about parental nutrition and hand-rearing practices.

Spondylolisthesis

This is a condition seen in poultry where the fourth thoracic vertebra displaces vertically, compressing the spinal cord and causing varying degrees of paresis. It is also known as 'kinky back'.

Tibial dyschondroplasia
Definition/overview

This is seen in turkeys, chickens and ducks, but not in companion birds.

Aetiology

The condition is characterized by the presence of a nonmineralized cartilage mass that extends distally from the growth plate of the metaphysis at the proximal end of the tibia and, occasionally, to the distal end of the tibia, the proximal end of the tarsometatarsus and the proximal ends of femur and humerus. It is a result of a defect in vascularization of the cartilage, resulting in an insufficiency of minerals and nutrients to the cartilage. This results in inadequate mineralization and cartilage necrosis. It has been associated with copper deficiency, toxins, excessive dietary cysteine and acidosis.

Clinical presentation

Bone deformity and lameness are seen in fast-growing chickens.

NUTRITIONAL/METABOLIC
Rickets
Aetiology

Rickets is a metabolic bone disease, usually seen in juvenile birds, predominantly caused by a vitamin D3 deficiency. (This can be due to inadequate nutrition, lack of exposure to sunlight, defective vitamin D3 activation, defective vitamin D3 receptors, hypoparathyroidism, renal failure, renal phosphate loss or gastrointestinal malabsorption.) Lack of adequate dietary calcium may also contribute to the development of rickets.

The result is impaired mineralization of osteoid tissue or epiphyseal cartilage, leading to thinning and weakening of the bones and excessive growth of cartilaginous structures.

Clinical presentation

There is deformity at the ends of the bones, particularly in the proximal tibiotarsus, the beak (rubber beak), the head of the ribs and, sometimes, the costochondral junction (rachitic rosary). There may be bowing and rotational deformities of the long bones.

Diagnosis

Radiographically there may be widening and distortion of the growth plates.

Management

Parenteral vitamin D3 should be given until the inciting cause is identified and corrected. Note that excessive vitamin D3 can promote soft tissue (especially renal) mineralization. An initial injection, followed by ultraviolet B exposure (preferably in the form of unfiltered sunlight) is a safe course of treatment.

Treatment of chronic nutritional deficiencies is by dietary change, usually to a formulated diet. However, owners should be made aware that the full clinical effect may take a year to be seen.

Leg deformities may require surgical correction (see Chapter 11, Disorders of the legs, feet and toes, p. 140).

Prognosis

Severe deformities carry a very poor prognosis.

Osteomalacia

Osteomalacia, or osteoporosis, is a similar condition to rickets, occurring in adult birds housed indoors and suffering from a vitamin D3 deficiency. There is a generalized thinning of the bone, with pathological micro- or gross fractures and resultant pain.

Nutritional secondary hyperparathyroidism
Aetiology

This condition is commonly seen in birds fed a diet that is either calcium deficient or has an excess of phosphorus (or both). For example, seed-only diets may have a calcium:phosphorus ratio as low as 1:10. Fruits, nuts and most vegetables are also calcium deficient. When these diets are fed exclusively, the parathyroid gland releases parathyroid hormone, which, amongst other effects, withdraws calcium from the bone to maintain normal serum calcium levels. The result is thin bones that bend or break easily, leading to malformations (**170**).

Management

Nutritional correction is necessary. Surgery or external coaptation may be required for fracture repair.

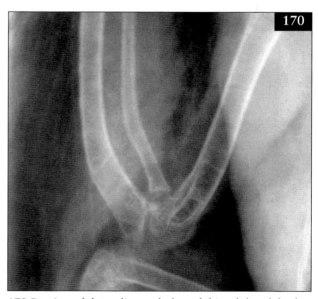

170 Bowing of the radius and ulna of this adult galah, due to osteomalacia, is the result of an all-seed diet.

Prognosis
Severe pathological fractures carry a poor prognosis (**171**).

Osteopetrosis or polyostotic hyperostosis
Definition/overview
Osteopetrosis is the development of bone in the medullary cavity of the femur, ulna, radius, pectoral girdle and vertebrae. It is seen as increased radiopacity of these bones (**172, 173**).

Aetiology
The deposition of this bone is stimulated by oestrogen. It may be nonpathological (a normal change in the reproductively active hen, as this bone is the primary source of calcium for the formation of the egg shell) or pathological (associated with hyperoestrogenic conditions such as ovarian neoplasia and cystic ovarian disease).

Management
Once the oestrogen levels return to normal, the bone density also returns to normal. In the normal reproductively active hen, no treatment is required. Pathological cases require treatment for the inciting cause (see Chapter 20, Disorders of the reproductive tract, p. 214).

OSTEOMYELITIS
Aetiology
Osteomyelitis may be a result of infection (localized or systemic disease) by bacteria (aerobic and anaerobic both implicated), fungi (*Aspergillus* (**174**) and *Candida*) or mycobacteria. It may also be the result of trauma or neoplasia.

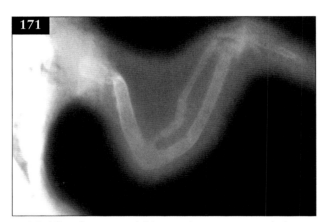

171 Folding fractures of this severity carry a guarded prognosis.

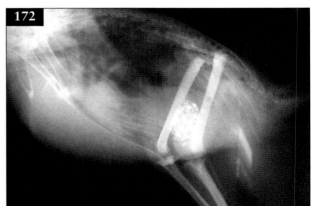

172 Osteopetrosis (polyostotic hyperostosis) in a reproductively active budgerigar hen.

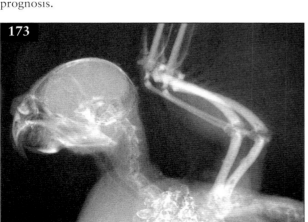

173 Osteopetrosis (polyostotic hyperostosis) in a reproductively active budgerigar hen.

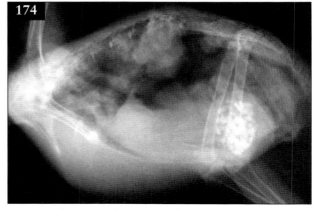

174 Spinal osteomyelitis in an African grey parrot due to aspergillosis.

Clinical presentation

There is soft tissue swelling around the lesion. The lesion is painful, sometimes shown as lameness or an inability to fly. There may be a fracture (and subsequent instability) associated with the infection.

Diagnosis

Radiographically there is usually clearly defined lysis of bone, as opposed to the more diffuse changes associated with neoplasia. (Note that mycobacterial infections can also be diffuse.) The pus is caseous and does not drain; if an abscess forms, it enlarges to form an expanded outline within the bone, especially if it has formed within the medullary cavity. There is often a marked proliferative periosteal reaction.

Haematologically there may be a leucocytosis, with heterophilia, monocytosis and basophilia.

Management

Surgical debridement of the lesion is usually required to remove the caseated pus and necrotic bones. Antibiotic-impregnated polymethylmethacrylate beads, placed into the cavity left by the abscess after debridement and lavage, allow antimicrobials to be delivered locally in high concentrations. Antibiotics used include gentamicin, amikacin, tobramycin, lincomycin, clindamycin, neomycin, ceftiofur and cephalothin. Bacterial and fungal culture and antibiotic sensitivity should be performed, ideally before beginning treatment, to guide the choice of antibiotic therapy. With the exception of intra-articular placement, implanted beads can be left in place indefinitely.

Systemic antibiotic therapy should be directed by culture and continued long term (2–3 months).

NEOPLASIA

Aetiology

Neoplasia of skeletal structures can be either primary (osteomas, osteosarcomas (**175**), chondromas, chondrosarcomas, osteochondroma, fibrosarcomas, haemangiomas) or metastatic (air sac carcinomas, other carcinomas).

Clinical presentation

The tumour usually presents as a firm swelling.

Diagnosis

Radiographically there are varying degrees of bone changes including proliferative lesions, osteolysis and pathological fractures (**176**).

Neoplasia must be distinguished from osteomyelitis. This may require deep bone biopsy using a fine needle aspirate or a bone biopsy needle (e.g. Jamshidi bone biopsy needle). In small birds an 18–22-gauge needle can be used to obtain a core sample: the needle is guided through the centre of the lesion from one side to the other, and then a stylet of sterile stainless steel wire is pushed through the needle to extrude the biopsy specimen. Care must be taken to sample the centre of the lesion, as proliferative bony reactions on the periphery of the lesion may mask the origin of the lesion.

Management

Treatment usually requires amputation, followed by adjuvant chemotherapy and/or radiation.

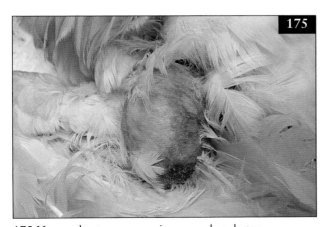

175 Humeral osteosarcoma in an aged cockatoo.

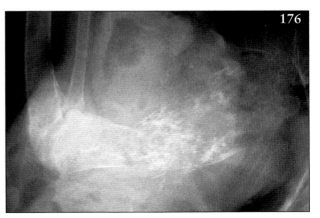

176 Radiographic view of the mass seen in the **175**. A poor prognosis must be given due to the likelihood of metastatic disease.

JOINTS
LUXATION
Definition/overview
All joints can be affected, but the knee and elbow joints are most commonly affected.

Aetiology
Luxation may be the result of trauma or a congenital condition.

Clinical presentation
Localized swelling, pain and reluctance to use the affected limb are seen.

Diagnosis
Diagnosis is based on the clinical signs referrable to luxation and radiography.

Management
Conservative therapy is often successful because of the joint anatomy and powerful contraction of flight or leg muscles.

Elbow
Closed reduction can be successful if the luxation is diagnosed soon after the injury. If the luxation is mild, suturing the triceps tendon to the common digital extensor tendon can be successful in stabilizing the joint.

Knee
Conservative therapy is unlikely to be successful. Several surgical techniques have been described:
- An appropriately sized pin or K-wire is introduced through the knee joint into the femur and another into the tibiotarsus, such that the ends protrude through the cranial aspect of the joint. The luxation is then reduced and the ends of the pins are locked together and stabilized with dental acrylic to hold the bones in normal apposition.
- A transverse hole is drilled through the distal femur and another through the proximal tibiotarsus. A nonabsorbable suture is then looped through these holes and tied so that, as it is tightened, it reduces and stabilizes the knee.
- External skeletal fixation (ESF) pins are placed in the femur and tibiotarsus, the luxation is reduced and then connecting bars are attached so that they bridge the joint. This stabilizes the reduced luxation.

After 1–2 weeks (depending on the age of the patient), the pins or sutures can be removed.

Shoulder
Luxation is often accompanied by an avulsion fracture of the ventral tubercle of the proximal humerus. A figure-of-eight bandage for 10–14 days may be successful in early cases.

Hip
Luxations generally occur craniodorsal to the acetabulum. Closed reduction and splinting of the leg to the body may be successful in early cases. Open surgical reduction and suturing are sometimes needed and are recommended in avian species with a gliding hinge-type coxofemoral joint (noncursorial species such as most psittacine birds and raptors).

Prognosis
The prognosis for full return to normal use of the joint is fair to guarded; however, a pain-free leg can usually be achieved even if it is not fully functional.

SWOLLEN JOINTS
See Chapter 11, Disorders of the legs, feet and toes, p. 141.

MUSCLES
CONGENITAL
Muscular dystrophy
This is seen in chickens and turkeys, but not in companion birds. Muscle fibres are lost and are replaced by fat.

Arthrogryposis
Congenital flexure or contracture of joints occurs secondary to atrophy of skeletal muscle and subsequent fibrosis of the muscle. This atrophy is due to congenital neurological defects, either anatomical deficits or following parental alkaloid plant toxicosis (e.g. lupines).

NONINFLAMMATORY
Atrophy
Aetiology
Atrophy may be caused by disuse (e.g. painful conditions of a limb, inability to fly, joint contraction following excessively long splinting of an injured limb or pressure on the sciatic nerve from a renal tumour). It may also result from ageing, and denervation caused by trauma or neoplasia.

Generalized chronic disease can cause muscle atrophy. Acute illness in birds sees a demand for energy greater than dietary intake. This triggers glycogenolysis, which quickly exhausts body stores of glycogen. Fat oxidation cannot meet the demands for energy and, after a few days, the process of gluconeogenesis using muscle protein (catabolism) begins. This results in muscle atrophy. The pectoral muscles are most noticeably affected, with the keel bone becoming more prominent. This condition is colloquially known as 'going light'. It is not a disease syndrome in itself, it is simply an indication of a chronic disease process.

Management
Disuse atrophy and denervation require identification and correction of the underlying problem, if possible.

Muscle atrophy due to chronic disease requires correction of the underlying disease problem, supplemental feeding (e.g. tube feeding for debilitated birds that cannot eat normally) and good-quality food (e.g. formulated diets to assist in the recovery and place the bird into an anabolic state). Recovery of the lost muscle mass is invariably slow, taking several days or weeks to return to normal.

Nutritional: vitamin E and selenium deficiency
Aetiology
This deficiency is seen in piscivorous species fed a diet of improperly frozen and thawed fish. Any species fed a diet containing rancid polyunsaturated fat can develop the same condition.

Clinical presentation
Vitamin E and selenium deficiency can result in cardiomyopathy and muscle lesions, showing as generalized weakness.

Management
Recovery is usually rapid once nutritional deficiencies are corrected.

Toxic: ionophores (monensin, lasalocid, salinomycin, narasin)
Aetiology
This condition is seen in nongallinaceous birds fed medicated poultry feeds.

Clinical presentation
Toxicosis is seen as generalized weakness and paresis due to damage to skeletal muscle.

Management
No specific treatment is available. The drug should be removed from the animal's diet and supportive care provided.

Plant toxins
Some plant toxins can cause muscle problems (e.g. gossypol, *Cassia* spp.).

INFLAMMATORY: NONINFECTIOUS
Trauma
Aetiology
Muscle inflammation may be caused by blunt trauma (e.g. flying into objects such as ceiling fans or aviary wire) or iatrogenic trauma (e.g. intramuscular injections, especially doxycycline and oxytetracycline).

Clinical presentation
Bruising and swelling can be seen and this may develop into necrosis or fibrosis with chronicity.

Management
Severe or painful muscle injuries (**177**) should be treated with an analgesic (e.g. meloxicam or butorphanol).

Exertional/capture myopathy
Definition/overview
This is usually seen in flamingos, crowned cranes, Canada geese, sandhill cranes and wild turkeys (USA) that have been recently captured or handled.

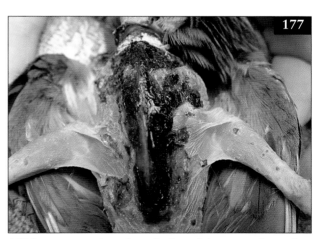

177 Severe necrosis and mutilation of the pectoral muscles of an adult quaker with quaker mutilation syndrome. The cause of this problem is still unclear.

Clinical presentation

Muscle necrosis and intramuscular haemorrhage are commonly noted, followed by fibrosis with chronicity.

Diagnosis

Diagnosis of exertional myopathy is based on history of recent capture or trauma, clinical signs and elevation of AST, ALT, CK, LDH and serum potassium.

Management

Treatment includes fluid therapy, vitamin E and physiotherapy. The use of corticosteroids has been advocated by some authors; its benefits must be weighed against possible adverse effects on the liver and immune system.

Prognosis

Prognosis in severe cases is poor.

INFLAMMATORY: INFECTIOUS
Viral

Viral myositis is uncommon. Acute polyomavirus infections may cause muscle pallor and haemorrhage.

Bacterial

Bacterial myositis is usually an extension of an infection in the skin or underlying bone; however, foreign bodies (e.g. microchips implanted without attention to sterility) can introduce an infection. The infection may be aerobic or anaerobic.

Fungal

Fungal myositis usually occurs as an extension of infection from air sacs or by haematogenous spread. It is similar in appearance to bacterial myositis and granulomas and can only be distinguished histologically.

Sarcocystosis
Aetiology

Caused by *Sarcocystis* spp., a parasite of many species of birds, with a worldwide distribution. There are believed to be six species of *Sarcocystis* that infect birds. It has an obligate two-host life cycle that alternates between a sexual intestinal phase in the definitive host and an asexual multiorgan (especially the lungs) and ultimately muscular cyst phase in the intermediate host. The definitive host is usually a carnivore that eats an animal (the intermediate host) with mature cysts in its muscles. The intermediate host is usually an herbivorous or insectivorous bird. Transmission to the intermediate host is usually mechanical, in the form of insects such as flies and cockroaches. There is no direct spread from bird to bird, although several birds in one collection can be infected simultaneously.

Clinical presentation

While some intermediate hosts have evolved with both the parasite and the definitive host (and therefore do not develop clinical illness) naïve species exposed to *Sarcocystis* often develop clinical signs.

Acute pulmonary disease, due to asexual reproduction in the lung, causes severe dyspnoea and often acute death. Encephalitis can develop in psittacines and raptors (posterior or unilateral paresis, intention tremors and head tilt). Cardiac disease can develop in some birds if cysts localize in the myocardium. Severe myositis can occur in some birds; other birds may have the cysts present, but display no clinical signs.

Diagnosis

Diagnosis in the live bird is difficult. Blood tests show elevated CK and AST, and leucocytosis. An immunofluorescent antibody (IFA) test is available in some countries. Muscle biopsy of the quadriceps muscles gives better results than the pectoral muscles because the muscular cysts there are less likely to degenerate before reaching maturity.

Management

For the surviving mate, pyrimethamine is given at 0.5 mg/kg orally q12h for 2–4 days then 0.25 mg/kg for 30 days.

Treatment for affected birds:
- Amprolium in drinking water for seven days.
- 500 mg sulfadoxine/25 mg pyrimethamine 0.5 mg/kg orally q12h for 45 days.
- Primaquine phosphate 1 mg/kg orally q24h for 45 days.

Control involves keeping definitive hosts out of the aviary or immediate surroundings and utilizing effective insect control.

Leukocytozoon
Aetiology

Leukocytozoon is a protozoan parasite of erythrocytes and leucocytes, but with schizogony occurring in tissues other than the blood. Usually the parasite is nonpathogenic, but in some cases it can cause disruption of skeletal and cardiac muscles.

Clinical presentation

Clinical signs can include anorexia, weakness, haemoglobinuria, depression and dehydration.

Management

Chloroquine, primaquine or pyrimethamine may be used for treatment. Exposure to biting insects should be prevented.

NEOPLASTIC

Muscle neoplasia is uncommon in companion birds. It can be primary (rhabdomyoma, rhabdomyosarcoma) or secondary (lymphosarcoma, melanoma). Metastatic disease is rare.

TENDONS AND LIGAMENTS

TENDON CONTRACTURE ('JOINT DISEASE')

Aetiology

Enforced immobility of a joint in a flexed condition (e.g. when a wing or leg is splinted) can lead to contracture of the tendons controlling that joint. This can result in a permanent reduction in the joint's range of movement.

Management

Treatment requires a programme of gradual extension and extension of the joint, performed under general anaesthesia, to break down the fibrous adhesions causing the contracture. The prognosis for return to normal joint flexibility is guarded.

To prevent this problem, joints should be immobilized for no more than two weeks, if possible. If this is not possible, weekly physiotherapy should be performed (e.g. passive flexion and extension of the joint through its normal range of movement). This usually requires a short general anaesthetic to remove the splint, perform the physiotherapy and then replace the splint.

SLIPPED TENDON (PEROSIS)

Definition/overview

Medial or lateral luxation of the gastrocnemius tendon occurs over the tibiotarsal condyles. It is most commonly seen in juvenile poultry, waterfowl and ratites (where it is associated with nutritional deficiencies), but has been seen in psittacines with leg deformities.

Diagnosis

Diagnosis is made on clinical signs and palpation of the joint and tendon.

Management

Surgical replacement of the tendon and repair of the tendon retinaculum is invariably unsuccessful, the repair often breaking down within hours or days when the bird attempts to use the affected leg.

Another technique involves placing a K-wire into the tarsometarsus on the medial side of the ligament, with the proximal end of the pin protruding from the bone and effectively preventing the ligament from slipping medially. This technique appears promising, although a degree of joint stiffness often results. Any bone deformities predisposing to the tendon luxation must be corrected.

This condition often requires arthrodesis of the hock joint.

TENDONITIS

Aetiology

Tendonitis may be infectious (may start in a joint and extend into the surrounding tendons) or noninfectious. Infectious causes include bacteria, *Mycoplasma* spp. and reovirus. Noninfectious causes include trauma, articular gout and tendon contracture (see above).

Clinical presentation

There is lameness or reluctance to use the limb, and localized swelling.

Management

Inflammation is reduced with NSAIDs such as meloxicam. Antimicrobial therapy is given if appropriate.

FURTHER READING

Quesenbery K (1997) Disorders of the musculoskeletal system. In: *Avian Medicine and Surgery*. RB Altman, SL Clubb, GM Dorrestein, K Quesenberry (eds). WB Saunders, Philadelphia, pp. 523–539.

Stanford M (2006) Calcium metabolism. In: *Clinical Avian Medicine, Vol 1*. GJ Harrison, TL Lightfoot (eds). Spix Publishing Inc, Palm Beach, pp. 141–151.

Villar D, Kramer M, Howard L, Hammond E, Cray C, Latimer K (2008) Clinical presentation and pathology of sarcocystosis in psittaciform birds: 11 cases. *Avian Diseases* **52(1)**:187–194.

CHAPTER 13

DISORDERS OF THE GASTROINTESTINAL TRACT

THE OROPHARYNX AND CROP
CANDIDIASIS
Definition/overview
Candidiasis is also known as thrush, moniliasis, sour crop and crop mycosis. It is most commonly due to the yeast *Candida albicans*, which can be part of the normal intestinal flora and is frequently isolated from droppings of normal bird. It is primarily a disease of the upper gastrointestinal tract (oropharynx, oesophagus and crop), but can be found lower in the tract on occasion.

Predisposing factors include: young birds that are not fully immunocompetent; prolonged antibiotic use; concurrent immunosuppressive conditions (debilitation, PBFD, malnutrition); poor hygiene in environment and food preparation, or failure to clean excess formula from the skin or mouth of hand-reared chicks; high concentrations of sugar in fruit and hand-rearing formulae providing an optimal medium for the growth of yeast; alkaline crop contents, seen when crop stasis occurs for other reasons, encouraging yeast overgrowth.

Clinical presentation
Affected birds show general malaise, weight loss and reduced growth rates. There may be regurgitation/vomiting. Crop emptying times are increased, the crop may be distended with fluid and mucus, and the crop wall becomes thickened. Diphtheritic membranes may be present in the oropharynx and crusty lesions are seen on the commissures of the mouth. Infection can extend through the choana into the sinuses, causing signs of upper respiratory tract infection. It can also become a dermatitis (see Chapter 7, Disorders of the skin and feathers, p. 109).

Diagnosis
Diagnosis is based on history, clinical signs and lesions, as culture alone may not distinguish between normal flora, dietary yeast and pathogenic overgrowth. Cytology (Gram stain) of throat swabs, crop washes and faeces may reveal the yeast in three different forms: oval nonbudding yeast, budding yeast and pseudohyphae formation:
- Oval nonbudding yeast are usually of dietary origin.
- Large numbers (>5 per high powered field) of budding yeast are significant.
- The presence of pseudohyphae may indicate tissue invasion.

Gross lesions (**178**) must be distinguished from pox virus, trichomoniasis, hypovitaminosis A and internal papilloma disease (IPD).

Management
Underlying factors must be addressed (e.g. environment, hygiene, husbandry, food handling, concomitant antibiotic therapy). Antifungal therapy includes nystatin, ketoconazole, fluconazole or itraconazole. Nystatin is not absorbed systemically and must therefore be given into the mouth (rather than by crop needle) as it requires direct contact with the yeast to be effective. Acidification of crop contents

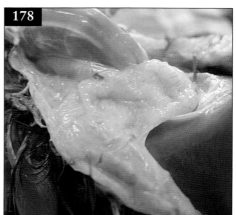

178 Thickening of the ingluvial wall in a lorikeet with candidiasis.

by adding apple cider vinegar to drinking water or hand-rearing formula (10 ml/litre of water) may decrease crop pH and discourage growth of yeast.

TRICHOMONIASIS
Definition/overview
Trichomoniasis is also known as canker (pigeons and budgerigars) or frounce (raptors). It is most commonly seen in budgerigars, lorikeets, pigeons and raptors, but has been reported in most species. It has a worldwide distribution.

Pathophysiology
Trichomonas gallinae has a direct life cycle, with the protozoa being passed from bird to bird via feeding (courtship behaviour, feeding young) or via contaminated drinking water (faeces, crop secretions). The organism dies quickly outside the host.

Aetiology
The causative organism is *T. gallinae*, a protozoan parasite with an undulating membrane and four anterior flagella (**78**).

Clinical presentation
Signs include unthriftiness and high mortality in young birds; gagging, regurgitation, vomiting; diarrhoea; ptyalism; weight loss; and diphtheritic membranes in the oropharynx, oesophagus and crop (**179**).

In raptors it may extend into the sinuses (causing a caseous sinusitis) or into the Eustachian tubes (causing a head tilt). Young pigeon squabs develop a visceral form of the disease involving the liver, gastrointestinal tract and navel.

Diagnosis
A crop wash or throat swab shows motile protozoa. Rarely, there is a single lesion in the thoracic oesophagus causing clinical signs, but the protozoa are not readily detectable. These cases are difficult to diagnose antemortem. Motile protozoa are occasionally found in the faeces.

Management
Treatment with a nitroimidazole (metronidazole, ronidazole, carnidazole) is usually effective. Some cases with severe ulceration and diphtheritic membranes will die despite treatment. In some raptors, surgical debridement of lesions may become necessary.

In pigeons, strategic treatment of the flock may be necessary (i.e. during the breeding season, at weaning, immediately prior to and after the racing season). The extent of treatment required in pigeons is the subject of some debate, as there is evidence that

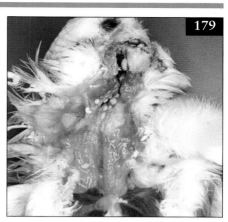

179 Ingluvial ulceration in a budgerigar with trichomoniasis. Note the seed extending from the mouth to the lesion — but not beyond. Starvation is a common cause of death.

infection by lentogenic strains of *T. gallinae* provides some protective immunity against velogenic strains.

HYPOVITAMINOSIS A
Definition/overview
Vitamin A is formed in the liver through the conversion of beta-carotenes (from vegetables and fruit) and retinol (from liver and fish oils). Deficiencies in vitamin A (or its precursors) result in keratinization of epithelial cells, causing squamous metaplasia of the mucous membranes of the oropharynx. The metaplasia blocks the ducts of the salivary and mucus glands, causing abscesses in these glands.

The author's experience is that birds that have evolved with high levels of beta-carotenes in their natural diet (i.e. fruit and vegetables) appear to more susceptible to hypovitaminosis A than birds that have evolved a much poorer quality diet (e.g. seeding grasses). Birds such as eclectus parrots, Amazon parrots, African grey parrots and lorikeets are more likely to show clinical signs of deficiency than cockatiels and budgerigars.

Aetiology
Hypovitaminosis A is caused by all-seed diets.

Clinical presentation
White or pale swellings are seen in the inter-ramular region, beneath the tongue or elsewhere in the oropharynx. There is blunting of the choanal papillae. Ptyalism occurs and sinusitis is common.

Diagnosis
History and clinical signs are very suggestive. Differential diagnoses include trichomoniasis, pox virus, candidiasis and IPD.

An aspirate of the swellings shows keratinized epithelial cells rather than inflammatory cells.

Management
Treatment includes parenteral vitamin A and diet correction. Surgical removal of masses may be required in extreme cases, but severe haemorrhage is likely to ensue.

POXVIRUS INFECTION
Birds with avian poxvirus infection may have diphtheritic membranes in the oropharynx. See Chapter 7, Disorders affecting the skin and feathers, for more detail.

INTERNAL PAPILLOMA DISEASE
Birds with IPD may have papillomas in the oropharynx. This condition will be discussed in more detail later in this chapter.

CROP STASIS
Definition/overview
Crop stasis, where the crop fails to empty, is commonly seen in preweaning chicks, but it can also be seen in adult birds.

Aetiology
There are several possible causes. Crop stasis may occur as a result of generalized ileus caused by systemic illness (e.g. severe renal disease), stunting, foreign bodies below the level of the crop, chilling, heavy metal toxicosis or dehydration. Conditions affecting the crop such as foreign bodies, an overstretched/atonic crop, infectious ingluvitis (e.g. *Candida albicans*, bacteria), fibrous food impaction or crop burns may also cause stasis. Dietary factors may also be involved (e.g. cold food, watery food, food that settles out, chronic overfeeding or overly dry food).

Clinical presentation
The crop fails to empty within six hours. It is palpably distended, often filled with fermenting food and water ('sour crop'). Regurgitation may occur, often on palpation of the crop. There are signs of dehydration.

Management
If possible, the aetiological agent should be identified and eliminated. The crop should be emptied (by surgery if necessary) and lavaged with warm saline. Parental fluids are given (to correct dehydration) until crop motility is restored, and antimicrobials are given as appropriate. Motility modifiers (metoclopramide, cisapride, fennel or cumin tea) may assist, but their efficacy is not universal.

Once the bird is rehydrated, small, watery meals should be given often. Predigesting hand-rearing formulae with pancreatic enzymes can liquefy the diet without diluting it.

Chronically distended, nonresponsive crops may require support with an elastic sling ('crop bra') or crop reduction surgery.

THERMAL INJURIES
Definition/overview
Thermal injuries are less common than in past years, as aviculturists have become aware of the problem. Novice hand-rearers, however, still present chicks with this problem.

Aetiology
The most common aetiology is a hand-rearing formula that has been overheated in a microwave oven and then fed before it has cooled sufficiently. 'Hot spots' (small foci of super-heated food) may be present in a mix and be overlooked when (if) the food temperature is checked. Some cases may be due to chicks coming into contact with incandescent light bulbs or heating pads, particularly while the crop is distended after a recent feed.

Clinical presentation
In the early stages (1–2 days) affected chicks may be lethargic and refuse feeding. Physical examination may reveal mild to moderate crop stasis and erythema of the most prominent part of the ventral crop. After the initial stage of erythema, blanching of the affected tissue develops. A crust then forms over the area; when it lifts off a fistula is usually revealed, often with food leaking from it (**180**).

Diagnosis
Thermal injuries must be differentiated from a crop perforation (see below).

Management
Surgical resection of the burn and repair of the crop and skin are necessary to effect a cure. However, surgery must be delayed until the fistula has formed and all devitalized tissue has become obvious (usually 4–7 days after the incident — see Chapter 26, Surgery, p. 259). The crop has an incredible ability to stretch and even large crop resections seem to be well tolerated by most young birds. Subsequent feedings will obviously need to be reduced in volume depending on the postoperative size of the crop.

While waiting for the burn to become clearly demarcated, the chick must be given supportive care, including analgesia and antibiotic coverage, and small

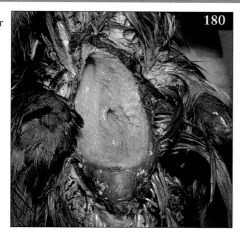

180 The outer wall of the crop of this chick has sloughed off following a crop burn.

feeds given frequently so as to avoid distending the crop. Placement of an oesophagostomy tube may be necessary in some cases.

CROP PERFORATIONS
Aetiology
Crop perforation usually occurs when using a metal feeding tube. The tube perforates the crop because either the chick has an unrestrained feeding response and thrusts up against the tube or the person feeding the chick does so roughly or impatiently. Food can be deposited outside the crop and under the skin, in some cases without being noticed.

Clinical presentation
Early cases may be presented because of blood on the feeding tube when it is withdrawn. These birds are usually asymptomatic. More advanced cases may be presented because of apparent crop stasis, often with severe systemic illness. Distension is palpable in the crop region, but food cannot be aspirated with a feeding tube.

Management
Surgical removal of the food deposited under the skin, followed by debridement and flushing of the subcutaneous tissues and repair of the crop injury, is essential. Prognosis is determined by the time lapse since the initial injury and the degree of sepsis present in the patient.

INGLUVIOLITHS AND OTHER FOREIGN BODIES IN THE CROP
Aetiology
Ingluvioliths are chronic concretions of starch and other materials that form in the crop. Other foreign bodies can be ingested by the bird or fed to it by its parents. They can include fibrous material, seed and nut husks, large pieces of food and pieces of wood.

Clinical presentation
Signs inlcude regurgitation, gagging, vomiting, weight loss, crop stasis and ptyalism.

Diagnosis
Diagnosis is based on palpation of the crop and plain and contrast radiography.

Management
Endoscopic retrieval through the mouth is feasible in some cases. Ingluviotomy may be required to remove some objects (see Chapter 26, Surgery, p. 258). Small ingluvioliths can be lubricated with liquid paraffin (mineral oil) and massaged until they break down into sludge or small particles that can pass through the digestive tract or be aspirated via a large-bore feeding tube.

PARASITES
Capillaria contorta (hair worm, thread worm)
Definition/overview
Capillariasis occurs in quail and pheasants. The worms burrow into the mucosa of the oesophagus and crop, creating tracts that fill with blood, producing hyperaemic streaks and some diphtheritic lesions. The life cycle can be direct or indirect.

Clinical presentation
Clinical signs include anorexia, dysphagia, diarrhoea and weight loss.

Diagnosis
Diagnosis is by finding double-operculated eggs on faecal examination.

Management
Treatment is with ivermectin or moxidectin.

Spiruroid worms (Spiruroidea)
Definition/overview
Spiruroid worms occur in wild corvids and strigiformes, and are also reported in passerines and parrots. They produce granulomatous lesions in the oropharynx, crop and proventriculus, with a worm protruding. The life cycle requires an arthropod vector.

Management
Treatment is with ivermectin or moxidectin, then the worms are removed manually if possible.

PROVENTRICULUS AND VENTRICULUS
FUNGAL INFECTIONS
Megabacteriosis
Definition/overview
Megabacteria is also known as avian gastric yeast or *Macrorhabdus*. It is an anamorphic ascomycetous yeast *Macrorhabdus ornithogaster*, a large, gram-positive, periodic acid–Schiff (PAS)-positive, highly pleomorphic yeast. It colonizes the gastric isthmus of many species of birds; in large numbers it can cause a maldigestion disorder and proventricular ulceration (**181**). It is probably transmitted by the ingestion of faecal material, although parent birds may pass it to their chicks when feeding them.

Clinical presentation
Megabacteriosis is most commonly recognized in budgerigars, but it has been diagnosed in most species including parrots, canaries, ostriches and poultry. Clinical signs include weight loss and weakness, and polyphagia, although often the bird is grinding its food and then letting it fall from its mouth. Some birds may regurgitate food and there may be blood staining around the beak.

Diagnosis
M. ornithogaster can often be detected on a plain faecal smear. Gram staining shows variably staining large 'cigar-shaped' organisms. Calcofluor stain is used in some laboratories to demonstrate the organism. Not all birds shed the organism consistently. A PCR test is available in the United States.

Autopsy findings include a dilated proventriculus (**182**), ulcerations of the proventricular–ventricular isthmus (**181**) and large numbers of the organism in mucosal scrapings.

Management
Amphotericin B is given at 100 mg/kg q12h or q24h for 30 days. Resistance may develop. Fluconazole may be effective in some cases; it is required for more than 30 days. Some birds will relapse after treatment.

Candidiasis
Candidiasis occasionally causes ventriculitis in small passerines (see above).

Zygomycetes and *Aspergillus* spp.
Definition/overview
These fungi will occasionally invade the mucosa and muscular layers of the proventriculus.

Diagnosis
Antemortem diagnosis is difficult, although endoscopic biopsy and brush cytology may be effective.

Management
Treatment with systemic antifungal drugs (fluconazole, itraconazole, ketoconazole) is required.

VIRAL INFECTIONS
Proventricular dilatation disease
Definition/overview
PDD is also known as macaw wasting disease, macaw fading syndrome, myenteric ganglioneuritis, infiltrative splanchnic neuropathy and neuropathic gastric dilatation. It has a worldwide distribution. It has been reported in most psittacine species, although suggestive lesions have been described in toucans, honey-creepers,

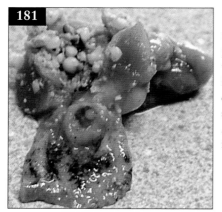

181 Ulcerations in the proventricular-ventricular isthmus are commonly seen with *Macrorhabdus* infection.

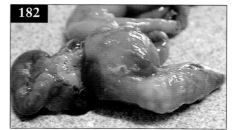

182 Enlargement of the proventriculus can be due to *Macrorhabdus* infection.

canaries, weaver finches, Canada geese and roseate spoonbills. It is usually adult birds that are affected, but it has been reported in chicks as young as ten weeks.

Aetiology

The exact aetiology is still not confirmed. Some authors believe it to be a togavirus. Paramyxovirus, adenovirus and other viruses have been isolated from affected birds. No consistent serology has been able to indicate that any of these viruses are always involved. Workers in the USA, Canada and UK have detected (by electron microscopy) an 80 nm enveloped virus-like particle in the fresh faeces of affected birds. This viral-like particle is unstable outside of the host, and is not detectable after three days. Recent work (2008) has raised the strong probability that this disease is due to a previously unreported avian bornavirus. Research is still continuing, but this looks to be the most promising finding in recent years.

Clinical presentation

PDD appears to be a segmental neuropathy, with clinical signs dependent on the organs affected. Most commonly, clinical signs are related to gastrointestinal dysfunction: passing whole food in droppings; regurgitation; weight loss; anorexia, lethargy and depression. Occasionally CNS signs are seen including ataxia, abnormal head movements, progressive paresis leading to paralysis, seizures, proprioceptive or motor deficit and self-mutilation.

Occasionally PDD causes sudden death due to an effect on the conduction pathways of the heart.

Secondary infections are common.

Diagnosis

With recent advances demonstrating the involvement of an avian bornavirus as the aetiological agent of PDD, it is likely that PCR testing will replace (to a large extent) other diagnostic modalities. However, PCR can only demonstrate the presence of the pathogen, not the disease. Some studies have already demonstrated avian bornavirus apparently healthy birds.

Biopsy remains the most accurate means of diagnosis, but the organ sampled will determine the degree of sensitivity. Biopsy specimens have been obtained from:

- Crop: the least accurate, but the easiest and safest to access (reports of its sensitivity vary from 66–72% to as low as 17%).
- Proventriculus: the most accurate, but sampling a dilated, thin-walled proventriculus is hazardous.
- Adrenal gland: accurate in cases affecting that area.

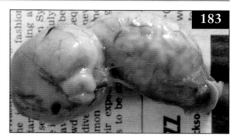

183 Proventricular dilatation in a bird with proventricular dilatation disease.

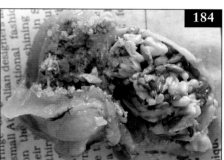

184 Proventricular dilatation in a bird with PDD. Note the thin wall of the proventriculus stretched over the contents.

The biopsy specimen must include a blood vessel and associated nerve. The myenteric plexus in the tunica muscularis of the proventriculus and ventriculus contains more lesions. The segmental nature of the disease means that the pathologist must examine stepped sections of the specimen to ensure lesions are not overlooked.

Histopathology shows a nonsuppurative lympho-cytic–plasmocytic ganglioneuritis of central and peripheral nerve tissue, with associated myositis and atrophy of the gastrointestinal tract, leading to dilatation and impaction. Adrenal glands show a lymphocytic–plasmocytic infiltrate. Immunohisto-chemical staining has been shown to demonstrate the presence of avian bornavirus in biopsies from infected birds.

Autopsy usually reveals the characteristic dilated, thin-walled proventriculus, often distended with ingesta (**183, 184**). Multiple tissues, including the brain and adrenal glands, should be submitted for histopathology.

Abdominal radiographs, with or without contrast media, show an enlarged proventriculus. Fluoroscopy demonstrates abnormal gastrointestinal motility.

Management

There is 100% mortality in untreated birds.

The use of celecoxib, a cyclo-oxygenase (COX)-2 inhibitor, to reduce the ganglioneuritis has apparently resulted in complete recovery in some birds, with return to normal function and biopsy showing resolution of the neuritis. Birds are given 10 mg/kg q24h for 6–24 weeks, with treatment cessation based on the bird regaining weight and resolution of lesions on biopsy. Some clinicians are concerned that this may result in a clinically normal bird that is still infectious to other birds. Until this is clarified, treated birds should remain isolated from other birds.

Cisapride, metoclopramide and high-fibre diets have all been used to assist gastrointestinal motility.

Aviary management is essential, involving hygiene and traffic flow.

Control

The mode of transmission remains unclear, but the faecal–oral route appears most likely. Transmission appears to be more likely in indoor aviaries with poor ventilation and insufficient attention paid to traffic control. Affected birds should be quarantined. At this time it appears that the best advice that can be given to aviculturists is to not sell in-contact birds for at least 2–3 years after the last diagnosis was made.

PARASITIC INFECTIONS

Finches, pheasants, quail and poultry are most commonly affected.

Acuaria spp. (gizzard worm)

Aetiology

Acuaria spp. (gizzard worm) are the most common worms involved. They include *A. skrjabini*, *A. humulosa* and *Dispharynx nasuata*. In canaries and finches these worms inhabit the proventriculus (causing swelling of the proventriculus mucosa) and under the koilin lining of ventriculus where they cause thickening of the ventricular wall. The intermediate hosts include weevils, grasshoppers, slaters and other insects.

Clinical presentation

Clinical signs are usually ill-thrift and death.

Management

Levamisole, moxidectin and ivermectin can be used, but resistance is common, so treatment efficacy must be monitored. Control of intermediate hosts is important.

FOREIGN BODIES

Definition/overview

A bird's curiosity and exploring nature will often lead it to ingest foreign bodies. The normal functioning of the ventriculus — the tougher koilin lining and the presence of grit, when combined with the grinding effect of the powerful ventricular muscles — effectively grinds up most of these foreign bodies within a few days. While the great majority of these foreign bodies cause little or no harm, others can cause gastrointestinal blockages, damage the gastrointestinal mucosa and release toxins such as lead and zinc, which are then absorbed and become a systemic problem.

Unless the bird is displaying clinical signs consistent with the foreign bodies causing a problem, most can be left and monitored to see if the body is removing them unaided. The administration of paraffin oil or pysillium may help to move smaller particles through the tract.

Clinical presentation

Clinical signs include anorexia, weight loss, regurgitation, decreased faecal output, melena and signs consistent with heavy metal toxicosis.

Diagnosis

Radiography, both plain and contrast, is useful. The entire tract must be evaluated; don't identify a foreign body in the crop and overlook the one in the proventriculus!

Haematology and biochemistry can be used to evaluate systemic changes.

Management

If a foreign body needs to be removed, it is easier to remove it from the crop or proventriculus rather than waiting until it is in the ventriculus or intestinal tract. Endoscopy, either through the mouth or via an ingluviotomy, can be used to remove foreign bodies in the crop or proventriculus.

A proventriculotomy can be used to remove foreign bodies in the proventriculus and ventriculus.

Smooth, nonpenetrating foreign bodies in the crop, proventriculus or ventriculus may be removed by flushing:

- Anaesthetize the patient, intubate and pack the choanal slit with gauze. Place the patient in either ventral or dorsal recumbency.
- Pass a flexible, large-bore feeding tube into the thoracic oesophagus through the exit from the crop in the right lateral dorsal corner of the thoracic inlet. This can be done blindly or with guidance from endoscopy.
- Tilt the bird head down at an angle of 30°.

- Flush the proventriculus gently and steadily with warmed saline. The flush can be allowed to run out or it can be aspirated with gentle suction.
- Collect the flush to identify and count the number of foreign bodies retrieved.
- Repeat the flush until all the foreign bodies have been retrieved.

NEOPLASIA
Definition/overview
The most common gastrointestinal neoplasia are papillomas associated with IPD (see below, Disorders of the cloaca) and gastric carcinomas, found at the proventricular–ventricular junction. Death from gastric neoplasia may be due to haemorrhage, gastric perforation and sepsis or endotoxic shock, or anorexia and subsequent catabolism.

Diagnosis
Diagnosis is by radiography, endoscopic biopsy or autopsy.

DISORDERS OF THE INTESTINAL TRACT
ILEUS
Definition/overview
Ileus is decreased motility or complete stasis of the intestinal tract.

Aetiology
Causes include foreign body obstruction, decreased or absent neurological function (e.g. lead toxicosis, PDD), enteritis, peritonitis, pancreatic disease (e.g. zinc toxicosis) and intussusception or torsion of the intestine.

Clinical presentation
Clinical signs include regurgitation, dehydration, lethargy and decreased faecal output.

Diagnosis
Radiography shows fluid or gas-filled loops of intestine, often with proventricular dilation.

Management
Dehydration should be corrected, and causative factors identified and rectified. Motility enhancers such as cisapride and metoclopramide may be of assistance.

PARASITES
Ascarids (roundworms)
Definition/overview
Species identified include *Ascaridia hermaphrodita*, *A. columbae* (shared between pigeons and psittacines),

A. galli (shared between gallinaceous birds and psittacines) and *A. platycercii* (restricted to psittacines). They are seen in birds with access to the ground, and are particularly common in budgerigars, cockatiels, quaker parrots and princess parrots.

Pathophysiology
The worms are found in the small intestine of the affected bird, particularly in the duodenal loop (**185**). They have a direct life cycle.

Clinical presentation
Clinical signs include lethargy, poor condition, diarrhoea and death.

Diagnosis
Diagnosis is by faecal examination (**186**).

Management
Most anthelmintics are effective. Ascarids are resistant to disinfectants and susceptible to desiccation, steam and flames.

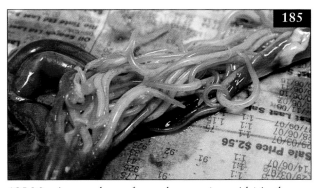

185 Massive numbers of roundworms (ascarids) in the duodenal loop.

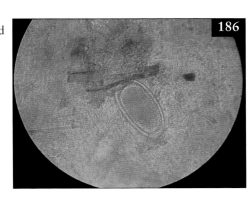

186 Ascarid egg in a faecal smear.

Capillaria (hair worm, thread worm)
Definition/overview
Species identified include *Capillaria annulata*, *C. contorta* (causes pseudomembrane formation in the oesophagus and crop [see above]) and *C. obsignata* (found in small intestine).

Pathophysiology
Capillaria imbed in mucosa, causing a marked thickening and inflammation of either the crop or the intestinal mucosa. The worms have a direct or indirect life cycle, using insect vectors. Eggs are infective in two weeks. They can remain infectious in the environment for several months.

Clinical presentation
Signs include anorexia, dysphagia, diarrhoea and weight loss.

Diagnosis
Faecal examination reveals a double-operculated egg.

Management
Ivermectin, moxidectin or levamisole can be used. Anthelmintic response needs to be monitored, as resistance is common. Access to insect vectors should be controlled.

Heterakis (caecal worm)
Definition/overview
Species identified include *Heterakis isolonche* in quail and *H. gallinarum*, which affects gallinaceous birds.

Pathophysiology
The life cycle is indirect, through earthworms.

Clinical presentation
There are usually no clinical signs, but the worms are significant because they transmit *Histomonas* spp. (see below).

Management
Most anthelmintics can be used. If possible, access to intermediate hosts should be controlled.

Cestodes (tapeworms)
Definition/overview
Species identified include *Raillietaenia*, *Choanotaenia*, *Gastronemia*, *Idiogenes* and *Amoebotaenia*. Tapeworms are commonly found in finches and Old World psittacines (African grey parrots, cockatoos, lorikeets and eclectus parrots). The life cycle is indirect. It may be complete in 3–4 weeks. Intermediate hosts include grasshoppers, beetles, ants, horseflies, earthworms, slugs, snails and crayfish.

Clinical presentation
Signs include catarrhal enteritis, emaciation and anorexia.

Diagnosis
Diagnosis is based on the finding, on faecal examination, of oncospheres (tapeworm embryos with six hooks).

Management
Praziquantel and fenbendazole may be used. Exposure to intermediate hosts should be controlled.

Coccidia
Definition/overview
Species identified are numerous, but include *Eimeria*, *Isospora* and *Caryospora* spp. This parasite tends to be host specific.
- *Isospora* oocysts have two sporocysts, each with four sporozoites. They are most common in parrots, passerines and Piciformes.
- *Eimeria* oocysts have four sporocysts, each with two sporozoites. They are most common in Galliformes and Columbiformes.
- *Caryospora* oocytes have one sporocyst and eight sporozoites. They are most common in raptors.

Pathophysiology
The life cycle is direct. The bird ingests the sporulated oocysts lying in its environment. Oocysts undergo schizogony in the intestine (asexual reproduction, producing multiple parts). If the schizonts produced are deep in the intestinal mucosa, they may damage the mucosa when they divide, causing enteritis. After schizogony, they differentiate into male (microgametocytes) and female (macrogametocytes) forms. They then undergo sexual reproduction (gametocytic), which is nonpathogenic. This produces nonsporulated oocysts, which are shed in faeces. Oocysts sporulate in a warm, moist environment to become infective.

Coccidia require 6–8 days to complete the life cycle, with clinical signs seen 4–6 days after infection.

Clinical presentation
Affected birds may not show clinical signs until stressed. Signs include lethargy, weight loss, diarrhoea (sometimes with blood and mucus), dirty vents and death.

Diagnosis

Oocysts can be found in faeces on smear and/or flotation. Note that clinical signs can be present before oocysts are detectable in the faeces.

Management

Anticoccidial treatments include amprolium, toltrazuril, ponzuril and sulphadimethoxine. Birds are treated daily for 2–3 days, then treatment is repeated after five days to treat those organisms that were in the prepatent period when the first treatment was given.

Access to infected faecal material is prevented by using concrete floors that are cleaned regularly, or having suspended wire floors. Food and water dishes should be kept off the ground.

Cryptosporidia
Definition/overview

Cryptosporidia are enteric coccidians that usually lie just inside the limiting membrane of the enterocytes. They can also attach to proventricular epithelium, the respiratory epithelium, the conjunctival sac, the urinary tract and the bursa. The oocysts are the smallest of any coccidia, with four naked sporozoites and no sporocysts in oocytes.

Pathophysiology

Cryptosporidia develop intracellularly at an extracytoplasmic location on the apical surface of the epithelial cells. They are often secondary pathogens. Although not very host specific, they appear to be infective only to other birds, not to mammals.

The life cycle is direct. The oocysts are sporulated when passed and, as such, are fully infective immediately.

Clinical presentation

Cryptosporidiosis is often asymptomatic. Clinical signs may include depression, dehydration, anorexia, persistent diarrhoea, malabsorption problems, abdominal pain, vomiting, coughing, sneezing and nasal discharge.

Diagnosis

Diagnosis is based on histopathology using modified (Kinyoun's) acid-fast stains. Infective cysts may be seen on faecal flotation.

Management

Treatment is with paromomycin sulphate.

Giardia
Definition/overview

Giardia has a wide geographic and host distribution. Its zoonotic potential is unclear. It has been reported in most avian species, although it has not been reported in finches and canaries. It has a direct life cycle, although cysts are shed only intermittently.

Clinical presentation

Signs include weight loss, depression, ruffled feathers and chronic diarrhoea. Persistent feather picking and pruritis may be seen in cockatiels (see Chapter 7, Disorders of the skin and feathers, p. 121). There are poor growth rates and neonatal mortality.

Diagnosis

Cysts or trophozoites can be detected in the faeces. As the trophozoites are not stable outside the bird, faecal examination should be performed on droppings within ten minutes of defecation.

Management

Nitroimidazoles are generally effective. Good hygiene is essential to break the life cycle. *Giardia* cysts may survive in chlorinated water, but are inactivated by quaternary ammonium compounds.

Cochlosoma
Definition/overview

Cochlosoma is a motile protozoan that is common in waterfowl and finches. In Australia it is common in cockatiels. Bengalese (society) finches can carry the parasite without clinical disease. It has a direct life cycle, with transmission due to the ingestion of infective trophozoites in faecal material and contaminated food and water.

Clinical presentation

Clinical signs include diarrhoea, weight loss and death.

Diagnosis

Diagnosis is made on examination of a fresh faecal smear.

Management

Drug resistance is common. Nitroimidazoles are used, but the treatment must be monitored for efficacy. Care must be taken when fostering gouldian finches with bengalese finches, as gouldians are very susceptible to this parasite.

Hexamita (*Spironucleus* spp.)
Definition/overview
This is a motile protozoa with eight flagella (six anterior and two trailing). It has been reported in pigeons (*Hexamita columbae*), game birds (*Hexamita meleagridis*), cockatiels, lorikeets, grass parrots and Australian king parrots. It has a direct life cycle. Concurrent disease and parasitism are common.

Clinical presentation
In pheasants and pigeons it is most commonly seen at 6–12 weeks of age. It causes decreased appetite, lethargy, emaciation and intractable diarrhoea.

Diagnosis
Diagnosis is made on examination of a fresh faecal smear; the parasite swims in a smooth linear fashion.

Management
Nitroimidazoles are used, but the treatment must be monitored for efficacy. Supportive therapy is essential, as many birds are hypoglycaemic on presentation.

Histomonas meleagridis
Definition/overview
Histomonas meleagridis is a motile protozoan that affects turkeys, quail, peacocks and pheasants. Chickens and guinea fowl may harbour latent infections. The disease in turkeys and peacocks is known as 'blackhead'. The life cycle is indirect, with transmission occurring through the ingestion of infected eggs of the caecal worm *Heterakis gallinarum*.

Clinical presentation
Clinical signs include weight loss, increased thirst, decreased appetite and brown–black to mustard-coloured diarrhoea. In chickens there may be blood in the droppings. There can be a high mortality rate, especially amongst juveniles.

Diagnosis
Diagnosis is based on clinical signs, identification of *Heterakis* eggs in droppings and autopsy findings (caecal cores [caecal necrosis] in game birds [this must be differentiated from coccidia and *Salmonella*] and hepatomegaly with multifocal yellow necrotic lesions).

Management
Treatment is with nitroimidazoles. Control of *Heterakis* is required (see above).

Microsporidiosis (encephalitozoonosis)
Definition/overview
Microsporidia sp. is an obligate intracellular protozoan, measuring only 1–2 µm, that is gram-positive and acid fast. It appears to have a direct life cycle, probably through oral transmission. The aerosol route is also thought to be feasible. *Encephalitozoon hellum* has been isolated from eclectus parrots, Amazons, lovebirds, budgerigars and finches. It has also been isolated from humans, so there is possibly a zoonotic potential.

Pathophysiology
There may be some element of immunosuppression involved in outbreaks (stress, overcrowding, concurrent disease [e.g. *Pasteurella*, PBFD]). Latent infections may exist.

Clinical presentation
Signs include anorexia, lethargy, weakness, diarrhoea, stunting, ruffled feathers, weight loss and neonatal mortality. Chronic conjunctivitis and sinusitis, as well as exophthalmos, corneal oedema and blepharospasm, were reported in a double yellow-headed Amazon parrot.

Diagnosis
PCR may be available. Histopathology using silver stain or acid-fast staining is necessary, as standard stains may not reveal the organism.

Management
Although not proven, microsporidiosis should be considered zoonotic.

Treatment is with albendazole (50 mg/kg orally q24h for 5 days).

MYCOBACTERIA
Definition/overview
Most avian infections are caused by *Mycobactrium avium* and *M. genevense*. *M. tuberculosis* and *M. bovis* are occasionally reported, but are considered rare.

Mycobacteriosis is most commonly an enteric infection, but it may be respiratory or disseminated. It is considered to be a leading infectious cause of avian deaths in many zoo parks with mixed species aviaries, where up to 14% of annual mortality can be attributed to mycobacteria.

Although not conclusively proven, it should be considered a potentially zoonotic disease.

Pathophysiology

Transmission is by ingestion of infected faeces, either directly or via contaminated food and water. Insects may act as mechanical vectors. Pulmonary disease by the aerogenous route is rare. The incubation period following infection can be months or years. Following ingestion, the mycobacteria penetrates the mucosa and colonizes under the serosa. It enters the blood supply and is removed from circulation by the liver, spleen and bone marrow. The lack of well developed regional lymph nodes in birds may be one reason for the ease with which this disease becomes systemic. Lesions therefore develop in the intestinal wall, liver, spleen and bone.

Clinical presentation

Weight loss and severe muscle atrophy are the most consistent clinical signs. Abdominal distension, hepatomegaly and dilated, fluid-filled, thickened intestines may be palpable. Lameness, due to arthritis or osteomyelitis, may be present. Nodular or diffuse keratinous skin lesions at the mucocutaneous junctions of the eyes and beak have been reported in parrots.

Diagnosis

Antemortem diagnosis in birds is difficult and often inconclusive, particularly in the early stages.

Diagnosis can be based on clinical signs, marked leukocytosis with monocytosis and elevations in AST and bile acids. Radiographs may show an enlarged liver, kidney and spleen, as well as focal, cloudy densities in the medullary cavities of long bones with osteolysis. Endoscopy and biopsy are used to confirm the diagnosis antemortem.

Faecal acid-fast stains may reveal the organism but, as it is only shed intermittently, this is not an effective screening tool. An intradermal test can indicate the presence of mycobacteria in a flock, but it is unreliable in an individual. It is probably unreliable in nonpoultry species. PCR performed on cloacal swabs may have value, but the results must be interpreted with caution. False positives and false negatives are not uncommon.

Autopsy usually reveals granulomas in the liver (187), spleen and subserosa of the intestinal tract. There may be hepatomegaly, splenomegaly and enlarged, thickened intestines.

Histopathology shows a spectrum of lesions from nodules of large foamy histiocytes packed with acid-fast bacilli to giant cell-containing granulomas that

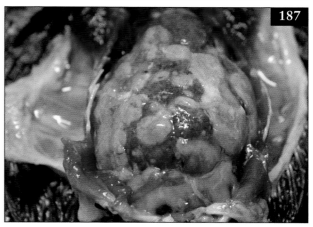

187 Mycobacterial infection in a parrot, showing disseminated granulomas throughout the liver.

are often caseous but not cavitated or calcified. Amyloidosis is seen in approximately 20% of cases.

Management

Consideration must be given to whether to treat because of the possible zoonotic implications.

Resistance develops rapidly, therefore combinations of drugs must be used. Treatment must be given for nine months or more, as the organism is only susceptible when replicating, which occurs every 16–20 hours, and even less in caseated lesions. One should aim to achieve the highest possible blood levels, not consistent levels, therefore once daily dosing is used. Commonly used combinations include isoniazid, ethambutol, rifampin and enrofloxacin.

Mycobacteria are resistant to typical physical and chemical destruction. They can survive for months to years in the environment.

BACTERIAL ENTERITIS

Several bacteria are commonly implicated in bacterial enteritis in birds. Most are secondary pathogens, although some can be primary. They include *E. coli*, *Clostridium* spp., *Salmonella* spp. and *Chlamydophila psittaci* (see Chapter 14, Disorders of the liver, p. 178). Many other species of bacteria can be involved, usually as secondary invaders.

Treatment is based on bacterial culture and sensitivity, and identification and elimination of predisposing factors and concurrent disease.

Escherichia coli

Definition/overview

E. coli is a gram-negative, nonspore-forming bacillus. It has a worldwide distribution and is a normal inhabitant of mammalian gastrointestinal tracts. Most *E. coli* strains produce endotoxins.

E. coli can be isolated from clinically normal parrots. It is debatable whether the isolation of *E. coli* from the cloaca of clinically normal parrots indicates a definitive pathogen, a potential pathogen or a commensal organism, or is merely transient. It is more common in cockatoos than in other psittacines.

Aetiology

Infection with *E. coli* is primarily the result of inadequate hygiene and faecal contamination of water sources, food, perches, floors and the general environment.

Clinical presentation

Signs vary from chronic diarrhoea to severe generalized septicaemia (lethargy, anorexia, weakness, ruffled feathers, diarrhoea and death). *E. coli* can also cause respiratory infections, infertility, ingluvitis and arthritis.

Clostridium spp.

Definition/overview

The clostridial organisms found in birds include *Clostridium perfringens* types A and C, *C. colinum* and *C. tertium*. They are anaerobic gram-positive bacilli.

Pathophysiology

An abrupt change in diet may disrupt the intestinal microflora, allowing clostridia to proliferate in the upper intestine. They can cause necrotic enteritis, 'gangrenous dermatitis' and malignant oedema.

Clinical presentation

Clostridial infection is often seen in juvenile cockatoos with concurrent enteric problems; they produce a characteristic foul-smelling diarrhoea.

Diagnosis

Spore-forming bacteria are seen on faecal Gram stains. Severe necrosis and petechial haemorrhages are found in the mucosa of the duodenum and jejunum.

Management

Addition of apple cider vinegar (10 ml/litre of water) has been effective in treating juvenile cockatoos with a simple enteritis. Penicillin derivatives and metronidazole are usually effective in more severe cases.

Salmonella spp.

Definition/overview

Salmonellae are a (usually) motile, gram-negative bacteria. *Salmonella* spp. are members of the family Enterobacteriaceae. There are over 2,100 serotypes, including the Arizona group. There are five subgenera; subgenus I is the most important to birds. Subgenus III (*S. arizonae*, *S. hinshawii*) is occasionally reported in birds, especially those in contact with reptiles. Two organisms are host specific and nonmotile: *S. pullorum* (pullorum disease) and *S. gallinarum* (fowl typhoid). *S. typhimurium* is the most common psittacine isolate. It is also the most common isolate in human beings with salmonellosis, making it important as a zoonosis.

Pathophysiology

Faeces of chronically infected carrier birds (often asymptomatic) are one of the most common sources of infection. Salmonellae can survive for extended periods in organic matter, faeces and dirt (up to two years). Ingestion of contaminated food or water or direct contact by aerosolization of faecal or feather dust is the most common mode of transmission.

Improper husbandry and sanitation can spread the infection through the contamination of seed, fruits, vegetables, drinking water and food containers.

Salmonella spp. can be a primary pathogen; some serotypes can penetrate the mucosal barrier. Virulent strains can penetrate intact intestinal mucosa, while nonvirulent strains require a mucosal lesion to enter the host. The incubation period can be as short as 3–5 days in acute cases.

Clinical presentation

The disease can be peracute, acute, chronic or subclinical depending on the number of organisms, their serotype and the age, species and condition of the host. Clinical signs include depression, lethargy, anorexia, weight loss, diarrhoea, a soiled vent, dehydration and crop stasis. Lameness and wing droop are associated with septic arthritis (swollen joints). In breeding birds with subclinical infections, there is often poor hatching or excessive fledgling mortality. Neurological signs may be seen, including convulsions.

Diagnosis

Diagnosis is based on autopsy findings: hepatomegaly, splenomegaly, air sacculitis and pulmonary congestion, caecal cores (caecal necrosis) in game birds, ulcerative enteritis, orchitis and oophoritis.

Bacteria are present on histological sections and there is focal necrosis in the affected organ, with organisms found within the necrotic areas. Culture of the digestive tract or liver sections, and faecal culture can be used for organism identification.

Antemortem diagnosis can be difficult because of intermittent shedding. A serological test is available for poultry.

Management

Antibiotics are given based on culture and sensitivity. Treatment must be given for 3–8 weeks.

Control of vectors (wild birds, rodents) and prevention of contamination of food and water are required. Good hygiene practices must be implemented. A vaccine is available for pigeons, but it may not be fully protective. Birds should be vaccinated four weeks prior to a show or race season. Autogenous vaccines may be produced from faecal cultures.

DISORDERS OF THE CLOACA
PROLAPSE
Aetiology
Cloacal prolapse can be caused by excessive straining: masturbatory behaviour in male cockatoos, sexual overwork in waterfowl and ratites, oviductal disease (egg binding, salpingitis), increased intra-abdominal pressure (fluid, organomegaly), cloacal disease (cloacoliths, cloacitis, IPD) or constipation or diarrhoea.

It may also be related to loss of cloacal tone, as a result of spinal cord disease or chronic trauma.

Clinical presentation
There is protrusion of the cloacal mucosa, with or without rectum or oviduct, through the lips of the vent (188). Phallic prolapse may be seen in waterfowl and ratites.

Cloacal prolapse is usually accompanied by straining and grunting while defecating, and blood around the vent or in the droppings. If the prolapse has been long-standing, the prolapsed tissue may be oedematous and superficially necrotic.

Diagnosis
Small prolapses need to be differentiated from papillomas (see below).

Management
Initial treatment is to stabilize the patient (if required), reduce the prolapse, hold it in place and treat any swelling and damage to the cloacal mucosa until the aetiology can be determined.

Under general anaesthesia, the prolapsed tissue is gently cleaned and (if possible) what is prolapsed is

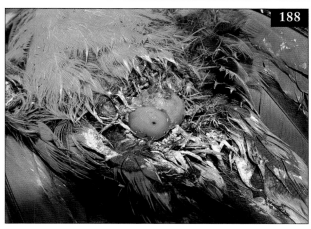

188 Prolapsed cloaca in a king parrot hen.

identified (cloaca, rectum or oviduct). If the prolapse is oedematous, the swelling can be reduced with the osmotic effect of sugar or glucose poured on to the mucosa. Once the cloaca is clean and normal sized, the prolapse should be gently reduced. Moistened cotton buds can be used to return the tissue to its normal anatomical position and it can be flushed with saline to inflate it and clean it. Instilling 1–2 ml of silver sulphadiazine cream has both a soothing and an antibacterial effect. As the vent is elongated rather than rounded, a purse-string suture is not recommended. Instead, one to two vertical mattress or simple interrupted sutures should be placed on both sides of the vent in order to reduce the size of the vent opening. This opening must be sufficiently large to allow the bird to defecate and urinate.

The cause of the prolapse is identified through a thorough history and physical examination, haematology and biochemistry, cloacal culture (caution must be taken interpreting this, as the possibility of contamination is high), whole body radiographs or cloacal endoscopy with/without biopsy.

Follow-up treatment is aimed at minimizing the possibility of recurrent prolapses by eliminating or minimizing the impact of the inciting cause and performing surgery to maintain the cloaca in place (cloacopexy or ventplasty) (see Chapter 26, Surgery, p. 263).

Long-term follow-up on cloacal prolapses indicates a reasonably high degree of recurrence, regardless of the techniques used. This must be communicated to the client before commencing any treatment.

INTERNAL PAPILLOMA DISEASE
Aetiology
The causative virus is psittacid herpesvirus 1 (PsHV1) genotypes 1, 2 and 3. This is the same virus that causes Pacheco's disease. It is thought that some birds with internal papilloma disease (IPD) have survived an initial episode of Pacheco's disease. PsHV1 genotype 3 may spread within a flock without causing overt disease, but result in IPD.

Pathophysiology
IPD has been reported mainly in macaws (green-winged, blue and gold, great green, scarlet, severe and military), Amazon parrots, conures and hawk head parrots. It has also been reported in cockatiels, budgerigars and African grey parrots, although the virus may not have been PsHV1.

The mode of transmission is unclear. Close contact appears to be essential. There is no evidence of egg transmission, although parent-reared chicks with IPD-positive parents have developed the disease.

Clinical presentation
The clinical signs depend on the site of the papilloma development:
* Cloacal. Often the first signs noticed are straining to defecate, pasting of the vent and blood on the droppings. The bird may develop enteritis and cloacoliths. There may be a red mass protruding from the cloaca (**189**). Cloacal examination reveals papillomatous lesions ('cobblestone' appearance). These will blanch with the application of 5% acetic acid (vinegar), but the appearance of the lesions is characteristic and blanching is not necessary.
* Oropharynx. Clinical signs of papillomas are rare, but may include dysphagia, dyspnoea, wheezing, anorexia and weight loss.

Lesions can extend into the oesophagus and crop, but rarely, if ever, into the proventriculus or ventriculus. Extension into the intestinal tract, nasal mucosa and nasolacrimal duct is extremely rare. Some birds may ultimately develop bile duct or pancreatic carcinomas, but this is variable.

Diagnosis
Gross findings are usually sufficient for diagnosis.

Cloacal or choanal biopsy shows a characteristic histological picture. There is proliferation of undifferentiated columnar epithelial cells arranged in a pseudostratified fashion, forming fronds of villi and papillae on a thin fibrovascular stalk.

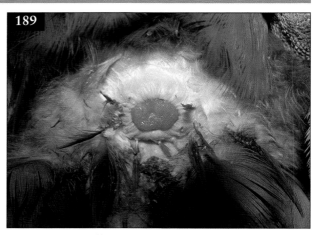

189 Internal papilloma disease affecting the cloacal mucosa.

Elevations in GGT may indicate development of bile duct carcinomas. (This may not be reliable in Amazon parrots.) AST and ALT remain unchanged. Ultrasonography may detect bile duct carcinomas before endoscopy.

A PsHV1 PCR is now available. All birds with papillomas will be positive on PCR, therefore there is only the need to test if the patient presents as an unusual presentation or when screening asymptomatic or in-contact birds.

Management
A variety of techniques have been tried for the removal of papillomas: cauterization with silver nitrate; cryosurgery; surgical debridement with radiosurgery or laser; cloacal mucosal stripping; imiquimod (Aldara) application (an interferon-immune response modifier). Mixed results have been obtained at this time.

Most birds initially respond to treatment, but later regress. Aggressive surgical debridement may result in strictures and should be reserved for severe cases only. Debridement of a small area may stimulate a (temporary) immune response and regression of the lesions.

CLOACOLITHS
Definition/overview
These are dried concretions of faecal material and urates in the urodeum or proctodeum. They are often adhered to the cloacal wall and, in extreme cases, can cause obstipation and intermittent ureter obstruction.

Clinical presentation
Signs include straining to defecate, decreased faecal output and fresh blood in droppings and around the vent. A flatulent sound is occasionally heard.

Diagnosis
Diagnosis is based on clinical signs and palpation of the cloaca. Radiography often reveals the cloacolith. Cloacal endoscopy may be used.

Management
Mild cases may respond to lubrication and gentle pressure to break the cloacolith into small pieces. Severe cases may require a cloacotomy to relieve the obstruction (see Chapter 26, Surgery, p. 264). Supportive care, especially fluid therapy and anti-inflammatory treatment, is essential.

CLOACAL ATONY
Aetiology
Cloacal atony can be due to loss of neurological innervation to the cloaca (spinal cord dysfunction or PDD) or loss of muscular strength of the cloacal sphincter. The latter may be a result of soft tissue trauma and swelling associated with egg laying, systemic illness and weakness or chronic cloacal disease (recurrent prolapses, cloacitis).

Clinical presentation
Signs include a flaccid appearing vent, faecal accumulation around the vent and loss of cloacal tone. When a normal cloaca is stimulated lightly with a cotton bud, the sphincter should close (in a manner similar to anal tone in a mammal). Faecal material, usually in large amounts, is easily expressed from the cloaca on palpation.

Management
Treatment includes NSAIDs and regular expression of the cloaca. Ventplasty may be necessary to reduce the size of the vent and prevent a prolapse.

CLOACITIS
Aetiology
Inflammation of the cloaca can be due to cloacal atony (see above), a retained egg in the distal oviduct, bacterial infection or trauma.

Clinical presentation
Signs include tenesmus, fresh blood in the droppings and faecal pasting around the vent.

Diagnosis
Cloacitis must be differentiated from IPD, cloacoliths and cloacal prolapse. Endoscopy, with or without biopsy, can help to determine the cause and nature of the cloacitis.

Management
Treatment includes NSAIDs and topical application of silver sulphadiazine cream into the cloaca. Topical flurbiprofen eye drops may assist when the pericloacal area is very inflamed.

NEOPLASIA
Definition/overview
Carcinomas, smooth muscle tumours and haemangiomas have been reported in the cloaca of birds.

Clinical presentation
Neoplasms produce similar signs to IPD and cloacitis.

Diagnosis
Biopsy is necessary to achieve an accurate diagnosis.

Management
A cloacotomy can be performed to resect a mass if necessary.

FURTHER READING

Doneley RJT, Miller RI, Fanning TE (2007) Proventricular dilatation disease: an emerging exotic disease of parrots in Australia. *Australian Veterinary Journal* 85:119–123.

Gelis S (2006) Evaluating and treating the gastrointestinal system. In: *Clinical Avian Medicine, Vol 1*. GJ Harrison, TL Lightfoot (eds). Spix Publishing Inc, Palm Beach, pp. 411–440.

Hadley TL (2005) Disorders of the psittacine gastrointestinal tract. *Gastroenterology*. TK Ritzman (ed.) *Veterinary Clinics of North America: Exotic Animal Practice* 8(**2**):329–350.

Hoefer HL (1997) Diseases of the gastrointestinal tract. In: *Avian Medicine and Surgery*. RB Altman, *et al.* (eds). WB Saunders, Philadelphia, pp. 419–453.

Reavill D (2007) Lesions of the proventriculus/ventriculus of pet birds: 1640 cases. In: *Proceedings of the Annual Conference of the Association of Avian Veterinarians*, pp. 89–94.

Chapter 14

Disorders of the liver

OVERVIEW OF LIVER DISEASE
Aetiology
Congenital

Extrahepatic biliary cysts have been reported in an African grey parrot. A congenital abdominal hernia involving the liver has been reported in Japanese quail.

Trauma

Trauma can cause tearing of the liver parenchyma and/or the capsule. This occurs when the bird is subjected to massive force (e.g. a moving motor vehicle) or when the liver is friable due to other problems (e.g. hepatic lipidosis). The severity of the liver rupture and resultant haemorrhage will determine whether the bird survives the initial trauma.

Metabolic/nutritional
Visceral gout

This is the deposition of uric acid crystals on and in organs. It is typically associated with renal disease, although dehydration and high-protein diets may be involved. In the liver, most of this deposition occurs on the capsule, but it can occur within the parenchyma where it is associated with necrosis and heterophilic inflammation.

Amyloidosis

Amyloidosis is most commonly seen in waterfowl and passerines. Amyloid A is a degradation product of inflammatory proteins and its deposition is commonly seen in birds with chronic disease. Affected livers are usually enlarged and friable and can be confused with hepatic lipidosis. Histologically, the amyloid is seen as a pale eosinophilic or amphophilic deposit between the cells, compressing them.

Hepatic lipidosis (fatty liver disease)

This occurs when excessive fatty acids are consumed (in the form of dietary fat), when there is increased lipolysis (e.g. diabetes mellitus or egg laying activity), decreased fatty acid oxidation in the liver, or when there is a decreased ability of the liver to secrete processed fatty acids back into the circulation (due to dietary deficiencies of lipotrophic factors such as choline, biotin and methionine). Affected livers are enlarged, pale yellow and friable. Histologically, there is vacuolation of the hepatocytes.

Iron storage disease (haemosiderosis)

This occurs when there is more iron in the circulation than is needed for erythrogenesis, allowing the iron to accumulate in the liver. It can result from excess iron intake, either dietary or via excessive blood transfusion. This condition is commonly seen in Sturnidae (mynahs, starlings), Paradisaeidae (birds of paradise), Ptyonorhynchidae (bowerbirds), Bucerotidae (hornbills) and Ramphastidae (toucans and toucanettes). It has also been reported in parrots, especially lories and lorikeets. Affected livers are enlarged and are usually golden-brown in colour, often with scattered dark foci. Iron can be seen histologically in the hepatocytes and Kupffer cells. There may be an associated inflammatory process with lymphocytes and occasional heterophils.

Lipofuscin

Lipofuscin pigment accumulates in hepatocytes secondary to a range of diseases. It is due to excessive biological oxidation at the cellular level. Vitamin E deficiency has been suggested as one possible cause.

Toxic

Toxic causes of liver disease include:
- Drugs: alcohol, dimetridazole, medroxyprogesterone.
- Plants: pyrrolizidine alkaloids, oleander, gossypol, avocado fruit.
- Aflatoxins, ergot.

- Heavy metals: lead, copper, iron.
- Pesticides: metaldehyde, phosphorus, vitamin D3 analogues.

Parasitic
Protozoa
Apicomplexa
Cryptosporidia may occasionally be found attached to biliary epithelium, causing proliferation of the epithelium and a mild chronic mononuclear reaction.

Atoxoplasma is primarily reported in passerines, especially canaries. It undergoes schizogony in the liver, causing a generalized inflammatory reaction composed of macrophages, plasma cells and lymphocytes. The organism may be found in macrophages and lymphocytes.

Birds infected with *Sarcocystis* and *Toxoplasma* are usually intermediate hosts. They produce a similar inflammatory reaction to *Atoxoplasma*. Organisms can be difficult to locate.

Haemoprotozoa
Plasmodium (avian malaria) is a widespread blood parasite. Some species, especially penguins, appear to be more susceptible. Schizogony occurs in the reticuloendothelial cells of many organs, with merozoites released to infect erythrocytes. Affected livers are enlarged, and in falcons often appear grey–black. There is infiltration of the liver with macrophages, plasma cells and lymphocytes, with the organism found in some of the inflammatory cells.

Haemoproteus is usually nonpathogenic, with schizonts occasionally found in the endothelial cells of the liver.

Leukocytozoon affects many species, with mortalities reported in ducks and geese. Where liver damage does occur it is usually acute and severe, with haemorrhage and necrosis, but minimal inflammation. Gametocytes can be found in peripheral blood smears.

Flagellates
Histomonas causes the disease known as blackhead in domestic poultry, especially peafowl and turkeys. It produces classical white–yellow granulomas throughout the liver parenchyma. The organism can be found in the lesions, although it may resemble macrophages and be difficult to detect.

Trichomonas is usually a gastrointestinal parasite, but heavy infections can spread to the liver. Necrotic lesions with the parasite found at the periphery are diagnostic.

Trematodes
Flukes of the family Dicrocoelidae inhabit the bile duct of many avian species, including psittacines, Anseriformes, Ramphastidae and ratites. Wandering flukes may be found in dilated bile ducts, and schistosomes can be found in dilated sinusoids. There is usually minimal inflammation unless there are degenerating eggs present. *Fasciola* flukes in emus provoke an eosinophilic response, with macrophages and lymphocytes present. Granulomas may form with giant cells and fibrosis.

Nematodes
Intestinal nematode larvae can migrate through the liver causing extensive fibrosis, bile duct hyperplasia and inflammatory cell infiltrates.

Infectious
Bacteria
Both gram-positive and gram-negative bacteria can cause liver disease, usually secondary to septicaemia or enteritis. *Salmonella* spp., *E. coli*, *Pseudomonas* spp., *Yersinia* spp. and *Campylobacter* spp. are common isolates. Affected livers are usually swollen, with grey–white foci throughout the parenchyma. Multifocal hepatocyte necrosis with a heterophilic inflammatory response is usually seen. Bacteria are usually seen in macrophages and Kupffer's cells. Additionally, endotoxins arising from bacterial enteritis can enter the portal circulation, damaging the periportal hepatocytes.

Viruses
Herpesvirus has been isolated from nearly all species of birds. Serotypes involved include Pacheco's disease virus (see below), pigeon herpesvirus, owl herpesvirus, falcon herpesvirus, crane herpesvirus, stork herpesvirus, quail herpesvirus and finch herpesvirus. Other strains of herpesvirus, while not specifically attacking the liver, may produce some degree of hepatic damage. Affected livers are enlarged, with variable yellow–grey mottling and haemorrhage. Histologically there is acute necrosis with variable inflammation, syncytial cell formation and intranuclear inclusion bodies.

Polyomavirus is primarily recovered from psittacines and finches, but may affect a range of birds. Affected livers are enlarged and friable, with the degree of severity often varying according to the species. There is multifocal or mid-zonal necrosis and haemorrhage, with characteristic inclusion bodies in the Kupffer cells.

Adenovirus rarely causes clinical disease unless there are other immunosuppressive factors at work. Many species of birds are affected including psittacines, poultry, pigeons and ostriches. Affected livers are discoloured, with scattered yellow–grey areas present (**190**). There is multifocal necrosis and haemorrhage, nonsuppurative cholangitis and large basophilic intranuclear inclusion bodies in the hepatocytes.

Paramyxovirus causes hepatomegaly in isolated cases, but its primary effects are neurological, gastrointestinal and respiratory. Histologically there is a lymphoplasmocytic infiltrate in the periportal area.

Circovirus is occasionally seen as an acute disease in young birds. In these birds, and in some adults with severe feather changes, there may be a mild necrosis and a lymphohistiocytic inflammatory reaction in the portal areas (**191**). Inclusion bodies can be seen in the Kupffer's cells.

Reovirus has been recovered from psittacines, Galliformes, Anseriformes, raptors, pigeons and chickens. Affected livers are enlarged with scattered grey–white or yellow foci. Histologically there is hepatocellular necrosis with minimal inflammation. Hepadnavirus is the cause of duck viral hepatitis, resulting in hepatic necrosis and periportal inflammation. Togavirus (eastern equine encephalitis) causes enlarged livers with some necrosis in many species of birds.

Fungi

Fungal infections involving the liver are usually opportunistic spread from other sites within the body. *Aspergillus* spp. affecting nearby air sacs have been reported to invade the liver locally, causing hepatic necrosis.

Chlamydophila

The obligate intracellular bacterium *Chlamydophila psittaci* is a common cause of liver disease in all species of birds. Affected livers are enlarged, discoloured and may show grey–yellow foci of necrosis. There is multifocal to confluent necrosis with a mononuclear inflammatory reaction. Organisms may be found in macrophages and hepatocytes (see pp. 178–181).

Mycobacteria

Mycobacterial infection in birds is primarily a gastrointestinal infection, with caseated tubercles occurring in the intestinal mucosa and the liver (**192**). Histologically, early lesions are comprised primarily of heterophils and macrophages, with only a few microorganisms. As the lesions progress, large epitheloid macrophages containing mycobacteria appear. These are best seen with an acid-fast stain

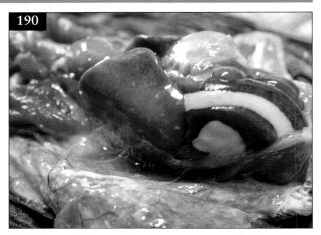

190 Adenoviral hepatitis seen on necropsy of a juvenile Malabar parrot.

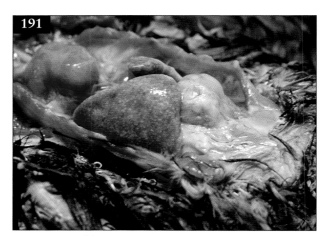

191 Circoviral hepatitis in a juvenile black cockatoo.

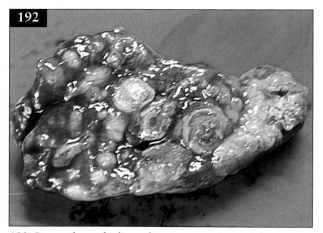

192 Cut surface of a liver showing mycobacterial granulomas.

(see Chapter 13, Disorders of the gastrointestinal tract, p. 167).

Rickettsia

Aegyptianella pullorum causes hepatitis in many species of birds, especially in the Mediterranean region. Intra-erythrocytic inclusion bodies can be seen with Giemsa stain.

Neoplastic

Hepatic neoplasia is usually primary, although metastatic neoplasia can occur. Primary bile duct tumours are more common than hepatocellular tumours. In psittacines these may be associated with IPD.

Idiopathic

Sometimes referred to as 'hepatopathy', 'chronic active hepatitis' or 'hepatic cirrhosis', this is a common condition in many species of birds. No one single cause has been identified, and it is probably multifactorial, possibly involving an immune-mediated component. Affected livers are often shrunken, pale and fibrotic. In the early stages of the disease there is hepatic vacuolization, a pleocellular inflammatory infiltrate in the periportal areas, bile duct proliferation and mild fibrosis. As the condition progresses, the fibrosis worsens and diffuse biliary hyperplasia develops (**193**).

CLINICAL SIGNS

Clinical signs seen in birds with liver disease can reflect any or all of the following malfunctions.

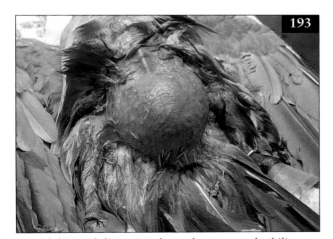

193 Abdominal distension due to hepatomegaly (biliary hyperplasia).

Cholestasis

Swelling of the hepatocytes and inflammatory infiltrates can cause occlusion of the biliary system. This results in the increased retention of bile and subsequent rise of serum bile pigment levels. Because of the lack of biliverdin reductase, it is uncommon for birds to produce bilirubin. Icterus is therefore uncommon in birds. However, increased levels of biliverdin in the blood due to cholestasis will result in biliverdin-stained urates and urine, giving these waste products a green discoloration. Decreased bile secretion into the intestine can result in maldigestion (weight loss, diarrhoea).

Inadequate conversion of ammonia to uric acid and urea

Failure to convert ammonia to uric acid and, to a lesser extent, urea leads to increased serum levels of ammonia and the onset of hepatic encephalopathy. Signs include weakness, depression, personality changes, behavioural disturbances, seizures and paresis. This is uncommon in granivorous birds because of the lack of dietary encephalopathic precursors.

Protein synthesis deficits

Inadequate production of clotting factors can lead to coagulopathies. This can be as subtle as mild haemorrhages in the rhinotheca or as dramatic as sudden death due to internal haemorrhaging. Decreased synthesis of ceruloplasmin can result in decreased iron mobilization and subsequent anaemia. Decreased albumin can be one factor in the development of ascites.

Abnormal carbohydrate and fat metabolism

Hypoglycaemia, weight loss and debility are frequently seen in birds with severe liver disease. Nutritional deficiencies resulting from liver disease may be the cause of the dermatological signs seen in affected birds. These include feather loss, skin changes and overgrown beaks and nails (**145**).

Failure of Kupffer's cell activity

Endotoxaemia and bacteriaemia may develop when the Kupffer's cells are unable to perform their function correctly.

Portal hypertension

Increased blood pressure within the sinusoids can result in the development of ascites, as oedema in the liver results in the movement of a modified transudate out of the liver into the peritoneal cavity.

Inadequate or inappropriate metabolism of drugs and chemicals

Decreased ability of the hepatocytes to modify or metabolize drugs and chemicals can lead to unexpected aberrant responses to administered drugs.

Other clinical signs

These result from other, less obvious, processes:

- Bile salts deposited in the skin may be the cause of some of the apparent pruritis seen in birds with liver disease.
- Pain from the stretching of the capsule over an enlarged liver can cause feather picking over the torso.
- Occlusion of the space normally occupied by the air sac by either the liver or ascites can result in dyspnoea.

DIAGNOSIS
Clinical pathology

See Chapter 4, Interpreting diagnostic tests.

Haematology, serum biochemistries

Test include plasma protein, enzymes (AST, CK, LDH, glutamate dehydrogenase [GDH], GGT), liver function tests (bile acids) and abdominocentesis. Ascites arising from liver disease is usually a modified transudate.

Diagnostic imaging
Radiography

Two views are required: lateral and ventrodorsal. Positioning is important; on the lateral view the two acetabulae should be superimposed, and on the ventrodorsal view the centre of the sternum (seen as a dark line) should be superimposed on the vertebrae. Both the size of the liver and the displacement of nearby organs should be examined.

Lateral view

On the lateral view the liver should not extend past the end of the sternum, and the proventriculus should slope down towards the ventriculus at an angle of 30–45°. There should be little or no space between the heart and the liver.

Ventrodorsal view

On the ventrodorsal view the liver shadow should not extend past a line joining the shoulder and acetabulum. Care must be taken in interpreting this view that the cardiac shadow or the proventriculus is not confused with liver.

Ultrasonography

This offers several advantages over radiography, in that it allows examination of the internal structure of the liver as well as examination of the nearby heart and pericardium, spleen and gastrointestinal tract. The avian liver is homogeneous, finely granular and contains transverse and longitudinal blood vessels throughout the parenchyma. The gall bladder, when present, lies to the right of the midline. Changes in echogenicity and size of the liver should be noted.

Endoscopy and biopsy

After using clinical pathology and diagnostic imaging to focus on the liver as the source of the patient's problem, the next step is to assess accurately the aetiology and pathophysiology of the disease process. To do this requires invasive technology; endoscopy to visually assess the liver and a biopsy to examine the histological basis of the problem. Several approaches have been described: through an incision behind the caudal ribs on either side; through the caudal thoracic air sac; and through a ventral midline incision (**194**).

TREATMENT

Treatment of an avian patient with confirmed liver disease should have three objectives: support of the patient and correction of the abnormalities caused by the liver disease; treatment of the specific condition; and creation of an environment within the liver most favourable to regeneration of normal liver tissue.

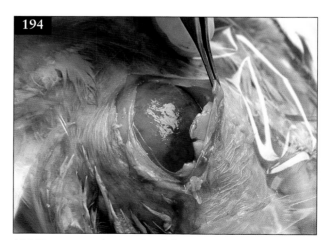

194 Hepatomegaly visualized during an exploratory laparotomy.

Support

Problems include dehydration, anorexia, weight loss, hypoglycaemia, hepatic encephalopathy, anaemia, septicaemia, dyspnoea (enlarged liver and/or ascites), bleeding disorders and diarrhoea.

Management

Fluid therapy is generally required. Blood transfusions can be used to treat both anaemia and coagulopathies.

Diet

Protein levels in the diet should be increased to allow for anabolic regeneration of the liver, but there may be the need to increase protein tolerance by feeding high-quality protein and the use of lactulose (in carnivorous birds). Diets high in simple and complex carbohydrates (such as vegetables, rice and pasta) offer many advantages to patients with liver disease. Vegetable protein appears to lack many encephalopathic components; the higher fibre alters the intestinal flora to minimize ammonia production; carbohydrate metabolism is useful for hypoglycaemic patients; and insoluble fibre (e.g. pysillium) binds many endotoxins and noxious bile acids. Fat levels in the diet can be left untouched unless cholestasis causes a maldigestion problem with subsequent diarrhoea, or in cases of hepatic lipidosis. Conversion to a formulated diet achieves all of these requirements and is the cornerstone of treatment for liver disease.

Vitamin supplementation may be given, but caution is needed with vitamins A and D to prevent toxicosis.

Treatment of the specific condition
Amyloidosis

Therapy for amyloidosis is aimed at correcting the underlying problem. Colchicine has been used in dogs to minimize further deposition and may be of use in birds. Other treatments used in humans and dogs have included immunosuppressive therapy, chemotherapy and dimethyl sulfoxide (DMSO) (oral or subcutaneous). No reliable treatment has been shown to work in all cases, and success is limited.

Hepatic lipidosis

Hepatic lipidosis in birds is most commonly due to the feeding of a high-fat, low-protein diet, where the fat becomes the major source of calories. All-seed diets are a typical example of this sort of diet, but hepatic lipidosis occurs in most avian species Treatment requires a reduction of dietary fat and an increase in dietary protein, as well as the provision of carbohydrates to replace fat as the main source of calories. Anorectic patients may need force feeding with such a diet until their catabolic state is reversed. Protein should not be restricted unless encephalopathy is present. Fluid therapy will be necessary for anorectic patients. Vitamin E (as an antioxidant) and B complex vitamins may also be beneficial.

Iron storage disease

Most cases of iron storage disease are believed to be associated with a high-iron diet. Treatment consists of feeding a low-iron diet, minimizing the absorption of iron from the intestinal tract and reducing the level of iron in the body. As the ascorbic acid found in citrus fruit reduces the ferric ion (Fe^{3+}) to the more easily absorbed ferrous ion (Fe^{2+}), citrus fruit should be eliminated from the diet. Commercial diets for susceptible species (Ramphastidae and mynahs) are now made with low iron levels (<100 ppm). Tannin added to the diet also binds iron in the intestine, reducing absorption. Iron levels in the body are reduced by weekly phlebotomy (1% bodyweight) and chelation therapy with deferoxamine.

Parasitic

Drugs used to treat hepatic protozoan infections are the same as those used for intestinal or systemic infections. Trematode infections are often difficult to treat. Praziquantel has been shown to reduce egg laying, but may not eliminate the parasite itself. Albendazole has been shown to eliminate *Fasciola hepatica* infections in emus.

Infections

Bacterial, fungal, viral, mycobacterial and chlamydial infections all have different treatments, according to the isolate and its sensitivity.

Neoplastic

Up until recently, hepatic neoplasia has been considered untreatable. Recent work suggests that some neoplasms may well respond to chemotherapy, and drugs such as carboplatin and cisplatin are been trialled for their efficacy.

Creation of an environment favourable to regeneration

Given the liver's ability to regenerate, treatment to maintain the acinar structure and minimize fibrosis will have a positive effect in patients with liver disease. Several drugs have been trialled in mammals to achieve these aims, and they show potential in avian medicine.

Ursodeoxycholic acid

Ursodeoxycholic acid (UDCA) is used as an adjunct in the treatment of cholestatic and necro-inflammatory liver disorders. Its use as a single agent therapy in mammals is relatively ineffective. Some of its effects include modifying the spectrum of noxious bile acids accumulating in the liver and blood of liver patients, thus minimizing their toxic effect on hepatocytes, a direct cytoprotective effect and minimizing the recruitment of hepatocytes and biliary epithelium into an inflammatory process.

Colchicine

Colchicine is used as an antifibrotic drug, although it does not appear to restrict the development of fibrosis. It is used concurrently with UDCA. Its effects include induction of collagenase activity, an anti-inflammatory effect and facilitation of excretion of hepatic copper.

Silibinin

Silibinin, the extract from milk thistle, is frequently recommended as a therapy for avian disease. To date, there are no proven benefits in its use, but experimental work in mammals indicates that it may have several effects: antioxidant; enhances protein synthesis and hepatocellular regeneration; protective effect against hepatotoxins; suppresses fibrogenesis; and promotes fibrolysis.

CHLAMYDIOSIS

Aetiology

As of 2000, the causative organism has been classified as a gram-negative, nonmotile, obligate intracellular bacteria of the order Chlamydiales, family Chlamydiaceae. There are two genera, *Chlamydia* and *Chlamydophila*. *Chlamydophila* is the genus of veterinary interest. There are six recognized species:

- *C. psittaci*: birds, cattle, humans.
- *C. abortus*: sheep, goats, cattle.
- *C. pneumoniae*: humans, reptiles, amphibians, horses, koalas.
- *C. pecorum*: ruminants, koalas.
- *C. felis*: cats.
- *C. caviae*: guinea pigs.

Chlamydophila psittaci

There are five serovars (A–E); different serovars infect specific species (e.g. A infects psittacines, E infects Columbiformes). Psittacines are most frequently infected with serovar A (genotype A) strains, but can also be infected with serovar B strains. Serovar A strains are considered to be highly pathogenic. The condition caused by *Chlamydophila* infection is also known as psittacosis and ornithosis. It has been a known zoonotic infection for about 100 years.

Clinical presentation

The virulence of the strain affects the clinical course, with clinical signs ranging from inapparent to severe septicaemia and acute death. Typically though, the disease affects either the respiratory tract, the gastrointestinal tract and liver, or both (**195, 196**).

Respiratory signs

These include conjunctivitis, often with loss or matting of periocular feathers, dyspnoea (tail bobbing, mouth-breathing) and sneezing with a purulent nasal discharge and sinus distension.

Gastrointestinal/hepatic signs

These include diarrhoea, biliverdinuria (green urates and urine), and a 'sick bird look' (fluffed, lethargic, anorexia and weight loss).

Other signs

There may be poor feathering and neurological signs (torticollis, tremors, convulsions). Polyuria is frequent due to the nephrotoxic effects of elementary bodies. Affected birds may be infertile.

Pathophysiology

This can be a highly contagious disease, with transmission occurring through ingestion (faecal material, mutual feeding and feeding chicks) or inhalation (respiratory secretions, aerosolized feather or faecal dust). Egg transmission may occur. Shedding of the organism can start 72 hours after infection, and birds may be shedding for up to ten days before they start to show clinical signs. The incubation period can be as short as four days, and up to 1–2 years.

The infection can be latent and activated during stress. There are indications that shedding in pigeons is greater in hot weather, possibly as a stress response to heat. A carrier state may exist.

Immunity to infection is short lived and birds are susceptible to reinfection shortly after treatment ends.

Diagnosis

Diagnosis can be difficult, as there is no single 'best' test. Testing can rely on antigen detection or antibody detection; ancillary testing can be used to support the

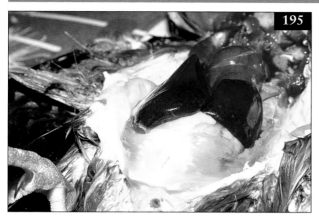

195 Hepatomegaly shown during necropsy of a bird that has died of chlamydiosis.

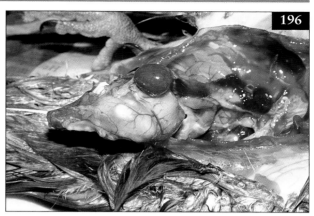

196 Splenomegaly in bird that has died of chlamydiosis.

presence of disease, rather than just the organism. The Centre for Disease Control (CDC) classifies the level of diagnosis as:

- Confirmed case: *C. psittaci* confirmed by isolation, fluorescent antibody (FA) of affected tissue, more than a fourfold increase in serological titre in paired samples collected two weeks apart and processed by same laboratory, or demonstration of the organism in macrophages via Macchiavelli's or Gimenez stain.
- Probable case: clinical infection consistent with *Chlamydophila* combined with one of the following: single high titre obtained after onset of illness; *Chlamydophila* antigen demonstrated by FA or ELISA in faeces, exudates or cloacal swab.
- Suspect case: clinical signs consistent with *Chlamydophila* in a bird epidemiologically linked to another case in a bird or human, but not laboratory confirmed; *or* an asymptomatic bird with a single high titre or antigen detected; *or* illness in a bird confirmed with a nonstandardized test; *or* clinical illness that is responsive to appropriate treatment.

Antigen detection
Respiratory epithelium (choanal/oropharynx) yields the most reliable samples for antigen detection:
- Isolation. Cell culture is the gold standard.
- Cytology. *Chlamydophila* inclusions are most easily demonstrated in serosal membranes, liver, spleen and affected air sacs. Smears are stained with Giemsa or Macchiavelli's stain to show intracytoplasmic inclusions. Negative staining does not rule out *Chlamydophila*.

- Immunofluorescence antibody testing. Commercial FA conjugate for detection of *Chlamydophila* spp. may cross-react with *M. avium* giving false-positive results.
- ELISA tests are available; however, be aware of false positives from *S. aureus* in the sample. ELISAs that detect the *Chlamydophila* lipopolysaccharide (LPS) should be avoided because it is serologically related to the LPS of Enterobacteriaceae. False positives result from the presence of cross-reactive antibodies in the serum; false negatives occur when *Chlamydophila* is shed intermittently.
- Latex agglutination tests (e.g. Clearview). A high number of false positives are seen due to bacteria.
- PCR tests. Be aware of false negatives: caused by presence of inhibitors of PCR reaction such as blood, serum, urine, faeces, sputum, hair shafts and lab reagents specifically haematin, DMSO, sodium chloride, phosphate-buffered saline, melanin, heparin, detergents and glove powder. DNA cannot distinguish between live organisms and dead organisms (which may be contaminants).

Antibody detection
Tests detect IgM or IgG, or both:
- Latex agglutination. Measures IgM. Note: False positives are found from *S. aureus*, *P. multocida* and *Sarcina* sp.
- Direct complement fixation (CF). Measures IgG. Only useful if paired serum samples are tested. CF is the most common serological test used in humans, but is not used in birds because they

produce mainly nonCF antibodies with *Chlamydophila* infection.
- ELISA (e.g. Immunocomb) (**73**).
- BELISA (blocking ELISA). This inhibitory ELISA is a very sensitive test; marketed in Germany.

Ancillary testing
Haematology shows anaemia, leucocytosis, absolute or relative heterophilia and monocytosis. Blood chemistry shows elevations in CPK, AST, LDH, total protein and bile acids if the liver is involved. Uric acid may be elevated if the kidneys are involved. Electrophoresis shows elevations in total globulins, beta and gamma globulins and a decrease in albumin.

Radiography may demonstrate hepato- and/or splenomegaly, air sacculitis and pneumonia. Biopsy of liver, spleen or air sac may also be helpful.

Acute lesions found at autopsy include fibrinous peritoneal exudate, air sacculitis (more frequent in psittacines than splenomegaly), perihepatitis, pericarditis, myocarditis, bronchopneumonia, catarrhal enteritis, nephrosis, orchitis, epididymitis and oophoritis. Chronic lesions include liver and kidney cirrhosis, pancreatic necrosis (budgerigar and pigeon) and nonpurulent meningitis.

Differential diagnosis
Differential diagnoses include herpesvirus, particularly Pacheco's disease, paramyxovirus and influenza A, and infection with Enterobacteriaceae.

Management
Tetracyclines
These inhibit *Chlamydophila* protein synthesis and are active only when intracellular reticulate bodies are actively replicating. Disadvantages include low intracellular concentration, immunosuppression, chelation with calcium (dietary calcium should be reduced to 0.7% or less) and inhibition of autochthonous flora. Duration of therapy is empirically set at 45 days, the average lifespan of a macrophage.
- Chlortetracycline. This is renally excreted and should be used cautiously in birds with renal disease.
- Doxycycline calcium. This is excreted extrarenally (faeces, bile). Adequate plasma levels are often achievable in medicated drinking water and seeds. It may cause hepatic necrosis with elevation of AST, which resolves with cessation of therapy.

Enrofloxacin
Clinical improvement and cessation of faecal shedding have been reported for five weeks post treatment. This is not fully documented, and enrofloxacin may not be effective clinically. Field trials indicate that it may not be as effective as doxycycline.

Azithromycin
This is a macrolide antibiotic, able to penetrate macrophages. There are anecdotal reports of effectiveness, but no clinical trials have been done as yet to confirm this. It is given orally once weekly for 3–6 weeks. The recommended dose is 40 mg/kg q24h for 30 days.

Disinfection
Free elementary bodies are unstable and can be inactivated in the environment within days. They are sensitive to heat, quaternary ammonium products, 70% ethanol and 3% hydrogen peroxide.

Clinical signs in man
Chlamydophila infection is a zoonosis, causing fever, chills, pneumonia, headache, weakness, fatigue, myalgia, chest pain, anorexia, nausea, vomiting and diaphoresis.

PACHECO'S DISEASE
Aetiology
Pacheco's disease is caused by PsHV. There are four genotypes of PsHV1 recognized. Different genotypes affect different species of birds. Herpesviruses are highly host-adapted, causing little or no disease (but lifelong infections) in the species that they have evolved with. Disease results when infection occurs in a species that has not adapted evolutionarily to the virus.

Clinical presentation
Sudden death is a common presentation (**197**). Birds exposed to virulent strains of PsHV usually develop clinical signs (lethargy, regurgitation, diarrhoea, biliverdinuria, neurological signs) or die within 3–10 days of exposure to the virus.

Pathophysiology
Asymptomatic carriers (e.g. conures, Amazon parrots and macaws) may serve as virus reservoirs. These carriers may shed the virus for life. The virus is shed in faeces and respiratory/pharyngeal secretions (**198**). Shedding may be triggered by periods of stress. Birds dying of Pacheco's disease will shed large amounts of virus into their environment. The incubation period may last five days to several weeks.

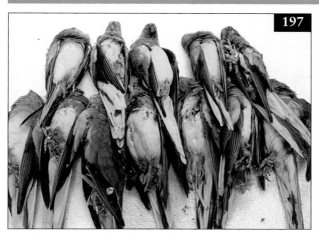

197 An outbreak of Pacheco's disease can cause devastating loss in a collection. This group of *Neophema* spp. parrots died acutely as a result of such an outbreak. (Photo courtesy B. Speer)

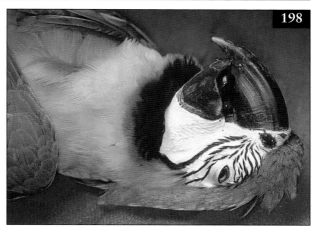

198 Haemorrhage from the nares and oral cavity in macaw that died of Pacheco's disease. (Photo courtesy B Dalhausen)

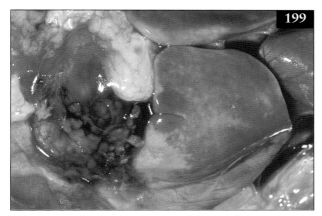

199 Haemorrhagic hepatitis in a bird that died from Pacheco's disease. (Photo courtesy R Schmidt)

Diagnosis

Autopsy may show no lesions or hepatomegaly and splenomegaly, with a mottled tan discoloration of the liver (**199**). Histopathology shows multifocal necrosis in the liver and spleen with intranuclear eosinophilic inclusion bodies.

Viral-specific PCR probes using oral and mucosal swabs have been developed to detect infected birds.

Management

Acyclovir, an acyclic purine nucleoside, can be effective. It works best in in-contact birds not showing signs of illness.

Prevention involves a PCR test (oral and cloacal) of all new birds and quarantine of new birds for at least 6–12 weeks and possibly for more than two years. Birds that have survived an outbreak should be regarded as carriers. An inactivated vaccine is available. The oil adjuvant has been associated with muscle necrosis in a number of birds, particularly cockatoos. The vaccine responsible for most of the reported reactions is no longer available. Side-effects are reported to be minimal when the currently available vaccine is administered subcutaneously and not intramuscularly.

FURTHER READING

Compendium of measures to control *Chlamydophila psittaci* infection among humans (psittacosis) and pet birds (avian chlamydiosis) (2009) http://www.nasphv.org/Documents/Psittacosis.pdf

Doneley B (2004) Treating liver disease in the avian patient. *Seminars in Avian and Exotic Pet Medicine* **13**(1):8–15.

Hochleithner M, Hochleithner C, Harrison LD (2006) Evaluating and treating the liver. In: *Clinical Avian Medicine, Vol 1*. GJ Harrison, TL Lightfoot (eds). Spix Publishing Inc, Palm Beach, pp. 441–449.

Tully TN (2006) Update on *Chlamydophila psittaci*: a short comment. In: *Clinical Avian Medicine, Vol 2*. GJ Harrison, TL Lightfoot (eds). Spix Publishing Inc, Palm Beach, pp. 679–680.

CHAPTER 15
DISORDERS OF THE PANCREAS

EXOCRINE
PANCREATIC INSUFFICIENCY
Aetiology
Pancreatic insufficiency may be caused by congenital pancreatic atrophy or end-stage chronic pancreatic disease with loss of exocrine tissue.

Clinical presentation
Clinical signs include weight loss and large, pale, voluminous droppings, often described as having a 'popcorn' appearance (200). Polyphagia is variable.

Diagnosis
Diagnosis is based in clinical signs and pancreatic biopsy.

Management
If possible, the causative agents should be identified and eliminated. The affected bird should be converted to a formulated diet, which can be supplemented with pancreatic enzymes, although palatability can be an issue in some birds.

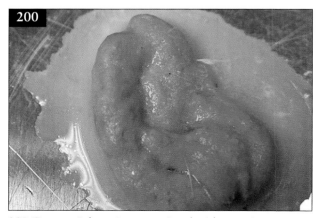

200 'Popcorn' droppings associated with exocrime pancreatic insufficiency. (Photo courtesy B. Speer)

PANCREATITIS
Definition/overview
The incidence of primary pancreatitis in birds is a matter for some discussion. However, pancreatitis secondary to other disease processes is probably underdiagnosed in avian medicine. This undoubtedly reflects on the lack of specific and sensitive tools to diagnose this disease. Our understanding of avian pancreatic disease is still in its formative stages.

Aetiology
Causes of pancreatitis include obesity, often when combined with high-fat diets or fatty meals; toxicosis, particularly zinc (see Chapter 21, Disorders affecting the urinary system), mycotoxins and selenium; trauma; viral infection (including paramyxovirus-3, adenovirus, avian influenza type A, infectious bronchitis and herpesvirus); chlamydiosis; bacterial infection; egg yolk peritonitis; and neoplasia.

Pathophysiology
Activation of the digestive enzymes (trypsin, protease and phospholipase) within the gland results in pancreatic autodigestion. Damage to the pancreatic cell walls allows the release of these enzymes into the intracellular space and ducts, and this in turn causes the production of unopposed free radicals, which cause even more damage. This again releases more enzymes, and the cycle continues.

Clinical presentation
Gastrointestinal dysfunction causes vomiting, ileus, weight loss, polyuria, polydypsia and abdominal distension. The condition is painful and signs of this include anorexia, lethargy, feather picking, aggression and obsessive chewing on the cage and other items.

Diagnosis
Clinical signs suggest a diagnosis. Significant elevations may be found in serum amylase and lipase

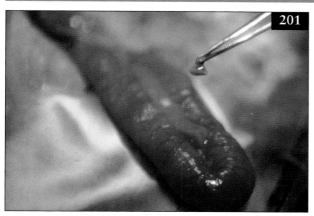

201 Pancreatic biopsy collected via a ventral midline coeliotomy.

concentrations. However, these biochemistries are neither specific nor sensitive for pancreatitis, and a diagnosis of pancreatitis based solely on hyperamylasaemia or elevated lipase can not be justified. Pancreatic biopsy can be used, either endoscopically or through a ventral midline coeliotomy (**201**) (see p. 262).

Management
If possible, the causative agent should be identified and eliminated (e.g. chelating zinc toxicosis, conversion from a seed diet to a lower fat formulated diet, surgical treatment of yolk peritonitis). Analgesia and fluid support are required and antibiotic therapy is given if indicated.

PANCREATIC NEOPLASIA
Definition/overview
Pancreatic neoplasia involves primary pancreatic carcinomas and adenocarcinomas. Secondary metastases are uncommon, but can be due to IPD.

Clinical presentation
Signs are similar to those seen with pancreatitis or pancreatic insufficiency.

Diagnosis
Antemortem diagnosis requires ultrasonography and biopsy.

Management
Chemotherapy has been used in a few cases, with variable degrees of success.

ENDOCRINE
DIABETES MELLITUS
Definition/overview
Diabetes mellitus is most commonly diagnosed in budgerigars, cockatiels and galahs. It has also been diagnosed in larger psittacines, toucans, mynahs and other species.

Aetiology
Diabetes mellitus in mammals, characterized by chronic hyperglycaemia and other metabolic abnormalities, is due to a lack of effect by insulin on glucose metabolism. This can be due to either an absolute lack of insulin or an inability of the insulin to lower blood glucose levels.

Understanding the pathogenesis of diabetes mellitus in birds is complicated by the role of glucagon and somatostatin in glucose metabolism in birds. In granivorous birds the pancreatic islets have a substantially higher percentage of glucagon-secreting cells compared with the mammalian pancreas. Correspondingly, the plasma glucagon:insulin ratio in these birds appears to be two to five times higher than that of mammals; it therefore appears that glucagon is the dominant hormone in glucose metabolism.

Glucagon is a powerful catabolic hormone that stimulates gluconeogenesis, lipolysis and glycogenolysis, thus increasing blood glucose. This process begins within hours of a meal, allowing continual production of glucose to meet the body's demands for energy. Insulin, on the other hand, is a powerful anabolic hormone, increasing the availability of glucose transport carriers, which allows easier transfer of glucose into the cell. It is antigluconeogenic. The effect of these hormones is modulated by somatostatin, pancreatic polypeptide, prolactin, thyroxine and growth hormone. It is therefore unclear whether diabetes mellitus in granivorous birds is due to an excess of glucagon or to a lack of insulin effect. The insulin:glucagon ratio and its regulation by somatostatin may be the critical factor in regulating glucose concentration rather than the actual concentration of the individual hormones.

Diabetes mellitus in mammals is classified as:
- Type I, which is characterized by destructive lesions of the pancreatic beta cells either by an autoimmune mechanism or by an unknown cause.
- Type II, which is characterized by combinations of decreased insulin secretion and decreased insulin sensitivity (insulin resistance), without any overt pancreatic disease.

- Type III, which is characterized by nonspecific destruction of pancreatic tissue associated with other pathological conditions or diseases, or diseases or drugs that cause insulin resistance.

No similar classification system has been applied to diabetes mellitus in birds and it may be that attempts to do so will be thwarted by the differences in glucose metabolism in birds compared with mammals. However, it would appear that the equivalents to these diabetes classifications do occur in birds.
- Type I diabetes, with selective destruction of pancreatic islets, has been seen in toucans and parrots.
- Type II diabetes is commonly associated with obesity. A link between iron storage disease and diabetes mellitus is being increasingly recognized.
- Type III diabetes is commonly associated with nonspecific pancreatic disease such as neoplasia and pancreatitis (see above), and the iatrogenic administration of megestrol acetate, medroxyprogesterone acetate or corticosteroids, hormones that inhibit the effect of insulin and lead to insulin resistance.

Clinical presentation
The principal signs are polyuria, polydypsia, polyphagia and weight loss. In some cases, especially those with concurrent disease, nonspecific signs such as depression, lethargy, vomiting or anorexia may be seen.

Diagnosis
Diagnosis is based on the finding of persistent hyperglycaemia and glucosuria. Birds normally have higher glucose levels than mammals, and can have stress-induced episodes of transient hyperglycaemia. Blood glucose levels consistently above 38–44 mmol/l are consistent with a diagnosis of diabetes mellitus. Fructosamine levels have not been fully evaluated in birds, as yet; it therefore remains an unproven but potentially useful tool for monitoring diabetic patients. Ketonuria is present in some avian patients, but is not consistently reported.

Management
The goal of treatment is to lower the patient's blood glucose levels and restore a more normal glucose metabolism. This is achieved by determining and correcting the primary disease process that is inducing the diabetes mellitus, stabilizing the unwell patient and correcting the hyperglycaemia. The latter may be achieved through the use of insulin or oral hypoglycaemic agents.

The immediate use of short-acting insulin (0.1–0.2 U/kg) can stabilize the patient initially, but long-term control at home usually requires longer-acting insulin (NPH or ultralente). Dose rates vary considerably and should be based on the observed effects. They range from 0.067–3.3 U/kg q12–24h.

Oral hypoglycaemic agents (sulphonylureas, e.g. glipizide) may assist. Sulphonylureas lower blood glucose concentrations in both diabetics and non-diabetics. The exact mechanism of action is not known, but these agents are thought to exert their effect primarily by stimulating the beta cells in the pancreas to secrete additional endogenous insulin. Extrapancreatic effects include enhanced tissue sensitivity to circulating insulin and reduction of the production of hepatic basal glucose. The mechanisms causing these effects are yet to be fully explained.

Monitoring the effects of either treatment can be difficult, as a measured glucosuria could reflect faecal contamination. Observing water intake and urinary output may be more practical measures for owners to take at home.

Conversion to a formulated diet is an important part of treatment. Not only does it correct many of the causative factors (e.g. obesity), it also provides a high-fibre diet that assists with regulating blood glucose. In many (but not all) cases, dietary conversion and treatment of primary disease processes can result in clinical resolution of the signs of diabetes mellitus, removing the need for ongoing insulin therapy.

FURTHER READING

Doneley B (2000) Acute pancreatitis in psittacine birds. In: *Proceedings of the Annual Conference of the Association of Avian Veterinarians Australian Committee*, pp. 261–267.

Gancz AY, *et al.* (2005) Diabetes mellitus in large psittacines: a possible relationship with excessive iron storage. In: *Proceedings of the Annual Conference of the Association of Avian Veterinarians Australian Committee*, pp. 267–269.

Gelis S (2006) Evaluating and treating the gastrointestinal system. In: *Clinical Avian Medicine, Vol 1*. GJ Harrison, TL Lightfoot (eds). Spix Publishing Inc, Palm Beach, pp. 411–440.

Hudelson KS, Hudelson PM (2006) Endocrine considerations. In: *Clinical Avian Medicine, Vol 2*. GJ Harrison, TL Lightfoot (eds). Spix Publishing Inc, Palm Beach, pp. 541–557.

Speer B (1998) A clinical look at the avian pancreas in health and disease. In: *Proceedings of the Annual Conference of the Association of Avian Veterinarians Australian Committee*, pp. 57–64.

CHAPTER 16

DISORDERS OF THE RESPIRATORY SYSTEM

UPPER RESPIRATORY TRACT

SINUSITIS

Aetiology

Underlying predisposing causes of sinusitis include the complex anatomy of the infraorbital sinuses; hypovitaminosis A causing squamous metaplasia of the epithelial lining of the sinuses and decreasing its normal function and resistance to infection; irritation of the sinuses (e.g. ammonia toxicosis in poorly ventilated, unhygienic cages and aviaries, cigarette smoke, other aerosol pollutants); extremes of humidity (too dry, too moist); and choanal atresia (see below).

Infectious agents may be primary or secondary and include: bacteria (*E. coli*, *Haemophilus*, *Klebsiella*, *Pasteurella*, *Pseudomonas*, *Mycobacterium*, spirochaetes in cockatiels); viruses (Amazon tracheitis, pigeon herpesvirus, poxvirus, reovirus, infectious laryngotracheitis, avian influenza); fungi (*Aspergillus* spp., *Candida albicans*, *Cryptococcus*, *Zygomycoses*); chlamydia; *Mycoplasma*; parasites (*Trichomonas*, *Cryptosporidia*).

Foreign objects (e.g. millet seed) and neoplasia (carcinoma, adenocarcinoma, fibrosarcoma, lymphosarcoma, malignant melanoma) may also result in sinusitis.

Clinical presentation

Clinical signs include oculonasal discharge, occlusion of the nares, exophthalmos (or enophthalmos in macaws — sunken eye syndrome) and distension of the sinuses (**202**). There may be matting or loss of the periocular feathering, and conjunctival hyperaemia or thickening. Affected birds may sneeze, shake their head and scratch at their face with their feet, or rub their face excessively on objects such as perches. There may be hyperinflation of the cervicocephalic air sac.

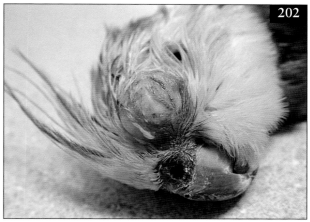

202 Sinusitis in a cockatiel. Note the yellow caseated pus distending the sinus dorsal to the eye, and the periocular feather loss.

Lockjaw syndrome may be seen in cockatiels aged 3–10 weeks. After an initial course of oculonasal discharge and sinus swelling, they are unable to open their beak and starve to death.

Diagnosis

Cytology and culture are helpful (see Chapter 3, Clinical techniques, and Chapter 4, Interpreting diagnostic tests). Diagnostic imaging, including contrast radiographs (using barium), CT and MRI, can be used to examine the anatomy and patency of the infraorbital sinuses and to localize a problem (e.g. a pocket of caseated debris). Endoscopy, via the choana, can be useful when a foreign body is suspected. Transillumination with an intense focal light can be used to examine the sinuses and rhinal cavity.

Management

The underlying cause must be identified and corrected. Nutritional modification and the use of parenteral vitamin A are particularly important in many cases.

If the nidus of infection is not found and removed, recurrence is common. Therefore, it is important to remove caseous exudate and other debris within the sinuses. Nasal flushing using normal saline or diluted acetylcysteine may remove some caseated material, but the complex anatomy of the sinuses makes it difficult to flush the infraorbital sinuses successfully. Infraorbital flushing and aspiration, using the same approaches as used for sampling, can achieve more than nasal flushing in some cases. Surgical debridement and drainage via trephination into the affected sinus is an aggressive, but often successful, therapy. Before attempting this surgery it is important to review the anatomy and consult surgical texts. It is extremely easy to damage underlying structures such as the eye or nerves.

Oral and/or parenteral antimicrobial therapy are given, based on cytology and culture. Topical therapy may also be helpful, using nebulization or application of drops into the nares.

RHINITIS

Aetiology

Causes of rhinitis are similar to those of sinusitis (see above). Occlusion of the nares can occur due to cere hypertrophy, *Cnemidocoptes* infection or rhinoliths. See Chapter 8, Disorders of the beak and cere.

Clinical presentation

Clinical signs include sneezing, rubbing at the face, nasal discharge and asymmetry in the size of the nares (203).

Diagnosis

Diagnosis of the causative organism may require cytology and culture.

Management

Rhinoliths can be removed with a small curette. Caseated debris is removed by nasal flushing. Topical or parenteral therapy is given based on culture and sensitivity.

RUPTURED CERVICOCEPHALIC AIR SAC

Aetiology

This condition may be the result of chronic sinusitis (see above), trauma or extension of air sacculitis or pneumonic conditions (see below).

Clinical presentation

The neck becomes distended with air (204).

Diagnosis

Physical examination and aspiration of air and radiography of the neck will indicate the diagnosis. Endoscopy of the air sac may help to localize the site of rupture, and biopsy of the air sac may better determine the aetiological agent. This condition must be differentiated from aerophagia.

Management

The underlying cause should be identified and treated. Lancing the distension with a scalpel or the bevelled edge of a needle, tearing through both skin and air

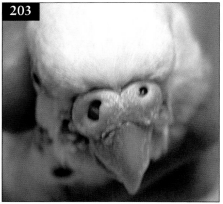

203 Chronic rhinitis in this budgerigar has led to asymmetrical nares.

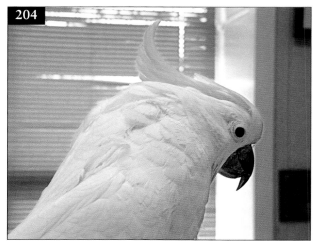

204 The cervicocephalic air sac in this cockatoo's neck has ruptured, leading to subcutaneous emphysema.

sac, will deflate the air sac. This may have to be done several times until the originating rupture has healed. Refractory cases may require the placement of an acrylic stent in the most prominent area of the distension. Purpose-made stents are available and are implanted surgically under general anaesthesia. An alternative technique has been developed that creates a shunt between the cervicocephalic air sac and the clavicular air sac, avoiding the maintenance of an external stent.

CHOANAL ATRESIA
Definition/overview
Failure of the choana to properly form during development results in a persistent membrane or bony plate at the palate of the nasal cavity, blocking the normal drainage of nasal secretions into the oral cavity. The condition is predominantly reported in African grey parrots and occasionally in cockatoos and Amazon parrots. There is no reason why it could not occur in other species. It is present at an early age.

Clinical presentation
Clinical signs include bilateral mucoid discharge and sinus swellings around the eyes. A choanal slit may be present, although not patent.

Diagnosis
Saline flushed into the nares fails to enter the mouth. Instead, the infraorbital sinuses swell. Rhinography using contrast media can be used to demonstrate the lack of communication between the sinuses and the choana.

Management
Surgical correction is required. An appropriately sized Steinman pin is used to bore a hole through each nare to the choanal slit. There may be some bone to pass through and, while haemorrhage is usually minimal, in some cases it may be significant and potentially fatal. An 8 Fr red rubber catheter is passed through each hole, leaving the ends long. Openings are cut into the sides of the tube at the nares to allow mucus to drain. The ends of the tube are tied behind the head and a chin strap is made of tape to prevent the tubes from slipping off the top of the head. The tubes are left in place for 4–6 weeks to allow the tracts to epithelialize, creating permanent openings. Once the tubes are removed, the nares are flushed twice daily for two weeks to help keep the openings free of debris.

LOWER RESPIRATORY TRACT
TRACHEITIS OR TRACHEAL OBSTRUCTION
Aetiology
Causes include:
- Foreign body. Cockatiels that have inhaled a millet seed are frequently seen, but other species and other foreign bodies are not uncommon (205, 206).
- Diphtheritic plaques due to bacterial infections (e.g. *Pseudomonas* spp.) are seen occasionally in cockatoos.

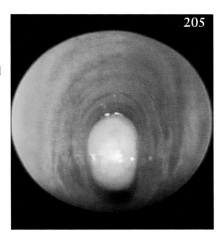

205 Endoscopy of the trachea of a dyspnoeic cockatiel revealed this millet seed obstructing the trachea. (Photo courtesy A Lennox)

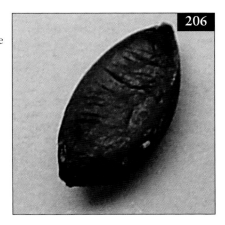

206 After removal, it can be seen that the millet seed is perfectly shaped for accidental inhalation and subsequent tracheal obstruction.

- Fungal granulomas usually develop in the syrinx, but can form in the trachea as well (**207**).
- Viral tracheitis (e.g. pigeon herpesvirus, Amazon tracheitis virus, paramyxovirus, adenovirus and cytomegalovirus).
- Parasitism (*Sternastoma tracheacolum*, *Trichomonas gallinae* or *Syngamus trachea*).
- Iatrogenic tracheitis and stenosis following intubation, especially in macaws.
- Extramural masses or compression (e.g. thyroid hyperplasia [goitre] associated with iodine deficiency in budgerigars, fractures of the coracoid bone, neoplasia, granulomas).

Clinical presentation

There is usually acute onset of dyspnoea, with open-mouth breathing, wing droop and tail bobbing. Occasionally, the neck will be stretched out. Respiration may be wheezing. Slower onset cases may present for a progressive change in voice.

Diagnosis

Tracheal endoscopy is helpful. The author prefers to visualize the trachea quickly following mask induction of anaesthesia. If tracheal obstruction, stenosis or severe tracheitis is obvious, an air sac catheter can be placed (see Chapter 3, Clinical techniques) to provide a secure airway while further diagnostic work and treatment is undertaken.

Radiography can be used to identify extramural compression of the trachea. Contrast radiography may be necessary in some birds to obtain a definitive diagnosis. A small amount of barium (0.5 ml/kg) is placed in the trachea using a catheter. Barium is inert and will not induce irritation or inflammation of the respiratory mucosa.

Management

In secure cases, a secure (temporary) airway can be maintained through the use of an air sac catheter (**98**) (see Chapter 3, Clinical techniques).

Foreign bodies, diphtheritic plaques and granulomas may require surgical removal or reduction. In large birds, endoscopic retrieval or debridement may be feasible. Care must be taken, as haemorrhage (and later iatrogenic stenosis) may result from aggressive debridement of plaques and granulomas. If the obstruction is located midway along the trachea, an intravenous catheter can be introduced caudal to the obstruction and advanced (with the metal stylet removed) rostrally. The tip of the catheter can be used to dislodge the foreign body and it can then be 'blown out' using air from a syringe attached to the catheter.

If neither of these techniques are feasible or succeed (e.g. syringeal obstructions), a tracheotomy may be required to access and remove the obstruction. The patient is positioned in dorsal recumbency with the shoulders elevated 45° to provide the surgeon with visual exposure to the thoracic inlet. A skin incision is made along the ventral midline, and the crop retracted if necessary (this may require some dissection of subcutaneous tissue). If the obstruction is located in the syrinx, the interclavicular air sac is entered to expose the sternotracheal muscles, which are transected with radiosurgery. This mobilizes the syrinx and allows it to be brought rostrally. Great care must be taken not to tear the bronchi off the syrinx. The tracheotomy is made through the ventral half of the annular ligament between the tracheal rings, rather than through them. If approaching the syrinx, the incision is made three to five rings rostral to the syrinx.

Closure of the trachea is achieved using a fine, synthetic, monofilament, absorbable material (e.g. 8-0 PDS) in a simple interrupted pattern. The sutures should be preplaced and positioned at 30° circumferentially so that a 50% tracheotomy is closed with two to three sutures. They should encompass at least two rings on each side of the tracheotomy and the knots are tied external to the tracheal lumen.

Tracheal stenosis can be treated by surgical removal of the stenotic section. The trachea is generally quite long in birds and removal of a section of trachea is easy to accomplish without placing undue tension on the anastomosis. The approach is as described above. The soft tissue surrounding the trachea is carefully dissected from the surface of the trachea to preserve the nerve and blood supply. The compromised area of trachea is then removed using a scalpel blade. Anastomosis is achieved using five to six simple interrupted sutures (8-0 PDS). The dorsal sutures are tied first, while the access is easier. The owner must be

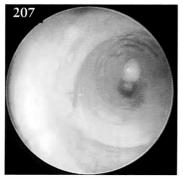

207 Endoscopy of the syrinx of a dyspnoeic grey parrot revealed a glistening white obstruction, an *Aspergillus* granuloma.

advised that a stricture can occur at the anastomosis site. This generally occurs during the contraction phase of wound healing, 3–6 weeks postoperatively.

Goitre (thyroid hyperplasia) can be treated by the use of thyroxine PO and Lugol's iodine as an in-water supplement.

Syringeal aspergillosis may respond to ultra-tracheal injections of amphotericin B, nebulizing with the same drug and oral antifungal medications such as itraconazole or voriconazole. The clinician must be aware that amphotericin B can be an irritant to the respiratory epithelium.

PULMONARY PARENCHYMA DISEASE

Aetiology

Infectious

Infections may be bacterial (*E. coli*, *Klebsiella pneumoniae*, *Pasteurella multocida* and *Pseudomonas aeruginosa* [208]), fungal (*Aspergillus*, *Cryptococcus*), chlamydial, mycobacterial, mycoplasmal, viral (paramyxovirus, herpesvirus, avian influenza, canary pox), or parasitic (*Sternastoma* spp. [air sac mite], *Sarcocystis* spp., *Cryptosporidium* spp., *Toxoplasma* spp., *Atoxoplasma* spp.)

Pulmonary hypersensitivity

This is seen in macaws housed with birds producing feather dander (e.g. cockatoos).

Inhaled toxins

These include smoke, polytetrafluoroethylene (PTFE—Teflon®), cigarette smoke, aerosol sprays, carbon monoxide, burning cooking oils, foreign bodies, aspirated food material, yolk embolism and fat embolism from bone marrow.

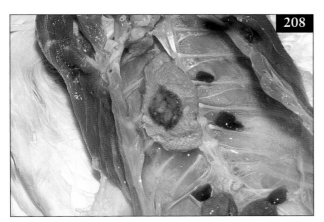

208 Pulmonary parenchymatous abscesses (bacterial, fungal, mycobacterial) are often found on the dorsal aspect of the lung, making surgical access difficult.

Pneumoconiosis

This is accumulation of dust-laden macrophages. It may arise from an incident that occurred months or years previously.

Neoplasia

Pulmonary tumours include fibrosarcoma, carcinoma and metastatic disease.

Clinical presentation

Signs include tachypnoea and/or dyspnoea, mouth breathing, voice change, exercise intolerance and general signs of illness.

Diagnosis

Haematology and biochemistries

Polycythaemia may be present in birds with chronic hypoxia due to pulmonary parenchymatous disease.

Radiography

Birds with pneumonia can have a variety of radiographic changes ranging from a diffuse to a uniform abnormal/thickened parabronchial pattern. Macaws with pulmonary hypersensitivity may demonstrate a more accentuated reticular pattern due to thickening of the interatrial septa.

Endoscopy

This is carried out via the cranial and caudal thoracic air sacs.

Tracheal/lung wash

This is performed using 0.5–1.0 ml/kg of 0.9% saline.

Lung aspirates and/or biopsy

These can be utilized for cultures, cytology or histopathological evaluation. Lung parenchyma biopsies can be obtained by two approaches: the cranial thoracic air sac (via endoscopy) or the intercostal approach (third intercostal space). The clinician needs to be aware of the potential for haemorrhage.

Management

Medications

Systemic antibiotic therapy is given as indicated by culture. Bronchodilation with albuterol (0.05 mg/kg q6–8h) may assist in some cases. Birds with acute onset of respiratory distress following exposure to smoke or PTFE may benefit from the administration of rapidly acting, short-duration corticosteroids (methylprednisolone sodium succinate, 15–30 mg/kg) and oxygen supplementation. Other than these cases, there is no role for corticosteroids in the treatment of avian respiratory disease.

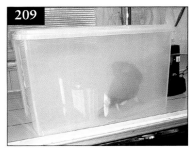

209 Nebulizing a grey parrot with amphotericin B for a syringeal *Aspergillus* granuloma.

Supportive care
Oxygen therapy can be beneficial, but prolonged exposure to oxygen can be dangerous. Oxygen concentrations should not exceed 35–50%. Nebulization using 0.9% normal saline with or without antibiotics is administered for 15–30 minutes three to four times daily for a minimum of three days beyond the resolution of clinical signs (**209**). Steam particles must be smaller than 3 μm to penetrate into the lung parenchyma. Mucolytics are not recommended in birds because they lack mechanisms to clear the exudates from their air sacs.

Surgery
Surgery (partial pneumonectomy) may be required to remove granulomas.

Ongoing care and prevention
The use of air filters is often necessary in poorly ventilated areas. Macaws should not be housed with cockatoos or African grey parrots.

AIR SAC DISEASE
Aetiology
Infectious causes include bacteria, fungi (*Aspergillus*, *Cryptococcus*), chlamydia, mycobacteria and parasites (*Serratospiculum* spp., *Splendidofilaria* spp.).

Air sac carcinomas may be seen.

Extramural pressure on air sacs may be the result of obesity, organomegaly (liver, oviduct, ovary [physiological enlargement, ovarian cysts]), neoplasia or fluid effusions (yolk-related peritonitis, ascites, heart failure).

Clinical presentation
Signs include increased respiratory effort, decreased exercise tolerance and weight loss. Auscultation may detect friction rubs.

Diagnosis
Radiographically, severe air sacculitis can often be documented by the appearance of 'air sac lines'. Size and position of internal organs can also be assessed to detect extramural pressure on the air sacs. Endoscopy can be used to both evaluate and biopsy the air sacs.

A blind air sac wash can be done by inserting an intravenous catheter between the last two ribs. The needle is inserted and the catheter advanced into the air sac. This will place the catheter into the caudal thoracic (shallow) or abdominal (deep) air sac. Sterile saline (1–2 ml/kg) is instilled and collected for evaluation.

Management
The causative agent should be identified and treated. Treatment is similar to that for lung diseases (see above).

FURTHER READING
Antinoff, N (2001) Understanding and treating the infraorbital sinus and respiratory system. In: *Proceedings of the Annual Conference of the Association of Avian Veterinarians Australian Committee*, pp. 245–260.

Hillyer EV (1997) Clinical manifestations of respiratory disorders. In: *Avian Medicine and Surgery*. RB Altman, SL Clubb, GM Dorrestein, K Quesenberry (eds). WB Saunders, Philadelphia, pp. 394–411.

Lichtenberger M, Orosz SE (2007) Acute respiratory distress (ARD) – from anatomy through treatment. In: *Proceedings of the Annual Conference of the Association of Avian Veterinarians Australian Committee*, pp. 151–159.

Simone-Freilicher (2008) Avian sinusitis: the sniffles, the sneezes, and the silent. In: *Proceedings of the Annual Conference of the Association of Avian Veterinarians Australian Committee*, pp. 251–260.

Tell LA (2005) Aspergillosis in mammals and birds: impact on veterinary medicine. *Medical Mycology* **43 Suppl 1**(0):S71–3.

Tully TN, Harrison GJ (1994) Pneumonology. In: *Avian Medicine: Principles and Application*. BW Ritchie, GJ Harrison, LR Harrison (eds). Wingers Publishing, Lake Worth, pp. 556–606.

CHAPTER 17

DISORDERS OF THE CARDIOVASCULAR SYSTEM

CARDIAC DISEASE

Definition/overview

It is thought that somewhere between 10% and 40% of companion birds have some form of cardiovascular disease. These estimates are based on retrospective pathology studies. It is relatively rarely diagnosed antemortem, but as diagnostic techniques improve, an increase in the incidence of diagnosed cardiovascular disease can be expected.

Predisposing factors for cardiac disease include restricted exercise, poor nutrition and keeping birds in a climate in which they did not evolve (e.g. keeping South American parrots in European winters).

Aetiology

Congenital heart disease

Intraventricular septal defects are becoming increasingly common, especially in umbrella cockatoos. Most are haemodynamically insignificant, but 2% will be associated with congestive heart failure. Blood is shunted from left to right, which leads to right ventricular failure and ascites secondary to valvular insufficiency. This is usually seen in birds aged 1–3 years. Duplicitas cordis, multiplicatis cordis and ectopia cordis have all also been reported.

Endocardial disease

Vegetative endocarditis of the aortic and mitral valves may cause vascular insufficiency, lethargy and dyspnoea. It is most common in birds with chronic infections (e.g. salpingitis, hepatitis and bumblefoot). Commonly implicated bacteria include *Streptococcus* spp., *Staphylococcus* spp., *E. coli*, *Pasteurella* spp., *Pseudomonas aeruginosa* and *Erysipelothrix rhusiopathiae*. Lesions consist of yellow irregular masses on any of the heart valves.

Myocardial disease

Myocarditis can occur secondary to viral, bacterial, mycotic and protozoan infections (**210**). Myocarditis has been reported with haemosiderosis, polyomavirus infection, chlamydiosis, PDD, *Sarcocystis* infections, pasteurellosis and mycobacterial and *E coli* infections.

Spontaneous turkey cardiomyopathy (STC) occurs in turkeys 1–4 weeks of age and is characterized by marked dilation of the right ventricle with extreme thinning of the ventricular wall. STC is also called 'round heart disease' and 'pulmonary hypertension and ascites syndrome'. Similar lesions can be induced in ducklings, chicks and turkey poults fed furazolidone. Cardiomyopathy has also been noted in young broilers (4–6 weeks old) selected for high meat yield. The oxygen demand by the large muscle exceeds what the heart/lungs can provide. This results

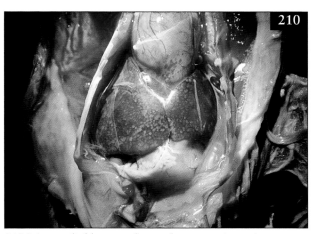

210 Myocardial haemorrhages due to septicaemia.

in polycythaemia, right ventricular dilatation/hypertrophy, valvular hypertrophy/insufficiency and right-sided failure. Vitamin E and selenium deficiencies cause cardiomyopathy in gallinaceous birds. It may also cause myocardial and skeletal muscle degeneration in ratites less than six months old and myocardial degeneration in cockatiels.

Ruptures of the myocardium may occur secondary to degenerative, inflammatory or neoplastic conditions of the myocardium or aneurysms of the myocardial vessels.

Myocardial infarctions are occasionally seen when an embolism originating from valvular endocarditis or heavy metal poisoning lodges in a coronary blood vessel.

Myocardial toxicity has been reported with avocado poisoning.

Pericardial disease

Pericardial effusion is a common finding in birds. It may result from cardiac or systemic disease and may be inflammatory (due to pericarditis or myocarditis) or noninflammatory. Transudative effusions may be due to congestive heart failure or systemic conditions causing hypoalbuminaemia.

Fibrinous pericarditis may lead to adhesions of the epicardium to the pericardium and subsequently to constrictive pericarditis. Serofibrinous pericarditis is most common with bacterial (*E. coli, Streptococcus* spp., *Listeria, Salmonella, Chlamydophila, Mycoplasma, Mycobacterium*) and viral (reovirus in Galliformes and polyomavirus in parrots) infections (**211**).

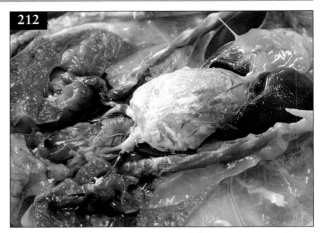

212 Visceral gout. Uric acid crystals have precipitated out over the pericardium.

Visceral gout may lead to a noninfectious pericarditis (**212**).

Arrhythmias

Arrhythmias can be normal (see below).

Sinus bradycardia can be induced by vagal stimulation and can be converted by the administration of atropine. Various anaesthetics and sedatives (e.g. halothane, methoxyflurane, xylazine and acepromazine) have been reported to cause sinus bradycardia when atropine is not given simultaneously. Hypothermia, which may accompany long-term anaesthesia, may potentiate this arrhythmia. Pathological conditions that may induce sinus bradycardia and sinus arrest include hypokalaemia, hyperkalaemia, thiamine deficiency and vitamin E deficiency. Several toxins have been reported to induce bradycardia, including organophosphorus compounds and polychlorinated biphenyls. Reflex vagal bradycardia may occur when pressure is exerted on the vagus nerve by neoplasms, and space-occupying lesions impinging on the vagal nerve should be considered when unexplained atropine-responsive bradycardia is seen. Atrioventricular (AV) nodal escape rhythm has been noted in ducks with sinus bradycardia from hyperkalaemia.

Atrial arrhythmias:
• Sinus tachycardia is considered nonpathological. The most common cause of sinus tachycardia is nervousness, but stress and pain may also precipitate the condition as well.

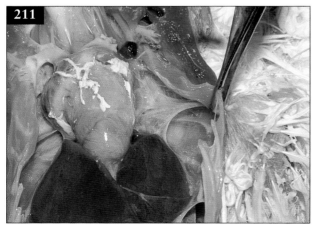

211 Pericarditis and air sacculitis.

- Atrial tachycardias may be seen as a result of pathological conditions of the atrium. Sinus tachycardia has been reported in chickens infected with avian influenza virus. When the heart rate is rapid, the P-wave may be superimposed on the T-wave (P on T phenomenon). This has been recorded in 16% of normal Amazon parrots and in 6% of African grey parrots.
- Atrial fibrillation occurs when electrical impulses are generated in the atrium in a rapid and irregular way, and the atrium is in a state of permanent diastole. Impulses reach the AV node in a high frequency and at irregular intervals, and hence the ventricular rhythm is irregular. The ECG is characterized by the absence of P-waves, normal QRS complexes (which may have an increased amplitude and duration because of ventricular hypertrophy) and irregular SS intervals.
- Supraventricular tachycardias may originate from the sinoatrial node (sinus tachycardia) or junctional area (junctional tachycardia). Differentiation between the two may be accomplished by measuring the PP interval. This interval is perfectly equidistant in atrial tachycardia, but may be irregular in sinus tachycardia due to vagal effects. Junctional tachycardias can be diagnosed by the presence of inverted P-waves in lead II.

Ventricular arrhythmias:
- Ventricular premature contractions (VPCs) are characterized by QRS complexes that are unrelated to the P-waves. Bigeminy is a rhythm characterized by alternating normal beats and VPCs, while in trigeminy two normal beats are followed by one VPC. VPCs in birds have been associated with hypokalaemia, thiamine deficiency, vitamin E deficiency, Newcastle disease and avian influenza viruses, myocardial infarction due to lead poisoning, and digoxin toxicity.
- Capture beats (normal P-QRS complexes in between VPCs) and fusion beats (a QRS complex intermediate between a normal P-QRS complex and a bizarre QRS complex that is formed by the simultaneous discharge of the ectopic ventricular focus and the normal sinoatrial node) are common with ventricular tachycardia.
- AV dissociation is a special form of ventricular tachycardia. The atrial and ventricular rhythms are independent of each other, whereby the atrial rate is lower than the junctional or idioventricular rate.

- VPCs, ventricular tachycardia and ventricular fibrillation may occur during periods of hypoxia and with the use of halothane. Changes in the configuration of the T-wave and ST segment should alert the clinician that myocardial hypoxia is present and more severe ECG abnormalities are imminent.

AV node arrhythmias:
- First-degree heart block occurs when the impulse through the AV node is delayed, resulting in an increased PR interval. This may be caused by halothane and xylazine, and the PR interval may increase to three to four times its normal value. This causes severe bradycardia that is reversible with atropine.
- Second-degree heart block is where some impulses do not reach the ventricles, but the majority of P-waves are followed by a QRS complex. Second-degree heart block Mobitz type 1 (Wenckebach phenomenon) has been reported as a physiological phenomenon in 5% of trained racing pigeons and is seen occasionally in asymptomatic parrots and raptors. In this form of AV block the PR interval lengthens progressively until a ventricular beat is dropped.
- Third-degree AV block is characterized by independent activity of atria and ventricles, where the frequency of the atrial depolarizations is higher than that of the ventricular depolarizations. The ventricular complexes may have a normal configuration or may be wide and bizarre, depending on the site of ventricular impulse formation. Complete AV block has been seen in chickens with hypokalaemia.

Congestive heart failure

This is defined as the compensated condition associated with fluid retention that results from a sustained inadequacy of the cardiac output to meet the demands of the body. The causes are numerous and include endocardial, epicardial, myocardial and combined diseases.

The pathophysiology of congestive heart failure involves both backward failure and forward failure. Backward failure involves increased atrial and venous pressure due to a failing ventricle, while forward failure involves decreased renal blood flow resulting in sodium and fluid retention. In response to low blood volume, renin is released from the juxtaglomerular cells of the kidney. Renin acts on circulating angiotensinogen to form angiotensin I, which is converted to angiotensin II. Angiotensin II stimulates aldosterone synthesis. Aldosterone causes sodium and fluid retention. Both mechanisms ultimately result in increased venous and capillary pressure, so that more fluid escapes by transudation into the interstitial spaces.

Pulmonary oedema predominates in isolated left ventricular disease. Systemic oedema with hepatomegaly and ascites will predominate in isolated right ventricular disease or when both ventricles are affected.

In birds, the right AV valve (muscular flap) thickens along with the right ventricle in response to an increased workload, and it has been postulated that this predisposes birds to right AV valvular insufficiency and right-sided heart failure.

Clinical presentation

Early stage signs include periodic weakness, syncope, lethargy and exercise intolerance. As the disease progresses, dyspnoea, coughing and coelomic distension due to ascites and hepatomegaly are seen.

Diagnosis

Auscultation of the heart

This is best performed on the left and right ventral thorax. Pleural or pulmonary fluid accumulation may cause muffled lung sounds or rales when a bird is auscultated over the back between the shoulder blades. Unique to birds, hepatomegaly can cause muffled heart sounds as the enlarged liver partly envelops the heart. Subtle murmurs may best be heard when a bird is anaesthetized.

Radiography

Radiographic detection of cardiovascular abnormalities may be difficult, although an enlarged cardiac silhouette or microcardia can often be visualized. The maximum width of the cardiac silhouette in a ventrodorsal radiograph should be 35–45% of the length of the sternum, 51–61% of the width of the thorax and 545–672% of the width of the coracoid.

Radiographic detection of an enlarged cardiac silhouette with muffled heart sounds is suggestive of pericardial effusion. An increased cardiac silhouette with normal heart sounds is suggestive of an enlarged heart. Microcardia is indicative of severe dehydration or blood loss that has resulted in hypovolaemia.

Other radiographic changes that suggest cardiac disease include congestion of pulmonary vessels, pulmonary oedema, pleural effusion, hepatomegaly and ascites.

Echocardiography

Echocardiography is the imaging technique that generally provides the most diagnostic information. Probes with small coupling surfaces and frequencies of at least 7.5 MHz are necessary, and the ultrasound devices should be able to produce at least 100 frames/second. Bipolar echocardiography is used to examine the heart in end-systolic and end-diastolic stage.

In small birds the echocardiographic image of the heart is best obtained by sweeping through the liver. B mode provides slices of the heart and allows anatomical evaluation of cardiac structures. M mode makes perpendicular slices of the B mode, allowing for quantitation of cardiac dimensions and timing of cardiac events. Colour Doppler facilitates identification of turbulence associated with valvular insufficiencies, stenoses and shunts.

Electrocardiography

This provides a graphic record of sequential electrical depolarization–repolarization patterns of the heart, detected on the surface of the body by changes in electrical fields (213). Electrocardiography may be useful for detection of cardiac enlargement from hypertrophy of any of the four cardiac chambers. It is indispensable for the diagnosis and treatment of cardiac arrhythmias and is also useful in monitoring changes in electrolyte concentrations during the treatment of metabolic diseases that alter electrolyte balance. Because the myocardium is very sensitive to hypoxia, electrocardiography can be a reliable indicator of oxygenation.

Leads are attached to both wings and both legs. In large or well muscled birds one may need the V electrode to the right or left of the sternum for greater amplitudes of all complexes. Needle electrodes placed subcutaneously are superior to alligator clips for use in avian patients. The Biolog® hand-held ECG machine has been used with one foot (lead) on the chest, one on the right wing and one on the right thigh. QRS complexes were larger than with standard machines, but they were comparable.

Different lead systems are used to record differences between different limbs:
- Standard lead system: leads I, II, III.
- Unipolar or augmented lead system: avR, avL, avF.
- Unipolar chest lead: V1–10.

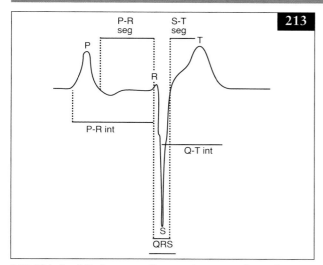

213 This lead II electrocardiogram is a recording of electrical currents generated during the depolarization and repolarization of the heart.

- The P-wave signifies that the atria have depolarized, causing contraction and ejection of their complement of blood into the ventricles.
- The PR segment indicates the short delay in the atrioventricular node that occurs after the atria contract, which allows complete filling of the ventricles before ventricular contraction occurs.
- The QRS complex represents ventricular depolarization and contraction with the ejection of blood into the aorta and pulmonary artery. The Q-wave is the first negative deflection, the R-wave is the first positive deflection and the S-wave is the first negative deflection following the R-wave.
- The ST segment and T-wave depict the repolarization of the ventricles. In clinically asymptomatic parrots, the ST segment may be very short or even absent, the S rising directly into the T-wave ('ST-slurring').

The sequence of depolarization and repolarization is recorded:

- Atrial depolarization: P-wave (the P-wave is positive on I, II, III and avF, and is negative on avR).
- Ventricular depolarization: QRS complex. This is negative in I, II, III and avF; there is no Q-wave in I, II and III (the negative mean electrical axis of ventricular depolarization in birds occurs because the depolarization wave begins subepicardially and then spreads through the myocardium towards the endocardium. Ventricular depolarization of the canine ventricles starts subendocardially).

- Ventricular repolarization: T-wave (positive on II, III and avF; negative on avR and avL; +/– or absent on I).
- T-P frequently overlap.

The paper needs to run at 50 mm/second or greater, as heart rates can vary from 100–1,000 beats per minute (bpm) (e.g. budgerigars: 600–750 bpm; cockatiel: 496–604 bpm). Some authors state paper speed needs to be at least 100 mm/s. For smaller species, paper speed may need to be set at 200 mm/second.

Determination of heart rate. The top of the ECG paper has a series of marks. The marks are 75 mm apart. The number of complexes that occur in three seconds are counted and multiplied by 20 to get beats/minute.

Determination of heart rhythm:

- Is the heart rate normal or abnormal for the species?
- Is the heart rhythm regular or irregular?
- Is there a P-wave for every QRS complex, and is there a QRS complex for every P-wave?
- Are the P-waves related to the QRS complexes?
- Do all the P-waves and all the QRS complexes look alike?

Determination of mean electrical axis:

- Find an isoelectric lead.
- Use the six-axis reference system chart and find which lead is perpendicular to the isoelectric lead.
- Determine if the perpendicular lead is positive or negative on the tracing and examine the angle value on the six-axis reference system. Compare these values with reference values.
- The average mean electrical cardiac axis is between 83° and –162°.

Measurements are all made on the lead II rhythm strip:

- P-wave. This signifies that the atria have depolarized, causing contraction and ejection of their complement of blood into the ventricles. With right atrial hypertrophy the P-wave becomes tall and peaked (P pulmonale), and with left atrial hypertrophy the P-wave becomes too wide (P mitrale). P pulmonale has been associated with dyspnoea induced by aspergillosis or tracheal obstruction. A tall, wide P-wave is suggestive of biatrial enlargement and is common with influenza virus in gallinaceous birds.
- PR interval. This indicates the short delay in the AV node that occurs after the atria contract,

which allows complete filling of the ventricles before ventricular contraction occurs. In the normal pigeon ECG, a small T_a-wave can be seen in the PR segment, indicating repolarization of the atria. This may also occur in some asymptomatic parrots and gallinaceous birds. This finding is considered normal.

- QRS complex. This represents ventricular depolarization and contraction with the ejection of blood into the aorta and pulmonary artery. The Q-wave is the first negative deflection, the R-wave is the first positive deflection and the S-wave is the first negative deflection following the R-wave. When there is no R-wave, the negative deflection is called a QS-wave. The largest wave in the QRS complex is depicted with a capital letter (i.e. Rs or rS). Two measurements are made on the QRS complex. The duration is measured from the beginning of the R-wave to the end of the S-wave. The second is the amplitude of the S-wave, measured from the baseline downwards. Low voltage ECGs often occur in birds with pericardial effusion. A QRS complex that is too wide or too tall indicates left ventricular hypertrophy or a bundle branch block. Prominent R-waves are suggestive of right ventricular hypertrophy.
- ST segment. Along with the T-wave this depicts the repolarization of the ventricles. In clinically asymptomatic racing pigeons and parrots, the ST segment is often very short or even absent. When present, it may be elevated above the baseline, which should not be interpreted as a sign of myocardial hypoxia, as it is in the dog.
- T-wave. In the normal avian ECG, this is always in the opposite direction to the main vector of the ventricular depolarization complex, and always positive in lead II. All measurements are made in lead II. When the T-wave changes its polarity, it suggests that myocardial hypoxia is occurring. The same is true for a T-wave that progressively increases in size (e.g. during anaesthesia). T-wave changes may also occur in association with electrolyte changes (e.g. increased T-wave amplitude with hyperkalaemia).
- QT interval. Prolongation might be associated with electrolyte disturbances (hypokalaemia, hypocalcaemia) and sedation, possibly due to a decreased heart rate. The QT interval may be prolonged in African grey and Amazon parrots.

Normal arrhythmias

Sinus arrhythmia, sinus arrest, sinoatrial block and wandering pacemaker have been reported in association with normal respiratory cycles and are considered physiological in birds.

The normal rhythm of the heart is established by the sinoatrial node. A normal sinus rhythm does not vary in rate from beat to beat. An increase in vagal activity may decrease the heart rate, while a decrease in vagal activity may increase the heart rate. Heart rate may increase during inspiration and decrease during expiration and hence the SS interval may not be equidistant. The associated rhythm is called sinus arrhythmia.

Sinus arrest is an exaggerated form of sinus arrhythmia and can be diagnosed if the pause is greater than twice the normal SS interval. Sinoatrial block occurs when an electrical impulse from the sinoatrial node fails to activate the atria. The pauses are exactly twice the SS interval. Wandering pacemaker refers to a continuous shifting of the pacemaker site in the sinoatrial node or the atrium, and an alteration in P wave morphology.

Blood pressure

The determination and monitoring of blood pressure has recently been recognized as a valuable diagnostic tool in the avian patient. Systolic blood pressure is the pressure exerted against the blood vessel wall during systole.

Direct arterial pressure measurement requires specific skills and is both invasive and expensive. Consequently, indirect blood pressure measurement techniques, based on the detection of blood flow beneath an inflated cuff, are more commonly used and have been found to correlate well with direct blood pressure measurements. The ultrasonic Doppler flow detector (Parks Medical Electronics Inc.) uses ultrasonic waves to detect arterial blood flow distal to a blood pressure cuff and produce an audible signal.

An appropriately sized cuff (depending on the size of the bird) is placed around the distal humerus or femur and taped in place. The Doppler probe is then placed above the radial carpal bone or tibiotarsal bone in order to detect arterial blood flow, and secured in place. The cuff is inflated until the Doppler signal is lost, and then slowly deflated. The pressure on the cuff when the first sound is heard is marked and recorded as the systolic pressure (see Chapter 25, Analgesia and anaesthesia).

Management
Congestive heart failure
Excessive neurohormonal activation is blocked by angiotensin converting enzyme (ACE) inhibitors (e.g. enalapril 0.5 mg/kg q12h). ACE inhibitors block the formation of angiotensin II, thereby blocking the renin–angiotensin–aldosterone system. They also have a diuretic effect. If the bird is on concurrent diuretic therapy, it may be best to start the ACE inhibitor at a low dose, while reducing the other diuretic therapy and then gradually increase the dose of the ACE inhibitor. Side-effects include hypotension, reflex tachycardia, gastrointestinal disorders, renal dysfunction and hyperkalaemia.

Myocardial function is supported with digoxin, 0.02–0.05 mg/kg q24h. This is indicated for myocardial dysfunction, chronic mitral insufficiency and chronic volume overloads. It is contraindicated for hypertrophic cardiomyopathy, ventricular tachycardia and sinus or AV node disease. Adverse effects relate to myocardial toxicity, therefore patients should be monitored for clinical improvement and via ECG for prolonged PR time. Serum concentrations should be measured after one week of therapy, or one week after the dose is changed. The dose can be increased if the serum concentration is <0.8 ng/l 8–10 hours after dosing.

Signs of congestion are treated with diuretics such as furosemide 0.15–2 mg/kg q12–24h. Overuse or high doses of diuretics can reduce the blood volume and trigger the renin–angiotensin–aldosterone system. Therefore, it is necessary to use the lowest effective dose.

Cardiac arrythmias
Treatment is not required unless the patient is clinically affected by the arrhythmia. The underlying cause should be treated.
- Supraventricular tachycardia:
  - Digoxin.
  - Beta blockers (e.g. propanolol 0.2 mg/kg q24h).
- Ventricular tachycardia: beta blockers.
- Bradycardia and AV blocks, limited therapy is available:
  - Atropine may be of some benefit
  - Ephedrine 0.5 mg/kg q8h.

Pericardial effusions
Diuretics are contraindicated because of the severe hypotension seen in many patients with reduced cardiac preload. Endoscopic pericardial fenestration may give temporary relief, but the effusion may return when the fenestration heals.

ATHEROSCLEROSIS
Definition/overview
Many avian orders may be affected, but Psittaciformes and Anseriformes appear to be particularly susceptible. Amazon parrots, macaws and African grey parrots seem to be particularly prone. Predisposing factors appear to include age (most affected birds are more than 8–15 years old), lack of exercise and high-fat diets (i.e. seed).

It is a diffuse or local degenerative condition of the internal and medial tunics of the wall of arteries. The degenerative changes include proliferation of smooth muscle cells and the deposition of collagen, proteoglycans and cholesterol. As tissue damage progresses, dystrophic mineralization occurs in the wall of the blood vessels. The resultant plaque protrudes into the aortic lumen and retards blood flow, increases surface tension and results in aortic aneurism and possibly aortic rupture. These changes are most commonly seen in the aorta, the brachiocephalic trunks and the pectoral and carotid arteries.

Aetiology
The accumulation of pathogenic material in the arterial wall has been explained by the insudative theory. Normally a transfer of plasma proteins occurs through the arterial wall, with subsequent removal from the outer coats by lymphatic vessels. During this process of permeation, fibrinogen and very low-density lipoproteins are selectively entrapped in the connective tissue of the arterial wall. Their presence stimulates reactive changes that give rise to the production of atherosclerotic lesions. Variations in vascular permeability and arterial blood pressure can explain the preference of atherosclerotic lesions for certain areas.

What triggers these changes is still the subject of debate, but it may include genetic predisposition in some birds, hyperlipaemia, endothelial inflammation, toxins, immune complexes and hypertension. The role of cholesterol and lipoproteins remains unclear.

Clinical presentation
Atherosclerosis is rarely reported in birds, and the condition is often associated with sudden death. Subtle and intermittent signs include dyspnoea,

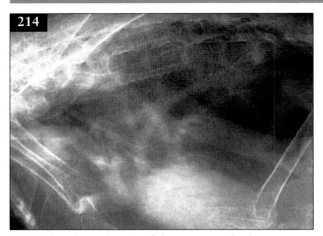

214 Early atherosclerosis of the great vessels above the heart.

weakness and neurological signs (e.g. seizures, tremors, paresis). Galliformes and Anseriformes may die acutely from dissecting aneurysms that result in aortic rupture secondary to hypertension and atherosclerosis.

Diagnosis

There may be elevated plasma cholesterol levels, but this is not consistent. Radiography may reveal an increased density and size of the right aortic arch (**214**).

Management

A variety of medical treatments have been advocated to lower cholesterol levels, but none appear to be consistent in their efficacy.

Beta blockers (e.g. propanolol, oxprenolol) may have a protective effect against the development of atherosclerotic plaques. Verapamil, nifedipine and diltiazem (calcium channel blockers) may decrease the extent and distribution of atherosclerotic lesions. These drugs have not yet been used in birds, but offer promise. Crocin, a natural carotenoid chemical compound that is found in crocus flowers, inhibits the formation of atherosclerosis in quails. Crocin exerts antiatherosclerotic effects by decreasing the level of oxidatively modified low-density lipoprotein, which plays an important role in the initiation and progression of atherosclerosis.

Change in diet to formulated foods and vegetables and a gradual increase in exercise play an important role in reducing obesity and increasing cardiovascular fitness.

HYPERTENSION

Definition/overview

Systolic blood pressures (measured with a Doppler) >200 mmHg (in conscious birds) or >160 mmHg (in anaesthetized birds) are considered to indicate hypertension in psittacine birds.

Blood pressure is determined by cardiac output and systemic vascular resistance. Cardiac output is determined by heart rate, preload and myocardial contractility. Tachycardia and increased myocardial contractility usually do not result in hypertension, as there is a corresponding decrease in systemic vascular resistance. Acute fluid overload can trigger a hypertensive episode.

The common denominator in the majority of hypertensive patients is an increase in systemic vascular resistance. This increase is mediated by increased levels of circulating catecholamines, increased alpha-adrenergic activity and activation of the renin–angiotensin–aldosterone system.

Aetiology

Primary or essential hypertension, although common in people, has been only occasionally documented in dogs. Its occurrence in other species, including birds, is unknown. It is due to excessive catecholamine release due to chronic stress.

Renal failure is relatively commonly associated with severe hypertension (through activation of the renin–angiotensin–aldosterone system) in dogs and cats, particularly in patients with protein-losing nephropathy (glomerular nephritis). The association between protein-losing nephropathy and hypertension in birds has not yet been documented, although glomerular nephritis is commonly found. Renal tumours may induce hypertension (through activation of the renin–angiotensin–aldosterone system) and are common in parrots. An association between renal tumours and hypertension has been documented in parrots.

Clinical presentation

Signs include ocular lesions (retinal haemorrhages, detachments, and/or papilloedema), neurological signs (depression, confusion, seizures), cardiovascular signs (ventricular hypertrophy and congestive heart failure) and renal system abnormalities (glomerulonephritis).

Diagnosis
Diagnosis is based on clinical signs and indirect (Doppler) blood pressure measurement.

Treatment
In patients without hypertension-related disease, treatment should be initiated cautiously with the goal of reducing blood pressure by 25% over several weeks. In patients with acute, severe hypertension-related disease, rapid reduction in blood pressure may be necessary.

Drugs used include ACE inhibitors (benazapril, enalapril). Calcium channel blockers (e.g. amlodipine) offer promise, but have not yet been trialled in birds.

FURTHER READING

Hanley SH, Helen GM, Torrey S (1997) Establishing cardiac measurement standards in three avian species. *Journal of Avian Medicine and Surgery* **11**:15–19.

Johnson HJ, Phalen DN, Kondik VH, Tippit T, Graham DL (1992) Atherosclerosis in psittacine birds. In: *Proceedings of the Annual Conference of the Association of Avian Veterinarians Australian Committee*, pp. 87–93.

Lichtenberger ML, Orosz S (2008) Cardiology: from anatomy to treatment. In: *Proceedings of the Annual Conference of the Association of Avian Veterinarians Australian Committee*, pp. 237–249.

Pees M, Krautwald-Junghanns ME, Straub J (2006) Evaluating and treating the cardiovascular system. In: *Clinical Avian Medicine, Vol 1*. GJ Harrison, TL Lightfoot (eds). Spix Publishing Inc, Palm Beach, pp. 379–394.

CHAPTER 18

DISORDERS OF THE LYMPHATIC AND HAEMATOPOIETIC SYSTEMS

The lymphoid organs are classified as primary (thymus and bursa of Fabricius) or secondary tissue (spleen, harderian gland, pineal gland, bone marrow and scattered aggregates of lymphoid tissue). The anatomy and function of these organs and tissues are described in Chapter 1, Clinical anatomy and physiology.

THYMUS
THYMIC CYSTS
Aetiology
The aetiology of thymic cysts is unknown, but they may be congenital abnormalities associated with persistent thymopharyngeal ducts, or acquired during thymic involution.

Clinical presentation
The cysts may fill with a colloidal fluid or gel and present as swellings on the neck

Management
Surgical removal of the cysts is recommended, but is often technically difficult because of extensive attachments to surrounding tissues.

PREMATURE THYMIC ATROPHY
The thymus normally involutes as a bird approaches maturity. Disorders associated with premature atrophy include viral infections, including circovirus, Pacheco's disease, avian influenza, Marek's disease, and infectious bursal disease, severe nutritional stress and iatrogenic corticosteroids.

The result is loss of the lymphocyte population (T cells) and subsequent immunodeficiency, leading to increased susceptibility to disease and some neoplasias.

NEOPLASIA
Definition/overview
Lymphosarcomas (**215, 216**) arise from lymphocytes; thymomas arise from the epithelial cells of the thymus.

Tumours may develop under the skin anywhere from the jaw to the thoracic inlet. They may be solid, cystic or haemorrhagic.

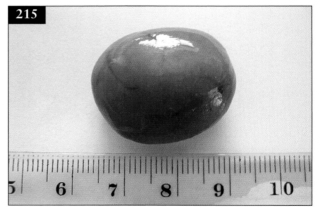

215 Lymphosarcoma in an African grey parrot. Massive splenomegaly due to neoplastic infiltration.

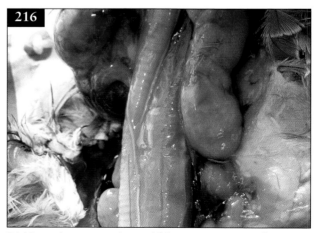

216 Lymphosarcoma in an African grey parrot. The lobulated masses running down the neck are the thymic gland infiltrated with neoplastic cells.

Management

Chemotherapy protocols for avian lymphosarcoma have been developed and have moderate degrees of success.

BURSA OF FABRICIUS
BURSAL ATROPHY

Definition/overview

Normal bursal involution occurs later in psittacines (18–20 months of age) compared with chickens. Premature bursal lymphocyte depletion can occur during incubation or post hatching.

Bursal atrophy results in an immunodeficient bird, particularly one that is deficient in humoral immunity (B cells). This is particularly important in young birds, making them more susceptible to many bacterial diseases and some fungal infections.

Aetiology

Causes include: acute or chronic disease (e.g. viral [circovirus, polyomavirus, avian pox virus, adenovirus, herpesvirus], bacterial, yeast and parasitic infections [*Cryptosporidium*]); toxins (oil, mycotoxins, pesticides); malnutrition (hypervitaminosis D3, hypovitaminosis A, calorie-deficient diets); and poor management leading to environmental stress (excessive temperatures, humidity and noise).

SPLEEN
SPLENIC ATROPHY

Hypoplasia or atrophy of the spleen may occur secondary to bursal disease. Lymphoid necrosis can be due to viral disease or other severe stress. Atrophy occurs due to age.

ENLARGED SPLEEN

Infectious causes include:
- Acute viral disease including polyomavirus, adenovirus and herpesvirus.
- Bacterial infections (especially *Salmonella* spp, and *Yersinia pseudotuberuclosis*) or septicaemia from gram-negative bacterial infections.
- Chlamydiosis.
- Mycobacterial infections.
- Mycotic infections.
- Parasites: *Atoxoplasma*, haemoparasites (e.g. *Plasmodium* spp.).

Splenic enlargement may also be caused by amyloidosis or neoplasia — primary (lymphosarcoma, fibrosarcoma, haemangiomas and haemangiosarcomas) or metastatic carcinomas.

BONE MARROW

The bone marrow is the main site of granulopoiesis (granulocyte production) and erythropoiesis (erythrocyte production). It is also a source of some long-lived lymphocytes. Various disorders can affect the bone marrow. Lesions can be hypocellular or hypercellular; granulocytic or erythroid. Evaluation of bone marrow aspirates requires comparison with peripheral blood.

Infectious diseases (bacteria, fungi, *Chlamydophila*, mycobacteria) usually trigger a hypercellular granulocytic response, leading to a leucocytosis. Some viral infections (herpesvirus, poxvirus, reovirus, polyomavirus), however, may have the opposite effect, inducing leucopenia. All infectious diseases have the capacity to cause a hypocellular erythroid response, leading to anaemia.

Various toxins can affect the bone marrow, causing a broad hypocellular response. These include ochratoxin A (produced by *Aspergillus ochraceous*), sulphaquinoxaline, cisplatin and fenbendazoles. Lead toxicosis induces a hypocellular erythroid response, leading to anaemia.

Myeloproliferative disorders (neoplastic proliferation of nonlymphoid haematopoietic cells in the bone marrow that subsequently invade the spleen and liver) cause anaemia. Haemangiosarcomas can be primary neoplasms of the bone marrow.

PRIMARY DISORDERS OF THE IMMUNE SYSTEM
IMMUNE SUPPRESSION

Immune suppression can occur either directly or indirectly.

Direct suppression is the inhibition of plasma cells, lymphocytes and macrophages, preventing antibody production, cell-mediated immunity or antigen processing. It occurs with:
- Drugs: tetracycline, tylosin and gentamicin can decrease antibody production.
- Aflatoxicosis: depresses complement activity and decreases phagocytic activity; also impairs cell-mediated immunity through inhibition of thymic-associated lymphocytes.
- Some viruses (e.g. influenza A virus) undergo antigenic variance wherein the surface proteins of the virus change and prevent immediate detection.
- Bursal disease (see above).
- Thymic disease (see above).

Indirect suppression occurs through the activation of the adrenal gland (by environmental stress) and subsequent production of corticosterone. This, in turn, inhibits antibody-forming cells and macrophage activity.

IMMUNE-MEDIATED DISORDERS
Allergies

Allergic dermatitis has been reported as a cause of feather picking and dermatitis in parrots. Confirmation can be difficult, as histological lesions are not definitive. Intradermal skin testing in birds is still to be completely validated, but it remains promising.

'Amazon foot necrosis' and other self-mutilating foot disorders are thought to be a delayed hypersensitivity to staphylococcal dermatitis or other allergens such as nicotine.

Allergic pneumonitis (respiratory hypersensitivity) is seen occasionally in macaws exposed to powder down/feather particles from other psittacines and organisms such as *Aspergillus* spp. See Chapter 16, Disorders of the respiratory system, p. 189.

Immune-mediated haemolytic anaemia
Definition/overview

Immune-mediated haemolytic anaemia occurs infrequently in poultry and is rarely documented in parrots.

Clinical presentation

Signs include weakness, polyuria and biliverdinuria.

Diagnosis

Blood samples show a strongly regenerative anaemia with a predominance of round, small erythrocytes (spherocytes), leucopenia and/or leucocytosis, and elevated plasma protein. There is splenomegaly.

Management

Immunosuppressive therapy is required (e.g. prednisolone).

Membranous glomerulonephropathy
Definition/overview

See Chapter 21, Disorders of the urinary system, p. 226. Glomerular disease is an important cause of end-stage renal disease in birds.

Aetiology

The cause of glomerulopathies is generally assumed to be immune-mediated, but the inciting aetiology is often unknown. PCR has been used to identify polyomavirus particles in the kidneys of many affected birds.

Diagnosis

Although proteinuria is the hallmark sign of glomerulonephritis in mammals prior to the onset of clinical renal insufficiency, avian leucocytes lack the proteolytic enzymes that would potentially damage the glomerular basement membrane (and allow protein leakage). Therefore, birds may not develop pathological proteinuria with glomerulopathies.

Renal biopsy is the best way to definitively diagnose glomerular (and other) kidney diseases in birds.

Management

Regardless of the possible causes, identifying and correcting underlying inflammation and/or systemic disease(s) are the first steps in managing renal disease.

Transfusion reactions

Transfusion reactions occur due to the incompatibility of donor red cells with host plasma. They have been reported in birds given multiple heterologous transfusions. Transfusion reactions may result in haemolysis of the donor red cells. Death may be the only sign associated with a transfusion reaction in a bird.

Reactions can be reduced by cross-matching individuals before giving a transfusion.

FURTHER READING

Gerlach H (1994) Defence mechanisms of the avian host. In: *Avian Medicine: Principles and Application.* BW Ritchie, GJ Harrison, LR Harrison (eds). Wingers Publishing, Lake Worth, pp. 109–120.

Ritchie BW (1995) Viral attack and avian response. In: *Avian Viruses: Function and Control.* Wingers Publishing, Lake Worth, pp. 47–82.

Schmidt RE (1997) Immune system. In: *Avian Medicine and Surgery.* RB Altman, SL Clubb, GM Dorrestein, K Quesenberry (eds) WB Saunders, Philadelphia, pp. 645–652.

CHAPTER 19

DISORDERS OF THE NERVOUS SYSTEM

INTRODUCTION

Birds showing neurological disorders, including loss of consciousness, seizures, abnormal mentation, ataxia, paresis or paralysis of legs and/or wings, cloacal atony, head tilt and nystagmus, are frequently presented to veterinarians.

Diagnosing neurological disorders requires a thorough examination in order to determine if the neuropathy is focal or diffuse. If the examination finds that dysfunction is present at more than one level, the lesion can be assumed to be either located at the highest location or multifocal. If the dysfunction is focal, an attempt is then made to localize the lesion to the head, cervical, thoracolumbar or lumbosacral spinal cord. If the examination fails to localize the lesion, a metabolic or generalized neuromuscular lesion should be considered.

As with any examination, a neurological assessment begins with a detailed history and involves a thorough physical examination before moving on to diagnostic testing to confirm a diagnosis or further localize the lesion.

HISTORY
The bird

The age of the bird is important: hereditary and inflammatory conditions are more common in the young bird, while degenerative and neoplastic conditions are more frequent in the older bird. Questions should be asked about diet, as malnutrition can be a primary cause of some neurological conditions. The bird's lifestyle should be determined with regard to access to toxins and likelihood of trauma. Reproductive activity may indicate the possibility of a yolk embolism. It is also important to ask the owner for details of any previous medical problems.

The problem

If the condition is of acute onset, one should consider toxicosis, trauma, vascular accident or generalized severe inflammation. If onset is more chronic, degenerative changes, neoplastic disease or low-grade inflammation is likely. If the disorder is progressive, a clear description of the chronological development of the clinical signs must be obtained.

The owner should be asked about the bird's mental state and demeanour, including changes to personality and behaviour. A precise description of the clinical signs is important (e.g. seizures may be difficult to differentiate from syncope). Generally, seizures are characterized by ataxia, disorientation, and falling off the perch, remaining rigid or having some form of motor activity for varying lengths of time.

DISTANT EXAMINATION
Mental status

If the bird is showing uncharacteristic aggression, a psychomotor-like epilepsy or a space-occupying mass in the forebrain should be considered. A depressed response to stimuli may result from lesions in the brainstem or forebrain. Semi-consciousness may be caused by acute encephalitis, forebrain trauma or neoplasia.

Posture

If there is a head tilt, lesions may be present in cranial nerve VIII. Tremor may be caused by lesions in the cerebellum or vestibular system, and falling or loss of balance may also be because of lesions in the vestibular system.

Flight

Uncoordinated flight or nonrhythmic fanning of wings may be related to a poor wing clip or lesions in the cerebellum, vestibular system or corpora striata. If the bird has poor obstacle avoidance, lesions in the eyes, cranial nerve II or the visual centre in the brain (neoplasia, abscess, granulomas) should be considered.

If the bird has poor take off or landing, one should consider a poor wing clip or lesions in the cerebellum, vestibular system, visual system, spinal cord or peripheral nerves. Paresis (flight not sustainable for lengthy periods) may be due to systemic disorders or lesions in the spinal cord or peripheral nerves.

Gait

Ataxia may be caused by lesions in the cerebellum or vestibular system. Dysmetria (inability to control or limit movement) may be due to lesions in the cerebellum. Circling can result from lesions in the vestibular system (unilateral) or corpora striata.

Poor obstacle avoidance may be due to lesions in the eyes, cranial nerve II or the visual centre, and poor righting reflex may be a reult of lesions in the vestibular system, corpora striata, visual or proprioceptive systems, cerebellum, spinal cord or peripheral nerves.

Other

Difficulties with prehension (abnormal tongue movement, reduced beak strength) may be a result of lesions in cranial nerves V and IX–XII. Reduced perching ability (not able to grasp a perch and support weight) can be due to lesions in the peripheral receptors, corpora striata, vestibular or visual system, cerebellum, spinal cord or peripheral nerves.

PHYSICAL EXAMINATION

A physical examination can be conducted after obtaining a thorough history and observing the patient from a distance. The examination should be performed methodically and logically. However, the order of the neurological examination depends on the clinical condition and cooperation of the patient. It is important to take into account the degree of cooperation of the patient when interpreting responses to neurological tests. Examination of the neurological system is detailed in Chapter 2, The physical examination, p. 52.

DIAGNOSTIC TESTS

Tests used in the diagnosis of neurological disorders include haematology and biochemistry, toxin analysis (especially blood lead levels), diagnostic imaging (radiography, CT, MRI), electroencephalograms (continuous recordings of the electrical activity of the cerebral cortex) and electromyograms (can be used to detect diseases of motor neuron cell bodies, ventral nerve roots, nerve plexuses, peripheral nerves, neuromuscular junctions and muscle fibres).

CENTRAL NERVOUS SYSTEM DISORDERS
CONGENITAL/HEREDITARY CONDITIONS

Hydrocephalus has been seen in older parrots, although possibly acquired rather than hereditary. Lafora body neuropathy has been reported, mainly in cockatiels. Glycoprotein-containing cytoplasmic inclusion bodies form within neurones, probably as a result of a defect in intracellular metabolism.

Teratogenic toxins such as dioxins can lead to asymmetrical brain development.

Lysosomal storage disease has been reported in emus, but not in companion birds.

VIRAL DISEASES
Paramyxovirus 1, 2, 3 and 5
Definition/overview

Paramyxovirus 1 (PMV-1, Newcastle disease) is seen in poultry, parrots and pigeons. PMV-2 is most commonly isolated from passerines. PMV-3 is the main paramyxovirus affecting parrots. Transmission of PMV-1 is horizontal through respiratory, faecal and oral secretions. Mechanical vectors (wind, insects, equipment and humans) may also spread the virus. Vertical transmission is possible. The incubation period may be between three and 28 days, depending on the strain. PMV-1 is a zoonotic disease. In humans (the only mammal to have clinical signs) there is mild acute granular conjunctivitis, general malaise and sinusitis, with recovery in 7–20 days.

Clinical presentation
PMV-1

PMV-1 may result in sudden death. Clinical signs can involve the CNS, respiratory and gastrointestinal systems, including depression, tremors, paralysis, a twisted neck, ataxia, opisthotonos, torticollis, conjunctivitis, nasal discharge, polyuria and diarrhoea.

PMV-3

PMV-3 may cause pancreatitis, lymphoplasmocytic myocarditis, otitis media and otitis interna. In neophemas, there is pulmonary oedema/congestion and hepatomegaly (high flock morbidity and low mortality). In nestling cockatiels there may be opisthotonos, tremors, leg paralysis, dyspnoea and a high mortality. In finches there may be initial conjunctivitis, anorexia, yellowish diarrhoea and dyspnoea.

Diagnosis
Diagnosis is made through serological testing (PMV-3 can cross-react with PMV-1) or viral isolation and culture.

Management
Vaccines (live or inactivated) are available, but may not be suitable for all species. The virus is inactivated by high temperatures (>56°C), sunlight, detergents, 1% chloramine, sodium hypochlorite, lysol, phenol and 2% formalin.

Proventricular dilatation disease
PDD can present as a primarily neurological disease (**217**) (see Chapter 13, Disorders of the gastrointestinal system, p. 161).

West Nile virus
Definition/overview
This is a flavivirus that is transmissible to birds, people and horses. Birds act as a reservoir for the virus, while mosquitoes act as vectors. The disease is seen in Africa, the Middle East, Europe, Asia and North America. In birds, death is caused by myocarditis and encephalitis.

Clinical presentation
Clinical signs include sudden death or depression, anorexia, weakness, weight loss and recumbency. Some birds show neurological signs, including abnormal head/neck posture, ataxia, tremors, circling, disorientation, paresis and impaired vision.

Management
Prevention revolves around vaccination and mosquito control.

Polyomavirus
Polyomavirus in budgerigars can cause cerebellar disease with marked intention tremors. It has also been observed in cockatoos with concurrent PBFD.

Herpesvirus
Pigeon herpesvirus can cause encephalomyelitis in pigeons. Parakeet herpesvirus affects *Neophema* and *Psittacula* parrots. They present with stargazing, stumbling, tremors, torticollis and dyspnoea. Marek's disease is seen in poultry, turkeys and quail.

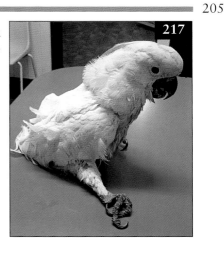

217 Leg paresis in a Moluccan cockatoo with proventricular dilatation disease.

Adenovirus
This rarely acts as a primary pathogen; one case the author saw was secondary to PBFD. Neurological signs have been noted in cockatiels and budgerigars. A nonsuppurative encephalitis is seen on pathology.

Togavirus
Togavirus causes eastern equine encephalitis and western equine encephalitis in emus, with clinical signs including ataxia, depression, anorexia, haemorrhagic diarrhoea and emesis, and ending with death. Togavirus is also considered to the cause of avian viral serositis, which can result in nonsuppurative meningitis and encephalitis in parrots.

Other viruses
A suspected viral encephalomyelitis is seen in lorikeets and *Polytelis* parrots presenting with progressive bilateral paralysis of the legs, with clenched feet (see Chapter 11, Disorders of the legs, feet, and toes, p. 145).

Avian influenza virus may cause loss of balance, ataxia and torticollis in some birds, although neurological signs are relatively rare.

BACTERIAL INFECTIONS
Bacteria identified as causing meningitis, encephalitis and myelitis include *Salmonella*, *Listeria*, *Staphylococcus*, *E. coli*, *Pseudomonas*, *Klebsiella* and *Mycobacterium*.

FUNGAL DISEASES
Aspergillus spp. can invade the brain, spinal cord and meninges via haematogenous spread or extension from the nasal cavity, sinuses or air sacs.

CHLAMYDOPHILA

Chlamydophila can produce a nonsuppurative meningitis (see Chapter 14, Disorders of the liver). This can result in seizures, tremors, torticollis and opisthotonos. In cockatiels, weakness or paralysis of the legs is occasionally seen.

PROTOZOAL DISEASES

Sarcocystis falcatula

This can cause an encephalitis in parrots and passerines (see Chapter 12, Disorders of the musculoskeletal system, p. 154).

Toxoplasma gondii

Definition/overview

Toxoplasma gondii infection is noted primarily in Galliformes and passerines, but has been diagnosed in parrots, raptors and owls. Cats shed the infective oocysts, which are then consumed by an intermediate host or by a bird.

Clinical presentation

Clinical signs include anorexia, diarrhoea, blindness, conjunctivitis, head tilt, circling and ataxia.

Diagnosis

Toxoplasmosis is diagnosed by serology or histopathology.

Management

Treatment is with pyrimethamine (0.5 mg/kg orally) or trimethoprim/sulphadiazine.

Leukocytozoon

This may form megaloschizonts in the brain (see Chapter 12, Disorders of the musculoskeletal system, p. 154).

NEMATODES

Baylisascaris procyonis

This causes ataxia, recumbency and other locomotor abnormalities in emus in the USA.

Filaria

Chandlerella quiscali is a parasite of grackles in the USA, transmitted by gnats. When emus are infected, adult worms develop in the lateral ventricles of the cerebrum, causing torticollis, ataxia, recumbency and death.

Wild-caught cockatoos from Indonesia are occasionally found to have microfilaria plugging the small vessels in the brain.

Migrating larvae of the rat lungworm (*Angiostrongylus cantonensis*) have been reported in the brain of yellow-tailed black cockatoos displaying neurological signs in Australia.

TRAUMA

Aetiology

Concussive head injuries are common in fully flighted birds that fly into ceiling fans, windows or aviary wire. They may also occur when a bird is attacked by another bird, either a cage mate or a wild predatory bird.

Clinical presentation

Clinical signs include depression, head tilt, circling and paresis of a wing or leg.

Diagnosis

Diagnosis is based on history and neurological examination, or on autopsy. Traumatic injuries usually result in haemorrhage in the meninges, extending into the brain parenchyma. There is often associated bruising and trauma to the skin and skull.

Postmortem pooling of blood in the venous sinuses of the calvarium is common with any cause of death, and must not be confused with traumatic injuries.

Prognosis

Prognosis improves with neurological improvement.

CEREBROVASCULAR ACCIDENTS

Aetiology

Thrombosis can lead to acute ischaemia and haemorrhage within the brain. A common cause of these emboli is yolk in reproductively active females.

Clinical presentation

Affected birds present with neurological signs that can be localized to the CNS. They may have a history of reproductive activity.

Diagnosis

Serum biochemistries usually support reproductive activity, particularly with hypercalcaemia and lipaemia.

Management

Reproductive rest is recommended. Meloxicam or other NSAIDs may be helpful.

TOXINS

Lead toxicosis

Definition/overview

There are two target organs of toxic lead intake: the nervous system and erythropoietic bone marrow. The source is often not determined. It may be lead shot, leaded petrol and oil, galvanized wire, lead-based paints, lead putty, solder, foil from some champagne and wine bottles, some welds on wrought-iron cages, lead weights (curtain and fishing), bells with lead clappers, lead-lighted glass, improperly glazed ceramics, batteries, bird toys with lead weights, costume jewellery or mirror backs.

Pathophysiology
Lead is solubilized in the ventriculus by the combination of its grinding action and the low pH (2–3.5). Once solubilized, lead is absorbed across the intestinal mucosa and is bound to metalloprotein for distribution around the body. Lead competes for calcium at the myoneurological junction, resulting in neuromuscular blockage, and it affects neuronal cell adhesion molecules and glucocorticoid receptors in neurones and glial cells. It also suppresses amino-leuvulinic acid dehydrase and heme synthetase, leading to an accumulation of aminoleuvulinic acid and protoporphyrin IX in erythrocytes, which inhibits the heme synthesis cascade. This leads to decreased erythrocyte production and anaemia.

Clinical presentation
Multifocal neurological signs include hyperexcitability, ataxia, paresis and paralysis (**218**), convulsions, wing droop and head tilt. Gastrointestinal signs include ileus, vomiting and abnormally coloured diarrhoea (green to black). There may be renal signs of polyuria and polydypsia, and haematuria in Amazon parrots and galahs. Anaemia causes lethargy, depression and weakness.

Diagnosis
Clinical pathology
Haematology reveals a hypochromic, regenerative anaemia. Erythrocytic ballooning is common, but not pathognomonic.

Biochemistry shows elevated LDH, AST, CK and uric acid concentrations, reflecting increased protein catabolism and renal dysfunction. In waterfowl, inhibition of delta-aminoleuvulinic acid dehydrogenase to levels <86 IU/l is suggestive of lead toxicosis.

Blood lead determination is a reliable indicator of toxicosis, as 90% of circulating lead is contained in erythrocytes. There is still debate as to what constitutes a 'normal' blood lead level. It might be better to say that below certain levels, clinical signs are unlikely to be seen. What effect these 'normal' levels are having on the patient is difficult to assess.

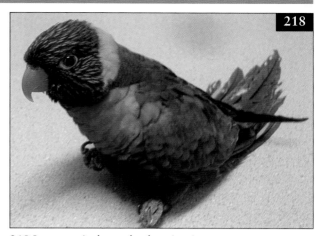

218 Leg paresis due to lead toxicosis.

- 'Normal' blood level is <0.7 $\propto$mol/l (14.5 µg/dl, 0.145 ppm).
- 0.7–1.7 $\propto$mol/l (35.2 $\propto$g/dl, 0.352 ppm) suggests exposure.
- >1.7 $\propto$mol/l confirms lead toxicosis.

Diagnostic imaging
Plain and contrast radiographs often show a dilated proventriculus and other evidence of ileus. Radiodense particles may be visible in the crop, proventriculus and ventriculus, but the absence of these particles does not exclude a diagnosis of lead toxicosis.

Histopathology
Acid-fast intranuclear inclusions are found in epithelial cells of proximal convoluted tubules and hepatocytes. There may also be neuronal degeneration (cerebral cortex, optic lobes, medulla oblongata) and Zenker's degeneration of the myocardium, the ventriculus, and pectoral muscles (hyaline degeneration and loss of muscle striations).

Management
Chelation
Calcium EDTA is given at a dose of 20–40 mg/kg IM q12h. There are reports of doses up to 100 mg/kg q12h being given without any evidence of nephrotoxicity. Metal ions displace the calcium in CaEDTA to form a water-soluble complex that is excreted in the urine. The author prefers to treat twice daily until the patient is asymptomatic (usually 3–5 days), then twice weekly until blood lead levels are in the 'normal' range (often up to six weeks). Response

is usually rapid, with a clinical improvement usually noticeable within 24–36 hours.

D-penicillamine is an effective oral chelator, but it may cause nausea and vomiting in some birds.

Removal of particles from the gastrointestinal tract

Most small particles will pass through the gastrointestinal tract in 4–5 days. Larger pieces may have to be retrieved endoscopically or by concurrent flush and suction with warmed water. As a last resort, a proventriculotomy can be performed.

Supportive care

See Chapter 5, Supportive therapy. Patients will require fluid support, nutritional support and thermal support. Blood transfusion may be required in very anaemic patients.

Botulism
Definition/overview

Botulism is most commonly a problem with game birds, ducks and pheasants, although it occurs sporadically in other wild or exotic species.

Aetiology

Botulsim is due to the ingestion of bacterial exotoxins produced by *Clostridium botulinum*, a widely dispersed saprophytic bacterium found in soil. This toxin (type C predominantly, although types A and E are sometimes identified) develops when *C. botulinum* grows in anaerobic conditions. It is present in vertebrate carcasses, decaying vegetation and dead invertebrates found in stagnant ponds, wetlands and marshes. Fly maggots and aquatic insects accumulate the toxin and are then ingested by birds. It is most often seen in late summer and early autumn when many ponds are drying out and water levels drop, exposing dead animals and rotting vegetation.

Pathophysiology

The toxin interferes with release of acetylcholine (ACH) at motor endplates.

Clinical presentation

Affected birds show ataxia and flaccid paralysis of the legs, wings and neck ('limber neck'). There may be diarrhoea, loose feathers, dyspnoea, gasping, conjunctivitis or sudden death.

Diagnosis

Diagnosis can be difficult, as there are few lesions found on autopsy. Botulinum toxin can be detected by a variety of techniques including ELISA, electrochemiluminescent (ECL) tests and mouse inoculation or feeding trials. The toxins can be typed with neutralization tests in mice.

Management

Treatment involves administration of antitoxin, if it is available, and supportive care. The prognosis is usually guarded to poor.

A vaccine is available in some countries. Prevention revolves around preventing access to decaying vegetation and dead animals by birds.

Organophosphates and carbamates
Definition/overview

Birds are 10–20 times more susceptible to acetylcholinesterase inhibitors than mammals. These chemicals are used as pesticides. Exposure is usually through inhalation of aerial spraying or cutaneous absorption through washing or dipping. Occasionally, wild birds are poisoned by ingesting grain laced in organophosphates or carbamates in an attempt to control wild bird numbers around grain silos.

Pathophysiology

Organophosphates and carbamates inhibit acetylcholinesterase, the enzyme that breaks down the neurotransmitter ACH. This results in ACH accumulating at nerve synapses and subsequent continued stimulation at cholinergic nerve endings and myoneural junctions.

Clinical presentation

Clinical signs include anorexia, diarrhoea, crop stasis, ptyalism, ataxia, tremors, seizures and paralysis. Death is usually due to respiratory failure.

Prolonged exposure to organophosphates may result in 'delayed neuropathy syndrome'. The organophosphate molecules bind to neuropathy target esterase; this binding then initiates degeneration of long axons in the peripheral and central nervous systems. The effects of this are seen 7–10 days after exposure as weakness, ataxia, decreased proprioception and paralysis. This syndrome is not associated with the inhibition of acetylcholinesterase.

Management

Atropine 0.2 mg/kg IM is given as needed until the clinical signs stop. Atropine has little or no effect on nicotinic receptors and used alone will not counteract neuromuscular paralysis. Pralidoxime 10–20 mg/kg

IM is administered every 8–12 hours as needed. It is only effective if used within the first 24 hours of exposure. It is contraindicated for carbamate toxicosis.

Chlorinated hydrocarbon(DDT)/organochlorines
Definition/overview
These chemicals have been used widely as pesticides since 1945. Exposure occurs through aerial spraying and ingestion of poisoned insects.

Pathophysiology
The mechanism of action is unclear, but it is believed to interfere with axonic transmission of nerve impulses.

Clinical presentation
Clinical signs include thin-shelled eggs and tremors and convulsions.

Diagnosis
Diagnosis is made by measuring levels of the chemicals in fat, brain and liver.

Management
Treatment is unrewarding

Dimetridazole
This causes convulsions, wing-flapping and opisthotonos in budgerigars, goslings, pigeons and ducks.

Levamisole
Definition/overview
Levamisole causes toxicity by stimulation of cholinergic receptors in the autonomic ganglia, neuromuscular junctions and CNS. However, in most studies the reported cause of death is asphyxia and respiratory failure. In poultry, toxic reactions only occur with doses in excess of 160 mg/kg and deaths at >480 mg/kg. This is why it has gained wide acceptance as a safe anthelmintic for poultry.

Clinical presentation
Levamisole causes regurgitation, ataxia, recumbency, catatonia, dyspnoea and death in parrots and poultry. Pulmonary oedema is a feature of levamisole toxicosis in a range of species whether given by injection or orally.

Nitrofurazone
Nitrofurazone causes screaming, convulsions, aimless running or flying and opisthotonos. There may be depression and growth retardation.

NUTRITIONAL DEFICIENCIES
Vitamins
Hypovitaminosis B1 (thiamine)
This causes anorexia, ascending paralysis and opisthotonos, polyneuritis with myelin degeneration and adrenal hypertrophy and skin oedema. Cases respond within hours to parenteral vitamin B1.

Hypovitaminosis B2 (riboflavin)
Hypovitaminosis B2 causes curled toe paralysis in poultry and nestling budgerigars, weakness, emaciation (despite a good appetite), diarrhoea, walking on hocks with toes curled inward and leg muscle atrophy; and demyelinating peripheral neuritis with nerve oedema. Chronic cases have irreversible damage.

Hypovitaminosis E and selenium deficiency
Vitamin E deficiency in young birds causes encephalomalacia, exudative diathesis and muscular dystrophy. It is particularly common in hatchling budgerigars.

Hypovitaminosis B6 (pyridoxine)
Hypovitaminosis B6 causes jerky, nervous walking progressing to running and flapping the wings. The bird then falls with rapid, clonic tonic head and leg movements, which usually lead to death.

Calcium
Definition/overview
Hypocalcaemic tetany is most common in adult African grey parrots.

Aetiology
It is usually associated with the long-term feeding of a diet deficient in calcium, combined with hypovitaminosis D3 (due to lack of UVB radiation or dietary supplementation). Initially the bird will maintain normal blood calcium concentrations by utilizing the calcium reservoir present in the bones, but eventually the homeostatic system fails and the blood calcium level will fall. In a normal adult grey parrot the blood ionized calcium concentration is kept within a very narrow range (0.96–1.22 mmol/l). Once the homeostatic system fails and the blood ionized calcium concentration falls below the normal level the bird will respond with a variety of neurological clinical signs.

Clinical presentation
Initially the bird may just twitch or flick its head. Ataxia develops and progresses to fits or convulsions.

Management

The clinical signs respond rapidly to parenteral calcium and vitamin D3 supplementation. Long-term therapy should involve improvement of the diet with respect to calcium and vitamin D3 content.

UVB radiation should be provided, either from natural sunlight or artificial full spectrum lights, particularly in birds exposed to low light levels kept indoors.

NEOPLASIA
Pituitary adenomas
Definition/overview

These are either adenomas or adenocarcinomas arising from chromophobe cells. They most commonly occur in young male budgerigars.

Clinical presentation

Clinical signs are related to compression of the brain and cranial nerves from the space-occupying mass. These signs include uncoordinated wing flapping, clonic leg twitches, seizures, circling, depression, somnolence, unconsciousness, exophthalmos, mydriasis, blindness and inappropriate behaviour responses.

If the tumour is functional, other clinical signs can include polydypsia and polyuria, feather abnormalities, cere colour changes and obesity.

Primary brain tumours

Primary brain tumours are rare. They include astrocytoma, glioblastoma multiforme, schwannomas, ganglioneuroma, neurofibrosarcomas, pineal body tumours, undifferentiated sarcomas and haemangiomas. Clinical signs are similar to those seen with pituitary tumours.

EPILEPSY/SEIZURES
Aetiology

Epilepsy/seizures can be due to a number of causes:
- Metabolic (e.g. hypoglycaemia, hypocalcaemia).
- Liver failure — hepatic encephalopathy.
- Kidney failure.
- Hypoxia.
- Nutritional deficiencies.
- Toxins (lead, organophosphates, organochlorines, chocolate, caffeine, some mycotoxins).
- Neoplasia.
- Infectious CNS disorders (viral, bacterial, fungal, parasitic, chlamydial).
- Cardiovascular disease including yolk embolism.
- Trauma.
- Heat stress.

- Storage diseases such as Lafora's disease.
- Idiopathic epilepsy has been reported in peach-faced lovebirds, red-lored Amazons and greater Indian hill mynahs.

Management

If possible, the cause of the seizures should be identified and eliminated.

Initial stabilization of the seizuring bird may require diazepam or midazolam. Longer-term stabilization requires phenobarbital, starting at 5–8 mg/kg orally q12h and increasing gradually to effect.

Monitoring the response to treatment is usually based on the patient's clinical signs. Serial measurement of blood phenobarbital levels may not be necessary, but liver function should be monitored.

OTHER CAUSES OF CENTRAL NERVOUS SYSTEM DISEASE

Atherosclerosis of the carotid arteries has been described as a cause of ischaemia and cerebral hypertension.

Xanthomatosis can appear in the brain associated with blood vessels.

Amyloidosis, due to chronic antigenic stimulation, can develop in the brain.

PERIPHERAL NERVOUS SYSTEM DISORDERS

Many of the disorders that are described above may present as peripheral neuropathies.

RENAL NEOPLASIA OF BUDGERIGARS
Clinical presentation

Progressive unilateral paresis occurs due to pressure exerted on the sciatic nerve by a renal tumour (carcinoma, adenocarcinoma, embryonal nephromas). There is normal flexion and extension of the hip joint, with decreased flexor/extensors and sensation, particularly below the knee (**219**).

Management

Chemotherapy has been tried, but with limited success at this stage. Prognosis is poor.

BRACHIAL PLEXUS AVULSION

The cause is usually traumatic. The bird may present with Horner's syndrome due to interruption of the sympathetic pathway from T1 and occasionally T2.

LEAD TOXICOSIS

This may cause a peripheral neuropathy with self-mutilation and feather picking as clinical signs (see p. 206).

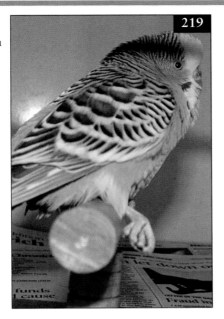

219 Paresis due to renal neoplasia in a budgerigar.

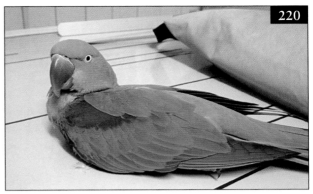

220 'Obturator' paralysis in an egg-laying hen.

OBTURATOR PARALYSIS
Clinical presentation
A form of 'obturator paralysis' is sometimes seen in egg-laying hens. After laying an unusually large egg, or after a difficult oviposition, the hen is paretic or paralysed in the legs (220).

Management
Rest, NSAIDs and calcium supplementation usually result in recovery, although this may take several weeks in severe cases.

MAREK'S DISEASE
Definition/overview
This is a disease of chickens, turkeys and quail caused by a herpesvirus. Affected birds are usually 2–16 weeks of age. Transmission is usually by inhalation of infected feather dust, debris and dust. The incubation period ranges from two weeks to several months.

Clinical presentation
Signs include paresis and paralysis due to lymphocytic proliferation in peripheral nerves, especially the sciatic nerve, visceral neoplasia and neoplasia in the skin, eyes, muscles and bones.

Diagnosis
Diagnosis is usually made on autopsy and histopathology.

Management
A vaccine is available, but the efficacy varies.

FURTHER READING
Antinoff N (2007) Stop the shakes! Diagnosing and treating neurological disorders in birds. In: *Proceedings of the Annual Conference of the Association of Avian Veterinarians Australian Committee*, pp. 201–215.

Platt SR (2006) Evaluating and treating the nervous system. In: *Clinical Avian Medicine, Vol 2.* GJ Harrison, TL Lightfoot (eds). Spix Publishing Inc, Palm Beach, pp. 493–518.

Rosenthal K, Orosz S, Dorrestein GM (1997) Nervous system. In: *Avian Medicine and Surgery.* RB Altman, SL Clubb, GM Dorrestein, K Quesenberry (eds) WB Saunders, Philadelphia, pp. 454–474.

Chapter 20

Disorders of the Reproductive Tract

THE MALE REPRODUCTIVE TRACT

Congenital

Abnormalities include abnormally shaped testes, fusion of the cranial poles, hypoplasia and agenesis. Usually there are no clinical signs, although aviary birds may be presented for infertility investigation. Diagnosis is by endoscopy, and no treatment is required.

Noninflammatory

Degeneration of the testes is associated with various drugs and toxins (e.g. furazolidone, copper fungicides and mercury). It is diagnosed by endoscopic biopsy or needle aspiration cytology.

Atrophy may occur as the end stage of degenerative changes.

Orchitis

Aetiology

Orchitis may be bacterial (*E. coli, Salmonella* spp. [221], *Pasteurella* spp.), fungal (extension from

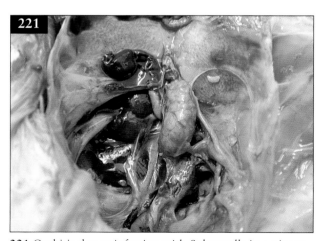

221 Orchitis due to infection with *Salmonella* in a pigeon.

fungal air sacculitis), mycobacterial (extension from systemic disease) or chlamydial (extension from systemic disease). Infection occurs by haematogenous spread or via an ascending infection from the cloaca/phallus.

Clinical presentation

No clinical signs are seen unless the bird is septicaemic.

Diagnosis

Diagnosis is by aspiration cytology or endoscopic biopsy.

Management

Antimicrobial therapy is given as indicated. Surgical orchidectomy may be required.

Neoplasia

Definition/overview

Neoplasia of the male reproductive tract is reported in numerous species. Tumours seen include Sertoli cell tumours (most common), interstitial cell tumours, seminomas, teratomas, lymphosarcoma, teratoma and leiomyosarcoma and carcinoma of the ductus deferens and epididymis.

Clinical presentation

Clinical signs include chronic weight loss, abdominal distension, unilateral paresis of the leg (due to sciatic nerve compression) and cere colour change in budgerigars (blue to brown). (Note: This colour change is not pathognomic for Sertoli cell tumours.)

Diagnosis

On endoscopic examination the testicles may appear cystic and can be confused with an immature ovary. Diagnosis is by endoscopic biopsy.

Management
Orchidectomy is indicated. There is a good prognosis if there is no metastatic disease.

PHALLIC PROLAPSE
Aetiology
Phallic prolapse is seen in ratites and waterfowl and is associated with sexual overwork. Inflammatory changes at the base of the phallus, occasionally associated with chronic bacterial infection, can maintain the prolapse even though the bird is sexually inactive.

Clinical presentation
The prolapsed phallus protrudes from the vent. The end of the phallus may become traumatized and/or necrotic from chronic exposure and contact with the ground.

Management
Sexual rest is required. The bird should be isolated from the hens and daylight hours reduced. A change in diet may be needed and one may consider GnRH agonists such as leuprolide acetate, human chorionic gonadotropin (HCG) and deslorelin. Anti-inflammatory treatment (e.g. meloxicam) and broad-spectrum antibiotics are indicated.

If the phallus is damaged, one may have to consider reducing the prolapse and placing lateral vent sutures to keep the phallus in the cloaca until healed. Phallic amputation can be considered, usually as a last resort.

THE FEMALE REPRODUCTIVE TRACT
THE OVARY
Congenital abnormalities
Congenital abnormalities include congenital atresia, retained right ovary and congenital ovarian cysts.

Both ovaries are frequently present in raptors and kiwis. All early embryos have bilateral ovaries and oviducts, but growth of the right ovary and oviduct is inhibited after the first trimester of incubation. Retained right ovaries are occasionally seen in species that would normally have only a left ovary. In poultry, 90% of enlarged right ovaries are the result of damage to the left ovary.

Congenital ovarian cysts are common in budgerigars and canaries.

Oophoritis
Aetiology
Infectious oophoritis can result from haematogenous spread of a bacterial (e.g. *Salmonella* spp.,

mycobacteria), fungal or viral infection (e.g. herpesvirus), or spread from adjacent air sacculitis or coelomitis. Noninfectious oophoritis may be caused by rupture of follicles and extrusion of yolk into the ovarian stroma or by toxins (e.g. aflatoxicosis).

Clinical presentation
Infectious oophoritis is often part of a systemic illness and many birds will present for generalized weakness. In milder cases there may be an infertility problem or increased embryonic deaths.

Diagnosis
Haematology may reveal a leucocytosis. Endoscopy may reveal abnormally coloured or shaped ovaries, often haemorrhagic and with abnormal follicles. The ovaries of birds with noninfectious oophoritis may appear enlarged, with multifocal yellow spots of varying sizes.

Management
Antimicrobial therapy is given as indicated. If possible, the abscessed follicle(s) should be drained completely, being careful not to contaminate the abdomen. Partial or complete ovariectomy may be required for chronically infected and caseated follicles.

Ovarian cysts
Aetiology
Ovarian cysts may be congenital (see above) or acquired, secondary to neoplasia or oophoritis.

Clinical presentation
If the cysts are small, there may be no clinical signs. Large cysts may cause abdominal enlargement and dyspnoea (through compression of the air sacs).

Diagnosis
This is based on ultrasonography, endoscopy and exploratory coeliotomy.

Management
Aspiration of the cyst may be carried out by ultrasound-guided transabdominal aspiration, endoscopic aspiration or surgical aspiration.

Ovariectomy (partial or complete) is difficult to achieve successfully because of the complex vascularity of the ovary. It should not be attempted without good magnification (e.g. an operating microscope).

Hormonal therapy (e.g. leuprolide acetate, HCG) has been suggested to reduce or resolve ovarian cysts in birds and offer a noninvasive treatment option. This, however, assumes that the cysts are primary in origin and are not secondary to other disease processes (neoplasia, oophoritis).

Neoplasia
Definition/overview
Tumours of the ovaries include granulosa cell tumours, ovarian carcinomas, dysgerminoma, arrhenoblastoma and teratoma.

Clinical presentation
If the tumour is small, there may be no clinical signs. Large tumours may cause abdominal enlargement and dyspnoea (through compression of the air sacs). There may be egg retention and oviductal impaction.

Granulosa cell tumours (and possibly other reproductive tract tumours) may be functional and cause increased plasma hormone levels. This can result in hormonal changes (e.g. polyostotic [medullary] hyperostosis **172, 173**).

Diagnosis
Diagnostic imaging (ultrasonography and radiography) helps to identify the presence of a tumour. Confirmation is by endoscopic or surgical biopsy.

Management
Treatment may include partial or complete ovariectomy, adjuvant chemotherapy or radiation therapy. The prognosis is guarded.

THE OVIDUCT
Congenital abnormalities
Congenital abnormalities include atresia, segmental aplasia and congenital cysts. The bird is usually presented for infertility investigation, yolk-related peritonitis (see p. 215) or salpingitis (see next column).

Cystic hyperplasia
Grossly visible cysts occur containing clear or cloudy fluid. They are probably endocrinal in origin, but this is not determined as yet. Birds are usually presented for either infertility investigation, yolk-related peritonitis (see p. 215) or salpingitis (see next column).

Neoplasia
Adenomas, adenocarcinomas and leiomyomas have been reported. Birds are usually presented for abdominal distension, yolk-related peritonitis (see p. 215) or salpingitis (see next column).

Salpingitis and metritis
Definition/overview
Salpingitis is inflammation of the oviduct and mesosalpinx and metritis is inflammation of the shell gland.

Aetiology
These are relatively common conditions in domestic psittacines and backyard poultry. Predisposing factors include age, malnutrition, excessive abdominal fat, excessive egg laying, egg-binding and other reproductive disorders.

Primary infections are uncommon in domestic situations; they may be caused by Newcastle disease virus or infectious bronchitis virus.

Secondary infection may follow yolk retention or prolonged/excessive egg laying. Haematogenous or ascending infections may occur. Bacterial species involved include *E. coli, Klebsiella* spp. and *Pseudomonas* spp.

Clinical presentation
Affected birds often have a history of extremely good egg production. They are often on a predominantly seed diet with inadequate vitamin and mineral supplementation. There may be a history of infertility or embryonic or neonatal mortality.

Clinical signs include weight loss, ruffled plumage, anorexia and lethargy. If the birds are still laying eggs, these eggs may be malformed (soft–shelled, stress lines (**222**), abnormal shape) or have streaking of blood

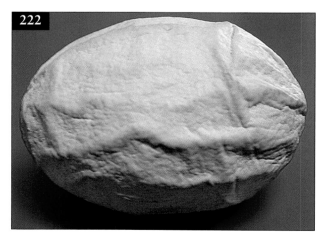

222 Stress lines in the egg of a hen with metritis.

on the shell. There may be chronic egg-binding, infertility, a distended abdomen, a flaccid vent and cloacal discharge.

Diagnosis

There may be a leucocytosis, either heterophilic or monocytic, depending on the chronicity of the problem. Clinical biochemistries may show a hypercalcaemia (if the bird is still reproductively active) and a hyperamylasaemia (if there is concurrent pancreatic disease associated with a yolk peritonitis).

Radiography may reveal retained eggs, an enlarged oviduct or the presence of abdominal fluid. Ultrasonography can distinguish between fluid enlargement and organ enlargement, and may reveal retained eggs or fluid in the oviduct. Endoscopy (if there is not free fluid in the abdomen) can demonstrate a swollen and inflamed oviduct. If abdominal fluid is present, abdominocentesis can help to differentiate the inciting causes.

Management

Conservative treatment may be attempted, but is usually unsuccessful. Recommendations include reproductive rest through environmental, nutritional and hormonal manipulation, NSAIDs (e.g. meloxicam) and antibiotics. If there is material in the oviduct (e.g. caseous pus, eggs or fluid), the use of prostaglandins may be indicated. Using PGE2 to relax the uterovaginal sphincter and stimulate oviductal contractility may assist in this regard. Caution must be exercised with this therapy, as chronic cases may have developed adhesions to the oviductal wall and strong contractions may lead to rupture of the oviduct.

In valuable breeding birds an attempt to combine the above therapy with a coeliotomy and retrograde flushing of the oviduct can be made. Definitive treatment may require salpingohysterectomy (see Chapter 26, Surgery, p. 264).

In all probability, a diagnosis of salpingitis or metritis indicates that the bird's reproductive life is almost certainly complete. If the patient is a breeder or egg layer, this must be communicated to the owner before commencing any treatment. Conservative treatment may give some short-term success, but the problem often recurs. Salpingohysterectomy often gives good long-term results, although some birds will continue to ovulate and develop yolk-related peritonitis (see below). These birds require environmental, nutritional and hormonal manipulation to minimize ovulation.

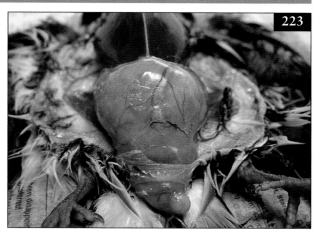

223 Coelomic distension due to yolk and fluid in a bird with yolk-related peritonitis.

Yolk-related peritonitis
Aetiology

Yolk-related peritonitis is caused by retropulsion of yolk from the oviduct into the abdomen, possibly associated with metritis/salpingitis, oviductal cystic hyperplasia or oviductal impaction, or with exuberant reverse peristalsis. It may also be caused by failure of the infundibulum to 'capture' ovulating yolk because of fat, trauma or disease.

Clinical presentation

The condition is usually seen in high-producing hens, especially cockatiels. It is usually sterile; if septic, signs are consistent with severe septicaemia.

Clinical signs are related to a fluid-producing inflammatory reaction in the coelom: dyspnoea, abdominal distension (**223**) and weakness. The bird may stop laying or may lay malformed eggs (elongated).

Secondary diseases may develop as a result of yolk-related peritonitis including neurological signs due to yolk emboli ('yolk stroke'), pancreatic disease (including diabetes mellitus), hepatitis, nephritis, splenitis and coelomic adhesions.

Diagnosis

There is a marked leucocytosis. Hypercalcaemia may be seen in reproductively active hens.

Abdominal ultrasonography confirms fluid distension of the abdomen rather than organomegaly. Caseous material (inspissated yolks) may be detected. Abdominocentesis reveals yellow–pink fluid and cytology shows mesothelial cells, leucocytes and pink yolk globules.

Management
Short-term therapy includes abdominal drainage, NSAIDs, antibiotics and hormonal manipulation to stop ovarian activity (leuprolide acetate or HCG).

Most cases will require surgery to lavage the abdomen and perform salpingohysterectomy. This is not always successful in preventing ovulation. Ovariectomy may be feasible, but it is fraught with danger due to the nature of the blood supply.

Egg binding (dystocia)
Aetiology
Predisposing factors include age (very young and very old birds are more frequently affected), malnutrition and obesity (it is particularly seen in birds on all-seed diets), excessive egg production, especially in cockatiels, budgerigars and backyard poultry, and lack of physical fitness in caged birds.

Causes include oviductal muscle dysfunction (calcium deficiency, myositis due to excessive egg production, concurrent salpingitis or metritis; excessively sized or malformed eggs) and systemic problems (concurrent illness, hypothermia, environmental stress).

Clinical presentation
Signs include excessive straining, a 'penguin-like' posture, dyspnoea, collapse and abdominal distension (224).

Diagnosis
This is based on the history of egg laying and the clinical signs (see above). Abdominal palpation usually reveals an egg, but soft-shelled eggs can be difficult to detect. Abdominal radiography (225) or ultrasonography may be required.

Management
If the bird shows no or only mild to moderate signs of discomfort and distress, confirm the time the last egg was laid; eggs are usually laid 23–26 hours apart and the patient may not be ready to lay. The bird should be placed in a heated hospital cage with adequate humidity and given calcium gluconate by intramuscular injections every 3–6 hours. Tube feeding highly digestible, high-sugar supplements may be given to provide a rapid source of energy. Stress and handling should be minimized, and the bird should be kept in a dark, quiet environment.

If the bird fails to respond to this treatment, oxytocin may be given, but there is controversy over its efficacy in birds, as it is not normally found in birds. Intra-cloacal PGE2 gel (226, 227) will usually produce uterovaginal sphincter dilation and straining within 5–10 minutes (228). If necessary, the egg can be manually manipulated into the cloaca and expressed. Caution must be taken not to push the egg up against the kidneys and spine.

If the bird is distressed or dyspnoeic, this is an emergency situation and ovocentesis and egg collapse may be necessary. A large gauge needle is introduced into the egg through the cloaca or abdominal wall and

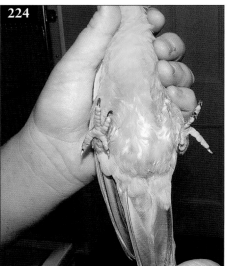

224 Abdominal distension due to egg binding in a sun conure.

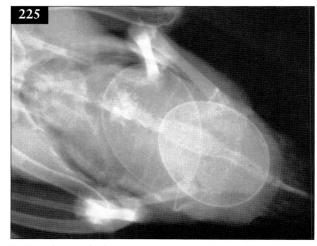

225 Radiograph showing two eggs in the coelom of a cockatiel presented for egg binding.

226 Prostaglandin E2 is the preferred prostaglandin for treating egg binding in birds.

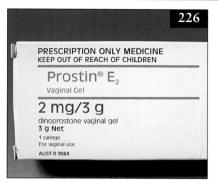

227 Prostaglandin E2 is introduced into the cloaca wih a syringe and absorbed rapidly across the cloacal mucosa.

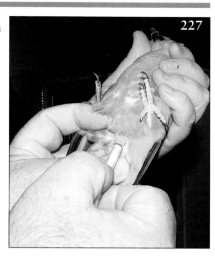

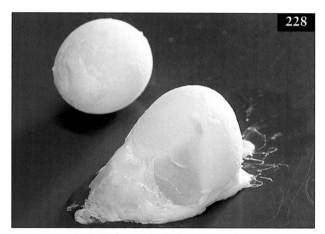

228 Two soft-shelled eggs laid almost simultaneously following prostaglandin E2 treatment of the bird in 225.

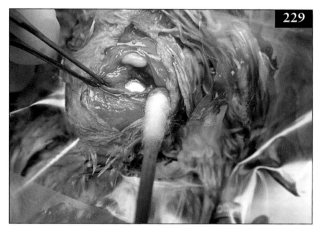

229 Occasionally a caesarean section is required to deliver an egg. This should be considered a last resort procedure.

the contents are aspirated, while the egg is simultaneously collapsed with digital pressure. The egg shell is usually passed within 48 hours of this procedure. It must be noted that while this procedure may be life-saving; damage to the oviduct usually requires a salpingohysterectomy at a later date.

In some cases it may be necessary to anaesthetize the bird (mask induction with isoflurane), intubate it and apply intermittent positive pressure ventilation (IPPV) while the egg is being manipulated through the cloaca. Coeliotomy and caesarean section may be necessary in some cases (**229**).

Prognosis
The earlier the case is presented, the better the prognosis. Simple cases have an excellent prognosis, while cases that have reached the stage where the bird is collapsed, dyspnoeic and unable to use its legs properly have a guarded prognosis.

Ectopic eggs
Definition/overview
These cases present clinically very similar to egg-bound birds, with the same aetiology and clinical signs. The hen fails to pass the egg, regardless of the treatment given. This is due to rupture of the oviduct at the level of the shell gland, leaving a fully shelled egg loose in the abdomen.

Management
Treatment requires a coeliotomy to remove the egg and repair the oviduct. Prognosis is good and some of these birds return to egg laying uneventfully, provided they are given several months to recuperate.

Retained eggs
Definition/overview
The egg may be retained in the oviduct, but it may have collapsed, leaving only the shell. Others may have the egg still intact, but are not straining to pass it. The egg is often located in the anterior coelom and usually does not cause dyspnoea.

Clinical presentation
These birds may present with abdominal distension (230) or they may be asymptomatic.

Diagnosis
Diagnosis is made radiographically.

Management
Treatment requires salpingohysterectomy.

Chronic or excessive egg laying
Definition/overview
This is most commonly seen in cockatiels (231), but any species can be affected. Left untreated, many of these birds deplete their calcium reserves and develop problems such as egg binding and pathological fractures. Many will develop salpingitis/metritis and subsequent yolk-related peritonitis.

Aetiology
Causes include readily available food and water, especially high-fat and sweet foods (e.g. seed and fruit), constant light (these birds are often housed indoors and do not have an appropriate diurnal rhythm), an 'appropriate' mate (this may not be another bird, in many cases it is the owner who has allowed an 'unnatural' bond to develop between themselves and the bird) and a secure nest site, which may be anywhere in the house or cage where the bird has established territoriality.

Management
Environmental modification
Normal diurnal rhythms need to be re-established. In some cases it may be necessary to drastically reduce daylight hours artificially (to eight hours or less) until the egg laying behaviour has stopped, and then bring the bird up to normal rhythms. Note that in species where daylength has little effect on breeding (e.g. zebra finches and budgerigars), changing daylength will have little effect on reproductive behaviour.

Nest sites should be removed (if possible). If the bird chooses an unconventional nest site (e.g. on the floor of the cage), re-arranging the area may effectively

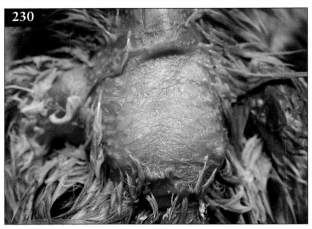

230 Coelomic distension in a bird with a retained egg.

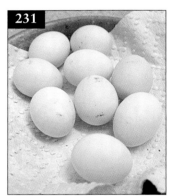

231 The eggs laid by one cockatiel hen in a one month period.

remove its attractiveness as a nest site. The bird's environment can be changed (e.g. new or re-arranged cage furniture, re-positioning the cage on an irregular basis). This induces a certain amount of environmental stress and reduces territoriality.

Behavioural modification
If appropriate (and possible), the companion bird can be removed. A normal relationship between human and bird should be established through the introduction of basic behavioural training and client education. The client must be taught what behaviours sexually stimulate the bird (e.g. stroking the bird's back).

Removing the eggs of an indeterminate layer, such as a cockatiel, will induce further egg laying. Leaving the eggs in the 'nest' or replacing them with artificial eggs will often result in a hen laying a normal sized clutch and then brooding the eggs. This shuts down (temporarily) the production of eggs.

Nutritional modification

Fat and sugar in the diet should be reduced by conversion to a formulated diet and removal of fruit from the diet. Foraging behaviour can be introduced. Typically, wild birds spend 80% of their day foraging for food, leaving 20% of the day to groom, socialize and 'nap'. In captivity, this time allocation is nearly reversed, with birds only having to spend a small amount of time looking for food. By introducing foraging activities, there is less time for pair bonding and other reproductive activities.

Hormonal manipulation

Hormonal therapy does not work in isolation. Unless the modifications in environment, behaviour and diet are instituted beforehand or concurrently, there will be minimal or no response to the use of hormones.

Drugs that have been used include:
- Leuprolide acetate, 100–700 µg/kg every 2–4 weeks.
- HCG, 500–1000 IU/kg every 2–4 weeks. Antibodies to HCG develop quickly, limiting its efficacy. It has been suggested that dexamethasone should be given concurrently to suppress the production of these antibodies, but this raises the spectre of generalized immunosuppression.
- Medroxyprogesterone acetate, 5–25 mg/kg every six weeks. Side-effects (diabetes, obesity and hepatopathies) limit its use.
- Deslorelin, a GnRH analogue available as an implant for dogs, is showing promise as a treatment of birds.

Surgery

Salpingohysterectomy has been proposed as a means of controlling egg production. Unfortunately, it appears that, by itself, it does not stop reproductive behaviour and subsequent ovulation, which then results in yolk peritonitis. Surgery should therefore be reserved as a 'last resort' therapy only.

INVESTIGATING REPRODUCTION PROBLEMS IN THE AVIARY
INTRODUCTION

Veterinarians are occasionally asked to investigate an apparent fertility problem in an avicultural collection. The problem is generally one of three types: lack of egg production, infertile eggs or poor hatchability.

Any investigation should start with a comprehensive review of the aviculturist's records including: the aviculturist's objectives and intentions; aviary design and construction; origin, age and species of birds; husbandry practices, traffic flow and nutrition; previous medical histories; production records; and description of the current problem.

In many cases it is appropriate to do this review before visiting the avicultural complex, utilizing written records, a map drawn by the aviculturist of the complex's layout and traffic flow, and photographs.

LACK OF EGG PRODUCTION

One should determine if the problem is generalized or is limited to a particular pair, a particular species or a particular part of the aviary.

Generalized problem

The following factors should be reviewed:
- Diet. The provision of high-fat foods at the start of the breeding season can stimulate reproductive activity. If these foods are fed all year round, that stimulus can be lost. Alternatively, the provision of a low-fat formulated diet will also often fail to stimulate activity. Feeding a formulated diet as the basis for the aviary nutrition and then using seed and nuts to stimulate reproductive behaviour when desired can be a powerful tool in reproductive management.
- Aviary design should reflect the height and space requirements for the species housed there.
- Privacy provision and stress reduction. Some birds will not feel secure enough to breed if they cannot access 'private' areas in the aviary where they can indulge in courtship and mating behaviours without feeling threatened. Stress from the surrounding environment (e.g. birds of prey, dogs, children, construction activities) must also be minimized.
- Species compatibility. Some birds will not breed if they can see or hear other birds of the same or different species during the breeding season.
- Local weather patterns and if 'artificial weather' in the form of artificial lighting or water sprinkling systems are being used to stimulate reproductive behaviour.

Representative birds should be examined for general body condition and health. Diagnostic tests should be aimed at screening for flock problems (e.g. chlamydiosis, parasites).

Problem is limited to one pair of birds

The veterinarian should determine:
- If they are a true pair. Sexually dimorphic species may require DNA or surgical sexing.

- If they are old enough to breed.
- If they are a compatible pair.
- If the aviary design, nest boxes and perches meet the birds' requirements for privacy, minimal stress, security and natural behaviours.

The health of the birds should be assessed.

Problem is limited to one species of birds

All the factors discussed above should be assessed. The known requirements for captive breeding of that species should be reviewed.

Problem is limited to one part of the aviary

All the factors described above should be assessed, with particular emphasis on aviary design, external stresses and environmental conditions in that area.

INFERTILE EGGS

The first step is to ascertain if eggs are infertile or are failing to develop. This requires several egg necropsies:
- Is the egg infertile or is the problem actually embryonic death?
- If the problem is embryonic death, at what stage of development did the embryo die?

Infertile eggs
Aetiology

There may be two female birds inadvertently paired together.

A properly formed egg usually, but not always, implies that there is not a medical problem with the hen, but that the cock bird is either not producing spermatozoa or is producing abnormal spermatozoa.

If the cock bird is producing healthy semen, it is not reaching the hen's infundibulum due to:
- Lack of successful mating: incompatible pairs, immature cock bird, inexperience on the part of either bird, inappropriate perches preventing normal mating (too small, too large, not fixed in place), or lack of privacy or external stresses (other birds, animals, humans) causing the birds to feel insecure.
- Physical impediments to successful mating (e.g. old leg injuries, excessively heavy feathering around the vent).
- Low-grade cloacitis or metritis inhibiting the passage of semen from the vent to the infundibulum.

Diagnosis

The author's preferred approach is to firstly determine that:
- The birds are, indeed, a true pair, through visual sexing, DNA sexing or surgical sexing.
- The birds are healthy, determined by physical examination, haematology, biochemistries, cloacal cultures and possibly radiography/ultrasonography.
- The cock bird is fertile, determined by semen collection (through cloacal massage) or endoscopic evaluation and biopsy/fine needle aspirate of the testicle.

If the birds' health and fertility can be shown to be normal, it is more likely that the aviculturist will accept that the problem lies with compatibility, immaturity, inexperience, husbandry or nutrition, and make critical evaluation of these areas more acceptable.

Embryonic death
Definition/overview

It is normal for up to 10% of all eggs laid to fail to develop normally. Normal embryonic mortality is as follows:
- First trimester: 3–4%.
- Second trimester: 1–2%.
- Third trimester: 4–5%.

Embryonic mortalities above these levels should be investigated (*Table 4*).

Aetiology

Parental factors include genetics, nutrition (calcium deficiency, excessive vitamin supplementation, especially vitamin D3) and health (oophoritis, metritis).

Incubation factors may be important:
- Natural incubation: nest box conditions (hygiene, humidity, temperature extremes) and parental factors (abandoning the nest, rough handling of eggs).
- Artificial incubation: temperature too high or too low, humidity too high or too low, ventilation inadequate, turning inadequate or poor hygiene.

Diagnosis

Egg necropsy should be carried out.
- The egg is weighed and weight loss (as a percentage of weight when laid) during incubation determined.

Table 4 Troubleshooting embryonic mortality.

Problem	Possible causes
Floating air cell	Rough handling of egg Parental nutritional deficiencies Genetics
Early embryonic mortality	Parental nutritional deficiencies Shaking/jarring of eggs Incubator problem: temperature, turning, ventilation Disinfection of eggs in first three days Formaldehyde fumigation of eggs Delayed egg collection Incorrect storage: temperature incorrect, stored too long
Mid-term embryonic mortality	Parental nutritional deficiencies Infection Inadequate turning Incubator problem: temperature, turning, ventilation Lethal genes
Late-term embryonic mortality	Malpositions Incubator problem: temperature, humidity, turning, ventilation Infection Parental nutritional deficiencies
Air cell pipped, fail to hatch	Hatcher problem: temperature, humidity, ventilation
Malformed chicks	Incubator temperature too high Parental nutritional deficiencies Genetics Teratogens
Oedematous chicks	Humidity too high Shell too thick Inadequate ventilation
Sticky chicks	Humidity too high Shell too thin
External yolk sac	Temperature too high Oedematous chick Inappropriate intervention to assist hatch

- Shell quality is assessed: surface texture, porosity and cleanliness.
- The egg is candled to identify the air cell, determine its size and mobility, and assess whether an embryo or infection is present. Hairline cracks in the shell can also be identified.
- The egg is placed vertically on to a support (e.g. a plastic ring or cup) with the air cell uppermost. The shell over the air cell is broken with a sharp implement, revealing the air cell. The shell is then removed down to the level of the inner shell membrane forming the base of the air cell. This membrane is then peeled away with fine forceps, revealing the egg contents.
- A swab (for culture of bacteria and fungi) can be taken from the albumen or inside the shell.
- If an embryo is not obviously present, the blastodisc on the yolk is examined. The yolk around this disc is less dense than the rest of the yolk, so it will float uppermost. In an infertile egg the disc will appear as a small white point. A very early embryo will appear as a small white

Table 5 Embryonic malpositions.

Malposition	Description	Possible causes (if known)
I	Head is down between the legs	High incubator temperature
II	Chick is rotated within the egg, with the head at the end opposite to the air cell	Egg position and low temperature during incubation
III	Head is rotated to the left, with the head under the left wing	Egg position, temperature and parental malnutrition
IV	Beak is away from the air cell, rest of the body is normally positioned	Egg position
V	Feet over the head	—
VI	Head over the right wing	Parental nutrition

'doughnut' with a translucent centre. Any blood vessel development at all is confirmation of fertility.

- If an embryo is present, the stage of development and the positioning of the embryo (if it is late-term) are determined.
- Embryonic position is observed before removing the embryo from the egg. The normal late-term embryonic position is: head next to the air cell, right side uppermost and turned to the right, with the beak adjacent to the right foot and shoulder; legs flexed on either side of the body and ventral to the shoulders; and the spine following the long axis of the egg. Any other position is classified as a malposition and may account for embryonic death. Descriptions and possible causes of classical malpositions are described in *Table 5*.
- Once the embryo has been removed from the egg, it can be either grossly examined and then fixed in formalin, or necropsied and tissues submitted in formalin.

FURTHER READING

Bowles HL (2006) Evaluating and treating the reproductive tract. In: *Clinical Avian Medicine, Vol 2*. GJ Harrison, TL Lightfoot (eds). Spix Publishing Inc, Palm Beach, pp. 519–540.

Joyner KL (1994) Theriogenology. In: *Avian Medicine: Principles and Application*. BW Ritchie, GJ Harrison, LR Harrison (eds). Wingers Publishing, Lake Worth, pp. 748–804.

LaBonde J (2006) Avian reproductive and pediatric disorders. In: *Proceedings of the Annual Conference of the Association of Avian Veterinarians Australian Committee*, pp. 229–238.

Orosz S, Dorrestein GM, Speer BL (1997) Urogenital disorders. In: *Avian Medicine and Surgery*. RB Altman, SL Clubb, GM Dorrestein, K Quesenberry (eds). WB Saunders, Philadelphia, pp. 614–644.

Schubot RM, Clubb KJ, Clubb SL (1992) *Psittacine Aviculture: Perspectives, Techniques and Research*. Avicultural Breeding and Research Center, Loxahatchee, Fl.

CHAPTER 21
DISORDERS OF THE URINARY SYSTEM

RENAL DISEASE
Aetiology
Inflammatory conditions
Causes of inflammatory renal disease may be infectious or noninfectious (**232**). Infectious causes include:
- Viruses: adenovirus, circovirus, coronavirus, herpesvirus, orthomyxovirus, polyomavirus, paramyxovirus, poxvirus, retrovirus.
- Bacteria (most bacteria, including mycobacteria).
- Chlamydiosis.
- Parasites: coccidia (waterfowl and raptors), cryptosporidia (rare in all species), microsporidia (lovebirds, budgerigars and finches), *Toxoplasma*, *Sarcocystis* (systemic infection), trematodes (waterfowl), schistosomiasis (waterfowl).

- Fungal infections: *Aspergillus* infections invading either from neighbouring air sac lesions or by haematogenous spread after fungal invasion of blood vessels.
- Immune-mediated: membranous glomerulonephritis following chronic antigenic stimulation (e.g. polyomavirus infection).

Noninfectious causes include egg yolk peritonitis and visceral gout.

Noninflammatory conditions
Causes include:
- Amyloidosis: most commonly seen in waterfowl, small passerines and raptors. Multiple organs, including the kidneys, are affected.
- Toxins: rodenticides (vitamin D3 analogues), aminoglycosides (gentamicin, amikacin), heavy metals (lead, zinc cadmium, mercury, arsenic), mycotoxins (aflotoxin, oosporein, citrinin, ochratoxin) and others (hypernatraemia, acetone, allopurinol, ethylene glycol, glycine, oxalic acid, selenium).
- Nutritional: hypercalcaemia, hypervitaminosis D3, hypovitaminosis A, hypervitaminosis A. A syndrome is seen in colour mutation varieties of cockatiels, budgerigars and lovebirds fed on a 100% formulated diet. Currently it is thought that these diets may contain excessive levels of vitamin A for these species, although this has yet to be proved.
- Metabolic: disseminated intravascular coagulation (DIC), haemachromatosis, haemoglobin deposits, lipidosis, nephrogenic diabetes insipidus.
- Genetic/congenital: renal cysts, agenesis, hypoplasia.
- Acquired: dehydration, hypovolaemia.
- Degenerative: renal mineralization, tubular nephrosis.

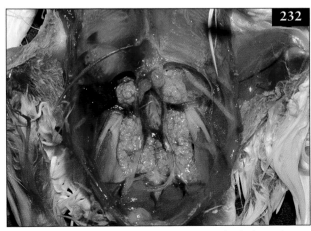

232 Nephritis in a cockatiel. By the time the kidneys have reached this advanced stage of disease, identifying the aetiology is difficult.

- Physical: obstipation due to egg binding, cloacoliths, uroliths.
- Trauma: general trauma or renal trauma during endoscopy or surgery.

Neoplasia

Kidney tumours include carcinomas, adenocarcinoma, round cell tumours, sarcomas and embryonal nephromas.

Clinical presentation

Signs include fluffed feathers, weakness, lethargy, anorexia, polyuria (**233**), polydipsia, gout (articular and/or visceral [in acute severe cases, uric deposits may be seen forming subcutaneously]) (**234**), vomiting and dehydration.

Diagnosis

Initial tests

Polyuria/polidipsia should be confirmed quantitatively if possible. Haematology and biochemistry can be helpful (see Chapter 4, Interpreting diagnostic tests). Blood lead and zinc levels can be assessed. While this is useful for lead toxicosis, it is doubtful if measuring zinc levels is of diagnostic value. This is because of natural diurnal variation in levels, the possible natural, but slight, elevation of zinc in unwell or stressed birds, the risk of contamination of the sample with zinc (e.g. from rubber stoppers on syringes) and the overdiagnosis of zinc toxicosis in cases with insignificant elevations.

Urinalysis

Urinalysis is indicated when there is persistent (not transient) polyuria. Interpretation of the results must be done with caution, as faecal contamination is the norm, and this must be taken into account. Factors to be checked include:

- Colour: biliverdinuria, haematuria (**235**).
- Urine specific gravity (USG). In normal birds there can be wide variation in specific gravity. In polyuric birds the USG has been reported as ranging from 1.005–1.020. The main value of USG, therefore, lies in cases with a persistently low USG and those where USG fails to increase with water deprivation.
- Dipstick evaluation:
  - pH: normally 6.0–7.5. Lower readings in psittacines may indicate acidosis. Higher values can indicate bacterial metabolism. Care must be taken to ensure that the colour of the urine does not influence the colour readings on the dipstick.

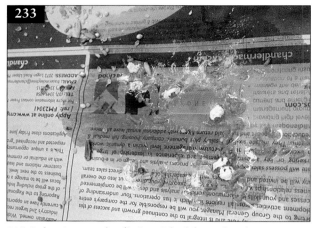

233 Polyuria must be distinguished from diarrhoea.

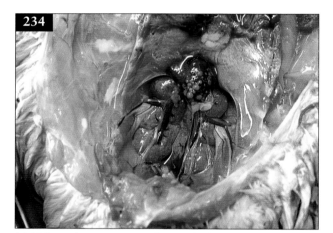

234 Visceral gout. Uric acid crystals deposited in the subcutaneous tissues.

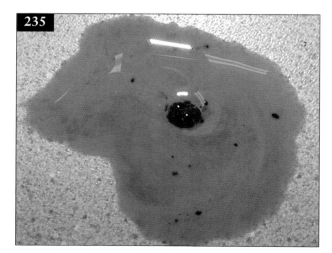

235 Haematuria is associated with severe renal disease or lead toxicosis.

- Protein: normally only trace amounts are recorded. Higher levels can indicate faecal contamination, renal disease, haemoglobinuria, haematuria, hyperproteinaemia or sepsis.
- Glucose: normally zero amounts are registered. Glucosuria indicates faecal contamination, diabetes mellitus or renal damage. Glucosuria without hyperglycaemia, in the author's experience, gives a guarded to poor prognosis.
- Ketones: ketonuria indicates severe catabolism or complicated diabetes mellitus. It also indicates a poor prognosis.
- Blood: haematuria/haemoglobinuria can indicate faecal contamination or severe renal disease, and warrants a sediment examination.

- Sediment can be examined under the microscope, at first unstained, and then stained with methylene blue. The following can be observed:
  - Desquamated epithelial cells from the cloaca.
  - Leucocytes and erythrocytes are rare in normal urine. More than two to three per high power field should be considered abnormal.
  - Casts (granular or cellular) can be seen with renal disease. Haemoglobin casts may account for positive haemoglobin readings seen on dipsticks and where no erythrocytes are seen.
  - Small numbers of gram-positive bacteria can originate from the faeces. Large numbers of bacteria should be considered abnormal. Comparison with a faecal Gram stain may help to determine their origin.
  - Uric acid crystals (small and spherical) are normal. Other crystals are occasionally seen, but their significance is unclear.

Radiography
Plain view radiographs allow visualization of the size and density of the kidneys. In a lateral view, with both acetabulae on the same plane, the normal kidneys lie in the sacral area and do not extend ventrally past the ventral rim of the acetabulae. Enlarged kidneys can often be seen below these limits. Radiodense mineralized kidneys can occasionally be seen. Both metastatic and dystrophic calcification can occur within the kidney as the result of renal disease, excessive dietary calcium or hypervitaminosis D3. Mineralization is not an indication of chronicity, as it can begin within days of the original insult. Radiodense metallic-like particles seen in the gastrointestinal tract can indicate lead or zinc toxicosis as possible causes of renal disease.

Endoscopy
The avian kidney is readily accessible using endoscopy. Renal gout, mineralization or physical anomalies can be visualized. Endoscopy also enables the clinician to biopsy the kidney. Biopsy is perhaps the single most important tool in the accurate diagnosis of renal disease. Haemorrhage is minimal and the resultant histology (and, if appropriate, culture) allows an accurate diagnosis, a more meaningful prognosis and a more concise treatment plan.

Water deprivation test
Once other possible causes of polyuria/polydypsia have been eliminated, a water deprivation test can be used to differentiate between psychogenic polydypsia and diabetes insipidus. The rationale behind a water deprivation test is that a bird with the ability to osmoregulate will concentrate urine in response to increased plasma osmolality, due in turn to water deprivation. A gradual water deprivation test is preferred to an abrupt water deprivation test in order to overcome the problem of renal medullary washout and cloacal concentration gradients. Water is gradually restricted by 10% per day over 3–5 days, and then deprived completely. This process gives the kidneys and the cloaca every chance to respond to gradually increasing plasma osmolality. Close monitoring is mandatory, as severe dehydration can result if the patient is unable to concentrate urine. Plasma proteins, PCV and weight should be monitored closely. The test should stop when the patient loses 5–7% of its bodyweight or is able to concentrate its urine. Failure to concentrate urine in the absence of other possible causes indicates diabetes insipidus. A vasopressin response test can then be performed to distinguish between neurogenic and nephrogenic diabetes insipidus.

Vasopressin response test
Diabetes insipidus (a deficiency of, or failure to respond to, arginine vasotocin [AVT]) has been recorded in birds. Birds that have had other causes of polyuria/polydypsia ruled out and have failed to concentrate their urine on a gradual water deprivation test are likely to have either neurogenic or nephrogenic diabetes insipidus. Desmopressin acetate (an AVT analogue) is given orally at doses of 0.02–0.2 mg/kg. A reduction in polyuria and polydypsia within 30 minutes of administration confirms the diagnosis of neurogenic diabetes insipidus. Neurogenic diabetes insipidus fails to respond to the desmopressin.

Management

Supportive care includes maintaining good hydration. Parenteral fluids given at 100 ml/kg/day for 3 days, followed by 50–75 ml/kg/day until uric acid levels return to normal and remain normal. Hyperuricaemia can be controlled with:

- Allopurinol: reduces the production of uric acid.
- Probenecid: in theory it increases the excretion of uric acid. However, it may exacerbate gout in birds, and is not currently recommended for use.
- Colchicine: reduces the inflammation and fibrosis associated with renal disease and uric acid deposition.

Dietary support (in theory, moderate protein restriction) is also an important part of supportive care.

Specific therapy can be given when a specific diagnosis is achieved by renal biopsy or other laboratory tests.

Membranous glomerulonephritis

This is commonly diagnosed in older birds. Therapy involves removal of the antigen responsible for the immune-mediated reaction, if possible, aspirin 1 mg/kg orally q24h and omega 3 and 6 fatty acid supplementation, mixed in a ratio of omega 6:omega 3 of 6:1 and given at a dose of 0.1 ml/kg.

Bacterial nephritis

Treatment of bacterial nephritis with appropriate antibiotics should be based on culture and sensitivity results when available. Otherwise, suspected bacterial-induced nephritis should be treated with broad-spectrum bactericidal antibiotics for a minimum of six weeks.

Dietary-induced renal disease

This can often be treated by discontinuing pellets and changing the diet to whole grains, seeds and vegetables. If after 3–6 months all signs of renal disease are gone, pellets (<50% of total diet) can be cautiously added to the diet.

Renal fibrosis

This can be treated with colchicine until the fibrosis resolves (and is conformed histologically). Otherwise, colchicine can be used for 6–12 months or until laboratory abnormalities normalize.

Articular gout

Colchicine and allopurinol are used together until all signs of gout and hyperuricaemia have resolved. The cause of the probable underlying renal disease should be diagnosed and managed appropriately. Aggressive fluid therapy should be used if articular or visceral gout is accumulating rapidly. The prognosis is guarded to poor.

Zinc or lead toxicosis

This can be treated with chelation therapy (calcium EDTA, d-penicillamine). Zinc toxicosis usually only requires treatment until the metallic particles in the gastrointestinal tract have been removed (approximately 4–5 days if left to pass naturally). (This needs to be confirmed radiographically before discontinuing treatment.) Birds diagnosed with lead toxicosis should be chelated twice daily until clinically normal, then twice weekly for 6–8 weeks. At the end of this period blood lead levels should be retested.

UROLITHIASIS

Definition/overview

The formation of ureteroliths in birds is rare. The stones are composed of uric acid crystals and a proteinaceous matrix. They are typically lodged in the ureters and may be unilateral or bilateral. Hypovitaminosis A may be a contributing factor.

Clinical presentation

Signs include nonproductive straining, depression and anorexia.

Diagnosis

Radiography reveals radiopaque obstructions of the ureter. Intravenous pyelography may help to define the obstruction and ureters. Endoscopic examination of the ureter may reveal a distended ureter proximal to the obstruction. If only one kidney is involved, it is unlikely that serum biochemistries will show elevations in uric acid (assuming the other kidney is normal).

Treatment

Diuretic therapy with fluids may help to 'flush' the stone out. The stone may be able to be milked along the ureter with an endoscope or during a surgical approach. If these techniques fail to relieve the obstruction, a ureterotomy may be required. Care must be taken to minimize postsurgical stricture formation.

OTHER CONDITIONS AFFECTING THE URINARY SYSTEM

Conditions arising from outside the kidney, but causing polyuria and or polydypsia, include:

- Liver disease.
- Pancreatic disease.
- Gastrointestinal disease.
- Septicaemia.
- Pituitary or pineal gland neoplasia is reported as a cause of polyuria/polydypsia, especially in budgerigars.
- Diabetes mellitus is frequently reported in psittacines, particularly budgerigars and cockatiels (see Chapter 15, Disorders of the pancreas, p. 182).
- Neurogenic and nephrogenic diabetes insipidus are rare, but have been reported in parrots. Diagnosis is based on exclusion of other causes of polyuria/polydypsia and failure to concentrate urine (i.e. continued polyuria/polydypsia) in response to a gradual water deprivation test.
- Hyperadrenocorticism due to adrenal neoplasia has been reported as a cause of polyuria/polydypsia.
- Renal phosphate flush seen with low-calcium, high-phosphorus diets (i.e. seed diets) is believed to be a cause of polyuria/polydypsia.
- Psychogenic polydypsia is a relatively rare condition, often associated with juvenile hand-reared cockatoos. Stress, excitement and fear may also be contributing factors.

FURTHER READING

Echols MS (2006) Evaluating and treating the kidneys. In: *Clinical Avian Medicine, Vol 2*. GJ Harrison, TL Lightfoot (eds). Spix Publishing Inc, Palm Beach, pp. 451–492.

Echols MS (2007) Avian kidney disease, Part I: types of renal disease. In: *Proceedings of the Annual Conference of the Association of Avian Veterinarians Australian Committee*, pp. 101–116.

Echols MS (2007) Avian kidney disease, Part II: diagnosis of renal disease. In: *Proceedings of the Annual Conference of the Association of Avian Veterinarians Australian Committee*, pp. 117–128.

Echols MS (2007) Avian kidney disease, Part III: treatment of renal disease. In: *Proceedings of the Annual Conference of the Association of Avian Veterinarians Australian Committee*, pp. 129–137.

Lumeij JT (1994) Nephrology. In: *Avian Medicine: Principles and Application*. BW Ritchie, GJ Harrison, LR Harrison (eds). Wingers Publishing, Lake Worth, pp. 748–804.

Orosz S, Dorrestein GM, Speer BL (1997) Urogenital disorders. In: *Avian Medicine and Surgery*. RB Altman, SL Clubb, GM Dorrestein, K Quesenberry (eds). WB Saunders, Philadelphia, pp. 614–644.

Raidal SR, Echols MS (2007) The advantages and disadvantages of excreting uric acid. In: *Proceedings of the Annual Conference of the Association of Avian Veterinarians Australian Committee*, pp. 87–100.

CHAPTER 22
BEHAVIOURAL PROBLEMS

INTRODUCTION
All bird behaviour originates from 'wild' behaviour, and can be either instinctive or learned. Companion birds need to effectively acquire learned behaviours that can make them socially acceptable as pets and companions. Common behavioural problems seen in clinical practice include behaviours such as:
- Attention demanding.
- Displacement behaviours.
- Territoriality.
- Biting.
- Feather damaging.
- Screaming.
- Reproductive issues.
- Phobias.
- Psychotic behaviour.

Many of these problems are often chronic by the time the bird is presented to veterinarians. Early recognition and treatment of these problems is more likely to result in successful treatment.

PRINCIPLES
Companion birds face many challenges. These challenges are directly attributable to a lack of knowledge — and sometimes ignorance — of a bird's requirements. The two most common presentations of chronic problems seen by avian veterinarians are malnutrition and behavioural problems. Malnutrition stems from the traditional concept of birds as seed eaters. The behavioural problems, however, stem from a lack of understanding of the unique nature of bird behaviour, and the owner's attempts to impose their own demands and expectations on their bird, expecting them to behave more like a dog or a cat, or even a child.

Understanding bird behaviour is a constantly evolving subject. What was accepted as fact 3–5 years ago has been debunked or disproved or, at best, modified. Pre-existing notions of bird behaviour and its 'modification' or 'therapy' need to be re-examined and, where appropriate, discarded.

UNDERSTANDING BIRD BEHAVIOUR
To understand bird behaviour it is necessary to go back and look at the behaviour of birds in the wild; after all, most pet birds are only a few generations removed from wild birds. However, to generalize and talk about 'bird behaviour' is akin to talking about 'mammalian behaviour'. There are some 9,000 species of birds; approximately 360 of these are parrots. Parrots have evolved in Australia, South America, Africa and Asia. Different environments and environmental pressures have shaped both the physical and psychological development of these birds, and to try and apply 'rules' across all 360 species is fraught with danger. However, there are some generalizations that can be made.

Avian behaviour can be categorized into two functional groups:
- Self-maintenance behaviours designed to accomplish a specific task to maintain the health of the individual. These include feeding, feather care, locomotion and concealment.
- Social behaviours designed to communicate information to another individual. These behaviours include territoriality, concern or fear and courtship.

Parrots are altricial; the young are hatched near-naked, blind and perhaps deaf. They live for the first weeks of their life in a quiet, dark hollow, completely dependent on their parents (236). Social interactions at this stage are limited, confined to their siblings and parents. After fledging, many parrots learn to socialize by contact with their parents, siblings and other birds (often their own age) in a flock (237). An example of this is the rose-breasted cockatoo (galah). In the wild, clutches of two to five chicks usually survive. Once they fledge, the chicks are taken to a nearby 'crèche', a tree or stand of trees where other galah 'families' are interacting. Here they learn early social skills before joining a nomadic juvenile flock where they remain until reaching sexual maturity. This socialization period teaches the juvenile birds food recognition (and how to locate it), predator recognition, sentinel duties, grooming behaviour, survival skills and early social behaviours.

As they reach sexual maturity, they learn new skills: how to select a mate, exhibit courtship behaviours and develop a pair bond; how to select, prepare and defend a nest site; and how to reproduce and raise their young.

Some of these behaviours are believed to be innate or instinctive; others are learnt. All are reinforced by the reaction the bird receives. Captive parrots, especially those hand reared as pets, may not have the opportunity to learn these behaviours. Their instinctive behaviours, particularly as they reach maturity, may bring them into conflict with their human flock.

HOW DO BEHAVIOURAL PROBLEMS DEVELOP?

Problems seen in clinical practice can be attributable to one of two causes. The first basic problem is a failure of the socialization process. This is usually the result of an individual bird being hand reared in isolation and not being taught basic social skills. Once weaned, the bird is often ignored as its novelty value wears off. This process often results in attention-demanding behaviour (begging calls, screaming, feather chewing) and displacement behaviours such as biting, feather damaging behaviour, phobias and sometimes even self-mutilating behaviour.

The second group of problems result as a failure of the human 'flock' to understand normal parrot behaviour, and expecting birds to 'fall into line' with their human expectations (**238**). It was once said that there are no abnormal behaviours, just normal behaviours expressed inappropriately. Behaviours such as screaming morning and night, displaying territoriality and certain reproductive behaviours are examples of normal behaviour that are inappropriate in a companion bird scenario.

So how do these problem behaviours develop?

The reinforcement of self-maintenance behaviours benefits companion birds, and abnormal self-maintenance behaviours are the most common behavioural disorders seen in these birds. They still have the same self-maintenance behaviours as their

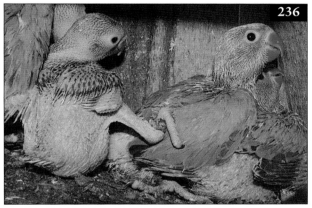

236 Indian ring-neck chicks (violet colour mutation) in the nest. Note the relatively cramped and dark conditions.

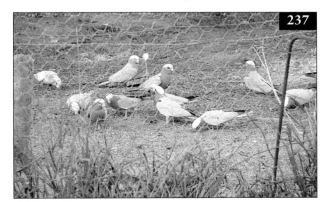

237 Flock of galahs feeding on seeding grass in Australia. Many parrots learn to socialize by contact with their parents, siblings and other birds (often their own age) in a flock.

238 Five-month-old Moluccan cockatoo. Many pet birds bond closely with humans at this age.

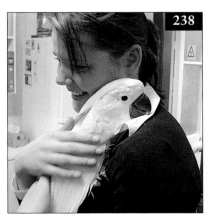

wild counterparts. However, they need less time for foraging and feeding behaviours (after all the food is in a dish in front of them every morning) and therefore feather care, social communication and displays make up more of their daily activities.

Young captive birds need continued mentoring and behavioural moulding and require guidance for the establishment of a normal bird–human flock relationship. This includes a range of normal social behaviours of flock interaction, with appropriate rules of conflict resolution and appropriate maintenance and social behaviours.

Failure to be taught — or learn — these behaviours means that many young birds are not prepared for a life in captivity, and may develop behavioural problems. In the absence of imposed rules, the bird will make its own rules based on immediate gratification and revolving around perceived value; however, these rules may not be socially acceptable. They eventually develop into behavioural problems and the bird becomes unable to interact socially with people without fear or social framework, and therefore a series of displacement or defensive behaviours develops (e.g. aggression, biting). As these behaviours develop, the bird may become even more isolated and therefore become more vocal in trying to re-establish contact with their 'flock'.

This is often reinforced when owners respond: the bird receives a positive response (e.g. talking, feeding) and it may augment the behaviour; if, on the other hand, the bird receives a negative response (e.g. covering cage, time-out, water pistols) that response may augment the feeling of isolation and the problem may worsen.

Unfortunately, these problems are often chronic by the time the bird is presented to a veterinarian. Early recognition and treatment are much more likely to result in successful treatment; prevention through education of bird owners is the most preferable approach. Techniques such incorporating behavioural training into annual wellness examinations are important steps in preventing problems, and they should be pursued vigorously by all those involved in the wellbeing of companion parrots.

HISTORICAL APPROACH TO TREATING BEHAVIOURAL PROBLEMS

Earlier attempts to treat behavioural problems in birds revolved around human concepts of 'discipline' and psychotherapy.

Humans are driven, in many cases, by fear of punishment and negative reinforcement. From early childhood people are made well aware of the consequences of inappropriate behaviour — corporal punishment or even just the disapproval of adults. Given that early thoughts on parrot IQ were along the lines of 'as intelligent as a 3–5-year-old, but with the maturity of a 2–3-year-old', it is not surprising that people expected birds could be motivated by the same fear of negative consequences.

And, if punishment did not work, surely drugs would! The use of hormonal therapies, anti-depressants, sedatives and even narcotic antagonists was advocated as the best therapy for 'misbehaving' patients. Conventional medicine sometimes dictates that for every disease or problem there is a drug. So, studies and trials were conducted that resulted in many a companion bird sitting on a perch in a drug-induced stupefaction, and everyone (except the bird) was satisfied.

Eventually, it was realized that neither of these approaches was successful in curing behavioural problems. They might have stopped for a while, but as soon as the threat of punishment or administration of drugs was stopped, the problem recurred.

NEW CONCEPTS

The first change in thinking on bird behavioural therapy came with the realization that drugs and physical restraint devices (e.g. Elizabethan collars) just did not work. Although they may have a limited, short-term role in selected cases, these therapies often worsen a situation and do not provide a long-term benefit.

A second change in thought was in dealing with the concept of dominance. It was long thought that a strict hierarchical structure existed within bird flocks, with dominance being reflected in advantages such as the highest perch, the best food and first choice when selecting a mate. It was further thought that in a human–bird 'flock' situation, a similar dominance had to be maintained, with the human at all times being the dominant member of the 'flock'. However, studies of wild birds has shown that dominance, while it does occur, is not at all strict; rather, it is a fluid arrangement with different birds being dominant at different times. A flock is inconsistent in its structures: members are lost to predators, family groups change between flocks, new members are constantly being added. This makes a straight-line hierarchy difficult to maintain, and too energy demanding to be compatible with survival in the wild. Therefore, the rigid dominance so often seen in human society does not readily transfer over to the bird world, and attempts to impose it usually involve 'flooding' a bird (overwhelming it with an imposed behaviour until it acquiesces) or using negative reinforcements and punishment as means of instilling discipline. The problem with these techniques is that the bird learns to perform a behaviour, or avoid exhibiting one, just enough to escape adverse consequences. Once these consequences are removed, the behaviour returns.

New concepts in behavioural therapy revolve around several principles:

- Birds are not people, or dogs, or cats.
- The best results are obtained when a bird wants to do the behaviour that the owner desires.
- A successful treatment may be a reduction in an unwanted behaviour, rather than a complete cessation of it.
- Successful behavioural change in companion parrots starts with behavioural change in the parrot owner.

BIRDS ARE NOT PEOPLE, OR DOGS, OR CATS

Imposing human values and emotions on to an animal (anthropomorphism) can hinder the behavioural modifications clinicians are trying to institute. Using terms such as angry, aggressive, jealous and happy implies a state of mind which, realistically, we cannot truly assess. By doing so, a set of expectations is created in the mind of the owners and perhaps in the clinician as well.

Parrots are animals that can:

- Learn to feed from seasonally variable food sources.
- Learn the specific call or 'dialect' of their flock.
- Interpret subtle nuances in body language of other members of their flock.
- Perform elaborate courtship displays.
- Learn to mimic sounds in their environment in order to manipulate an environmental condition or maintain a pair bond.
- Develop monogamous pair bond relationships.
- Rigorously defend breeding territory.
- Develop flight skills advanced enough to avoid/escape predatory attack.
- Successfully rear young and make decisions about resource availability that influence fledgling mortality.

They are not little children with feathers, nor are they similar to mammals such as dogs and cats. They are unique and deserve to be treated as such. It is important to attempt to replicate the environment in which they evolved, providing them with opportunities to exhibit normal behaviours such as foraging for food, flying, interacting socially and just having fun.

THE BEST RESULTS ARE OBTAINED WHEN A BIRD WANTS TO DO THE BEHAVIOUR THAT THE OWNER DESIRES

Reinforcing behaviour can be either positive or negative. Negative reinforcement involves applying a noxious consequence to a behaviour in the expectation that the bird will cease the behaviour to avoid the consequence. Examples of this include time out, covering a cage or squirting the bird with a water pistol. The problem with negative reinforcement is that the bird will do only just enough to avoid the consequence, and no more. In fact, as soon as the consequence is removed, the behaviour usually returns. Undesired consequences of negative reinforcement can include escape/avoidance behaviour, aggression, apathy (a decreased responsiveness in behaviour) and fear, leading to phobic behaviour.

Positive reinforcement, on the other hand, involves providing a favourable consequence (or reward) for a behaviour. This increases the likelihood that the bird will repeat the behaviour in the expectation of the reward. The motivation used to stimulate a desired behaviour must be evaluated from the bird's perspective, and this can be influenced by several factors:

- The relationship between the bird and the person. This relationship must be built on trust, respect and prior positive experiences. Good communication must exist between the two: both must understand the other's body language in order to know what they want (**239**).
- The bird's confidence and ability to perform the behaviour.

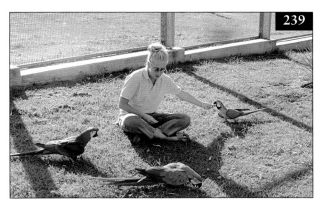

239 Macaws in a large free flight aviary choosing to interact with humans.

- The bird's past experiences in training and motivation.
- Natural influences such as social interaction, breeding season, comfort and height.
- The bird's hunger state or preference for certain feed items.

Some examples of good motivators include favourite food items, praise, and petting, proximity to people, a familiar object and even out-of-cage time.

Care must be taken to prevent inadvertently reinforcing a behaviour while trying to use negative reinforcement. The classic example of this is shouting at a screaming parrot. Parrots are naturally noisy animals that seem to thrive on noise and drama; it is, after all, a natural part of their life and normal social interaction. While the owner thinks he/she is 'punishing' an undesired behaviour, they are, in fact, giving the bird positive reinforcement and guaranteeing that the behaviour will be repeated.

Positive reinforcement can be used to increase or decrease the likelihood of a behaviour being repeated. It can also be used to establish and encourage other behaviours. These new behaviours can either be alternative behaviours or behaviours that are incompatible with the undesired behaviour. Either way, it can lead to extinction of an undesired behaviour.

A SUCCESSFUL TREATMENT MAY BE A REDUCTION IN AN UNWANTED BEHAVIOUR, RATHER THAN A COMPLETE CESSATION OF IT

Many behavioural problems are often chronic in nature by the time the bird is presented to a veterinarian. Feather picking is a classical example: by the time the owner has waited to see if it goes away, then consults the Internet and tries a variety of pet shop remedies, it may be many months or even years before the bird is presented to a veterinarian. Obviously such behaviours, now deeply ingrained and with their own set of positive motivators (perhaps only known to the bird), are going to be difficult to eradicate. This must be made clear to the owner from the beginning (i.e. that success in these cases may simply be a reduction in the behaviour, rather than its complete elimination).

SUCCESSFUL BEHAVIOURAL CHANGE IN COMPANION PARROTS STARTS WITH BEHAVIOURAL CHANGE IN THE PARROT OWNER

There is no doubt that the owners of many birds are directly attributing to the problems they are experiencing, and directly or indirectly reinforcing them. As mentioned earlier, people grow up in a 'punishing' environment, where transgressions are punished and human behaviours have evolved to avoid such punishments. Birds are not like this, and do not learn well in this manner. People who wish to interact and socialize with birds, preventing or overcoming behavioural problems as they do so, must change their own behaviour in order to better understand and work with their bird.

These principles call for a re-assessment of how humans think of, and interact with, birds. Until we do so, our success in modifying their behaviour will be limited.

BASIC STEPS TO IMPLEMENT IN A BEHAVIOUR-MODIFICATION PROGRAMME

There are some basic steps to implement in a behaviour-modification programme when dealing with problem behaviours. They include:
- Basic training.
- Normalization of social interaction.
- Avoidance of unwanted behaviours.
- Replacement of unwanted behaviours with acceptable behaviours.

BASIC TRAINING

Many pet birds are hand reared and seem to recognize and accept people as 'members' of their flock. This recognition,and the interaction that comes with it, is what helps to make parrots such enjoyable companion birds. Normally, other flock members would teach the juvenile bird what social behaviours are appropriate through a system of examples and trial and error. With companion birds, the role of mentor and teacher has to be filled by the owner of the bird. It is essential to have the basic requisites for training in place first in order to provide a solid foundation for acceptable social behaviours. These basics include step-up and step-down, and staying on a perch where placed.

Step-up

Stepping up onto an offered hand is a foundational manoeuvre upon which most training and behavioural guidance relies. In light of what is discussed above, it is important that the bird does this behaviour because it wants to, not because it has to. By using a food reward and the cue words 'step up', a bird can be taught to step up on to the owner's hand and stay there.

Step-down

Stepping down allows the owner to guide the bird's movement. Once again, positive reinforcement (e.g. a food reward) and the cue words 'step down' can be used to teach the bird to step off the owner's hand and on to a suitable perch.

Stay

Staying on a perch is important for a bird to experience 'normal' flock social interaction while outside of its cage with its 'flock members', without getting into mischief or requiring constant supervision. The free-roaming pet parrot is at a much greater risk of traumatic injuries and household poisonings. It is also more likely to develop pair bonded interactions with one person, and less likely to interact with other people. Portable table-top perches are suitable for this training since they can be put anywhere. The bird is stepped down on to the perch and rewarded (verbally or with a food reward) for remaining there. If they climb down and walk around, avoid inadvertently rewarding this behaviour; simply put them back on to the perch without any verbal cue or other reward. If they stay there, offer another reward. It is usually necessary to gradually extend the time between placing the bird on the perch and offering the reward.

NORMALIZE SOCIAL INTERACTIONS

This has to be done on two levels:

- The interactions between the parrot and the person to whom the bird has bonded have to be modified. Interactions such as picking up the bird, scratching its head and body and playing with it have to be stopped or reduced dramatically while the modification programme is being implemented. The bonded person can clean the cage and put in fresh food and water; however, the less interaction the better.
- Other members of the household need the opportunity to interact positively with the bird. To avoid distracting the bird or triggering protective or territorial aggression, it is best if the bonded person is not around while this is being done and, when 'out of cage' training is being done, the bonded person should bring the bird to a place in which it does not exhibit territorial behaviours. The bird should learn to interact with other people using a combination of positive reinforcement and incremental exposure. For example, the new person can drop

a preferred food reward in the bird's food bowl and then walk away. If this is done often enough, eventually the bird will look forward to seeing the new person. This person can then try offering the reinforcement to the bird through the cage bars. Eventually the reward can be offered for stepping up on the hand as well as other cooperative behaviour. Alternatively, working in a neutral territory, the other members of the household can cue the bird to perform simple behaviours the bird already knows how to do. This gives the bird an activity on which to focus, while at the same time receiving rewards from people other than the one the bird has bonded to. This can help build a positive relationship with the rest of the household.

The goal with these two levels of modification is to limit the positive experiences with the bonded person and, at the same time, increase the positive experiences with the new person. However, it may never be possible for the new person to interact at the same level the bonded person can with the bird, and it is unlikely positive interactions can occur while the bonded person is in the room.

AVOID UNWANTED BEHAVIOURS

Analysis of a problem behaviour should follow the ABC of behaviour, where:

- A = Antecedent: the situation which led to the behaviour.
- B = Behaviour: the actual behaviour displayed by the bird.
- C = Consequences: what the bird got out of the behaviour. Consequences can be positive or negative.

The consequence will determine whether a behaviour will be repeated or not. If it is not possible to alter the consequence (and therefore the bird's likelihood of repeating the behaviour), it becomes necessary to change the antecedent. For example, if a bird screams loudly each morning until it is fed, the behavioural analysis is as follows:

- The antecedent is that there is no food in the bird's bowl first thing in the morning.
- The behaviour is that the bird screams.
- The consequence is that the owner hurriedly feeds the bird, positively reinforcing its behaviour.

The bird still has to be fed each day; therefore, the consequence cannot be changed. However, if the owner places food in the bowl after the bird has gone to sleep the night before, and therefore food is available to the bird as soon as it wakes up, the antecedent has changed and the behaviour should change (or stop).

Sometimes it is necessary for the owner to change his/her behaviour in order to change the bird's behaviour.

REPLACEMENT OF UNWANTED BEHAVIOURS WITH ACCEPTABLE BEHAVIOURS

Most birds, captive or wild, spend their time during the day performing daily maintenance behaviours that are essential for survival (**240, 241**). These behaviours include foraging, social interaction and feather care. Wild birds spend approximately 80% of their waking life foraging for food, with the remaining 20% of their time devoted to socializing and grooming.

If 'normal' social interaction with members of the household is limited, as is often the case when owners are at work or school, the other maintenance behaviours (foraging and grooming) must be increased to fill the time (**242**). Companion birds, with their food provided in the same dish, in the same place and at the same time each day, do not have to spend so much time foraging in order to survive. This deficit in activity may be replaced with abnormal behaviours such as stereotypical behaviours, feather-damaging behaviour (through overgrooming, **243**) or screaming. It may also heighten the bird's anticipation of the owner's presence and lead to problems with pair bonding.

By increasing the daily foraging activities available to a bird, its lifestyle can be enhanced significantly. Interestingly, several studies have confirmed that when a bird is given a choice between foraging for food or eating it out of a dish, most birds prefer to forage. Foraging activities that can be implemented include:

- A piece of nontreated wood (e.g. pine) is drilled with holes into which nuts, seeds or other treats fit tightly. The reward should be visible but not accessible without chewing down through the wood. The wood can be used as a perch in the cage, hung in the cage to increase the challenge, or used as a toy outside the cage (**244**).
- Wrapping the food bowls with newspaper or cardboard to make the bird chew through it to get at the food. A starter hole may be necessary to encourage the bird to begin chewing.

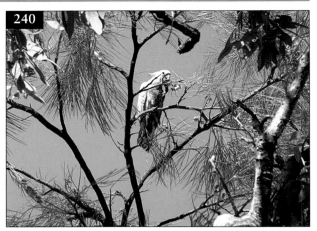

240 Wild cockatoo foraging for food, an activity that takes up nearly 80% of their normal day.

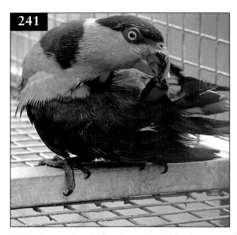

241 Grooming behaviour in a black-capped lory. Grooming takes up a relatively small amount of time in the wild, but captive conditions leave more time to groom and, sometimes, to overgroom.

- Wrapping food items in small pieces of paper, corn husks or other materials. Not all wrappings need to contain a reward.
- Mixing food with inedible items (e.g. wood buttons or other items) so that the bird has to dig through to find its food. Some parrot species can be particularly stimulated into new foraging behaviours by having a large box full of different items in which some desired food items or treats can be found.
- Puzzle toys that require birds to unscrew parts or manipulate components to get at their reward (**245**).

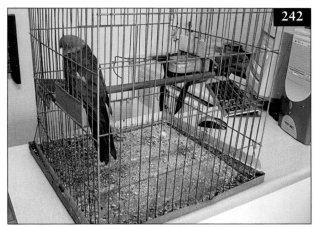

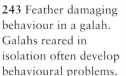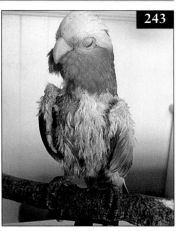

243 Feather damaging behaviour in a galah. Galahs reared in isolation often develop behavioural problems.

242 An undersized cage, with no relief from boredom or room to move.

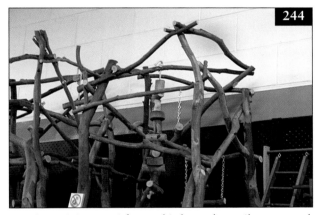

244 An activity 'gym' for pet birds can be easily converted into a 'foraging tree' to keep birds actively looking for food during the day.

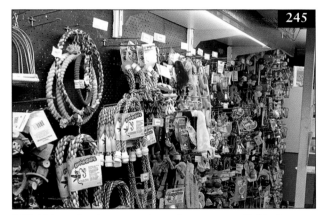

245 Although a large number of toys are available for birds, in some cases the bird has to be taught in stages how to use them.

Other activities that can be implemented to encourage normal behaviours include:
- Lightly spraying the bird with water will dampen the feathers and encourage the bird to groom normally.
- Providing items for the bird to chew and destroy (e.g. nontoxic tree branches, cardboard boxes, wooden toys).

Bird behaviour is complex and, as mentioned earlier, our understanding of it is still evolving. There is no simple approach to dealing with individual cases but, by applying the principles and strategies outlined above, clinicians should be able to have a positive impact on the relationship between bird and owner.

FURTHER READING

Briscoe JA, Reisner IR, Rosenthal KL (2004) Incorporating the veterinary behaviourist: a new model for the diagnosis and treatment of a feather damaging pet parrot. In: *Proceedings of the Annual Conference of the Association of Avian Veterinarians*, pp. 293–296.

Echols MS (2005) Practical use of foraging as a means of behaviour modification. In: *Proceedings of the Annual Conference of the Association of Avian Veterinarians Australian Committee*, pp. 185–194.

Friedman SG, Edling TM, Cheney CD (2006) Concepts in behaviour. Section I: The natural science of behaviour. In: *Clinical Avian Medicine, Vol 1*. GJ Harrison, TL Lightfoot (eds) Spix Publishing, Palm Beach, pp. 46–59.

Heidenreich B (2005) Addressing aggressive behaviour in birds. In: *Proceedings of the annual conference of the Association of Avian Veterinarians*, pp. 127–138.

Heidenreich B (2005) Solving companion parrot behaviour problems. In: *Proceedings of the annual conference of the Association of Avian Veterinarians*, pp. 219–228.

Heidenreich B (2006) How to train medical behaviours. In: *Proceedings of the annual conference of the Association of Avian Veterinarians*, pp. 135–148.

Luescher AU (2004) Rearing environment and behavioural development of psittacine birds. In: *Proceedings of the annual conference of the Association of Avian Veterinarians*, pp. 297–298.

Luescher AU (2006) *Manual of Parrot Behaviour*. Blackwell Publishing, Oxford.

Speer BL (2002) Practical clinical applications for the exam room. In: *Proceedings of the Association of Avian Veterinarians Australian Committee*, pp. 155–164.

Wilson L, Lightfoot TL (2006) Concepts in behaviour. Section III: Pubescent and adult psittacine behaviour. In: *Clinical Avian Medicine, Vol 1*. GJ Harrison, TL Lightfoot (eds) Spix Publishing, Palm Beach, pp. 73–84.

Wilson L, Greene Linden P, Lightfoot TL (2006) Concepts in behaviour. Section II: Early psittacine behaviour and development. In: *Clinical Avian Medicine, Vol 1*. GJ Harrison, TL Lightfoot (eds) Spix Publishing, Palm Beach, pp. 60–72.

CHAPTER 23
INCUBATION OF EGGS

WHY INCUBATE EGGS?

Incubation allows increased production, particularly in rare or valuable species. Removing an egg shortly after it is laid often induces the hen to lay a replacement. Poor parenting by some birds means that eggs and/or chicks can be lost in the nest. Removing and artificially incubating the egg can also reduce this risk.

It was thought that hand rearing birds made them bond closer to people; therefore, artificial incubation was (and still is) widely practised to provided 'bonded' chicks for the pet market (see Chapter 22, Behavioural problems, p. 233).

In some cases, artificial incubation is used as a means of disease control. Pathogens that are not vertically transmitted through the egg, but can be horizontally transmitted, can be reduced or eliminated by artificial incubation.

WHEN TO COLLECT EGGS

Artificial incubation is rarely as efficient and effective as natural incubation. The eggs of small species (e.g. conures, cockatiels, lovebirds, budgerigars) do not do well when incubated from day 0; it is thought that vibrations from the incubator may cause decreased hatchability. In these birds, incubation should start after two weeks of natural incubation. Large birds also benefit from natural incubation for the first 2–2.5 weeks.

However, it may, in some circumstances, be necessary to collect eggs immediately (or shortly after) being laid (e.g. when the parents are destructive to the eggs or when it is desired to increase egg production — if the hen broods for 2–3 weeks, she may not lay another clutch in that breeding season).

STORING EGGS PRIOR TO INCUBATION

Some aviculturists prefer to store eggs prior to beginning incubation in order to synchronize hatching and hand rearing. However, it is usually preferable not to store eggs, as hatchability reduces on a daily basis when stored. This loss of hatching viability is species dependent. If there are no other options (and the aviculturist accepts the risk of decreased hatchability), eggs can be stored as follows:

- Temperature in the storage area should be kept between 12.8°C and 18.3°C to prevent embryonic development.
- The relative humidity should be maintained between 80% and 90%.
- The eggs should be turned 90° at least twice daily.
- Eggs should not be stored for more than seven days.

SANITATION OF THE EGGS

Eggs should not be cleaned if at all possible. Routine washing is not recommended, as this can reduce hatchability. Dry cleaning with a soft brush is the preferred means of cleaning eggs. If it is necessary to wash the eggs, a 10% quaternary ammonia or 4.2% chlorine solution can be used. The water used should be warmer than the egg, so as to prevent the egg drawing in the washing solution through its pores. Detergents must not be used on very porous eggs.

Fumigation using formalin and potassium permanganate is sometimes recommended (20–30 minutes contact with egg), this but may be harmful/carcinogenic to humans. Formaldehyde gas is also teratogenic in chickens.

EQUIPMENT

Forced air incubators are better than convection heating incubators, as they give more uniform temperature control and air flow (**246**). Accurate humidity control is essential. Automatic turning controls are recommended, but must be checked for serviceability and vibration. As very few incubators can either cool air drawn in or dehumidify it, it is recommended that the incubator be kept in a clean, biosecure, air-conditioned and dehumidified room whenever possible.

INCUBATION PARAMETERS

TEMPERATURE

Temperature determines the rate of embryonic growth. The correct temperature should see the egg hatch at the same time a naturally incubated egg does. Larger eggs need lower temperatures; smaller eggs need higher temperatures. Typically, psittacine eggs develop normally if incubated between 36.9°C and 37°C. The room temperature in the incubator room must be cooler than the incubator, allowing the incubator to warm the egg rather than trying to cool it.

HUMIDITY

Eggs lose weight during incubation due to water loss through the shell (transpiration). The rate of water loss is dependent on shell thickness, porosity and water vapour concentration of the atmosphere. The expected weight loss is 16–22% over the incubation period. To achieve this, it is usually necessary that the relative humidity in the incubator should be 38–46%.

As incubators cannot dehumidify air, the relative humidity in the incubator room should be lower than in the incubator, allowing the incubator to add water to increase the relative humidity around the eggs.

VENTILATION

Oxygen and carbon dioxide are exchanged across the shell (respiration). If the carbon dioxide builds up in the incubator, the chicks may suffocate. Therefore, there must be a continual infusion of fresh air into the incubator (forced air incubators are more effective than convection incubators).

TURNING AND POSITIONING

This allows proper development of the embryo and the blood vessels in the egg, and allows better

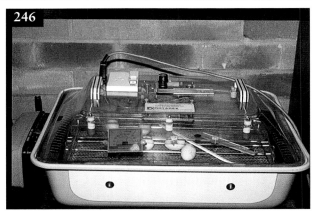

246 Forced air incubators are more effective and efficient than convection heating incubators.

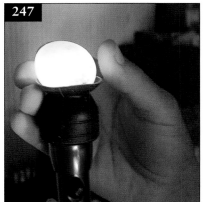

247 Candling an (infertile) egg.

distribution of nutrients in the albumen. The old theory of the embryo 'sticking' to the shell is no longer considered valid. Poultry and ratite eggs are incubated vertically, with the air cell up; psittacine eggs are incubated horizontally with the air cell end slightly elevated. The eggs should be turned a quarter turn along the long axis every 4–5 hours.

MONITORING

Embryonic development can be monitored by candling (examining the egg in a darkened room with an intense focal light to transilluminate it) (**247**). Candling at 7–10 days will indicate if the egg is fertile and developing properly. Clear yolks showing no signs of blood vessels or development by day 7 are infertile or died early, and should be removed. Occasionally a 'blood ring' (extravasated blood in a ring surrounding the remnants of the embryo and embryonic circle of blood vessels) is seen. This indicates early embryonic death.

Weight monitoring is also carried out. Eggs should lose 13–22% of their weight between setting and removal to the hatcher. They may lose another 3% during hatch, although excessive weight loss at this time may dehydrate the chick, making hatch difficult.

EMBRYONIC DEVELOPMENT

Embryonic growth is divided into three, approximately equal, phases.

EARLY TERM

In poultry the following events occur:
- Day 1: blastoderm develops, becomes doughnut-shaped as cellular division occurs.
- Day 2: brain, eyes and spinal cord develop.
- Days 2–3: heart and blood vessels grow, and the extra-embryonic membranes form:
  - Amnion (from the body wall, cushions embryo in amniotic fluid).
  - Yolk sac membrane (from gut, envelops the yolk).
  - Allantois (from hind gut, acts initially as bladder).
  - Chorion (an extension of the amnion). It fuses with the allantois to form the chorioallantoic membrane (CAM), the primary respiratory organ of the embryonic chick.
- Days 3–4: body wall and viscera grow.
- Days 4–5: limbs develop.

MID TERM

There is growth with little further differentiation. Feathers begin to form.

LATE TERM

The yolk sac is drawn up into the embryo and the albumen is actively drunk by the chick. Finally, the chick positions itself and hatches.

HATCHING

Hatching is stimulated by the chick converting to pulmonic respiration from CAM respiration.

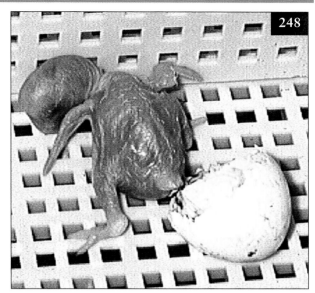

248 An Indian ring-neck chick hatching in an incubator.

Increasing carbon dioxide concentration causes the neck muscles to twitch and the chick becomes more active. The air cell expands and extends down one side of the egg 24–48 hours before internal pipping. This process is known as 'drawing down'.

The chick then penetrates the air cell (internal pipping) by rubbing its beak against the inner shell membranes until they tear. The chick is now able to breathe the air in the air cell. As the chick is jerking inside the egg, it rotates 360°, cracking the shell circumferentially (**248**). This is known as the 'external pip'.

The hatch time, the interval from internal pip to hatch, is usually 36–48 hours in most species. Hatching times less than 24 hours, or more than 80 hours can indicate a problem.

Requirements for a hatcher in which an egg can be placed to hatch are:
- A lower temperature than the incubator, usually 36.4–36.9°C.
- A higher humidity, up to 70%.
- No turning.
- Adequate ventilation.

PROBLEMS WITH INCUBATION

Embryonic mortality should not exceed 10% of fertile eggs set for incubation. This normal 10% mortality is made up of:

- Early-term deaths, 3–4%.
- Mid-term deaths, 1–2%.
- Late-term deaths, up to 4%.

Losses above these figures require investigation. The two most common causes of mortality/morbidity in the egg are malposition (the most frequent cause — see below) and inadequate moisture loss (see *Table 4*, p. 219).

MALPOSITIONING

The normal hatch position is as follows: the chick is orientated along the long axis of the egg, its head lies under the right wing in chickens and close to the right wing tip in psittacines, and the egg tooth is pointing towards the air cell. (See *Table 5*, p. 222).

FURTHER READING

Jordan R (1989) *Parrot Incubation Procedures*. Silvio Mattacchione and Co., Pickering.

Jordan R (2001) Incubation of psittacine eggs. *Seminars in Avian and Exotic Pet Medicine* **10**(3):112–116.

Joyner KL (1994) Theriogenology. In: *Avian Medicine: Principles and Application*. BW Ritchie, GJ Harrison, LR Harrison (eds). Wingers Publishing, Lake Worth, pp. 748–804.

Olsen GH, Clubb SL (1997) Embryology, incubation and hatching. In: *Avian Medicine and Surgery*. RB Altman, SL Clubb, GM Dorrestein, K Quesenberry (eds). WB Saunders, Philapdelphia, pp. 54–72.

Schubot RM, Clubb KJ, Clubb SL (1992) *Psittacine Aviculture: Perspectives, Techniques and Research*. Avicultural Breeding and Research Center, Loxahatchee, Fl.

CHAPTER 24
PAEDIATRICS

INTRODUCTION

Most companion birds (e.g. psittacines and passerines) are altricial (i.e. when hatched they are blind, deaf and not feathered, and therefore totally dependent on their parents or rearer) (**249**). As juveniles, their health status is determined by:

- Pre-laying factors:
  - Parental health.
  - Parental nutrition.
  - Parental maturity.
  - Parental genetics.
- Incubation factors:
  - Artificial vs. natural incubation.
  - Temperature, humidity and hygiene in the nest box or incubator.
  - Care in handling of the eggs by either the parents or the incubator operator.
  - Frequency and degree of rotation during artificial incubation.
- Post-hatch factors. If the chick has been hand reared, the following parameters in the rearing environment play important roles in the health of the chick:

- Temperature.
- Hygiene.
- Humidity.
- Nutrition.
- Management.

Detailed knowledge of hand-rearing practices, including weaning ages, can be obtained from reputable aviculture literature.

EXAMINATION OF THE CHICK
HISTORY

Factors to consider include:

- Parents: genetics, diet, health status.
- Siblings (if any): any problems or deaths within the group.
- Incubation: artificial or natural? Hatchability of fertile eggs is a key indicator of incubation performance.
- Hatching: if artificially incubated, were there any problems with hatch?
- Nursery management: hygiene, biosecurity, source of eggs and/or chicks.
- Diet: type of food, how prepared, volume and frequency of feeding.
- Records: hatch weights, growth rates, mortalities, medications, previous medical problems.

PHYSICAL EXAMINATION
Weight

The chick should be weighed and its weight compared with the expected weight range found in growth charts (if available).

Posture

It is important to be aware that chicks sleep and rest in what seems to be 'awkward' positions. These positions change as the chick moves; one should look for postures that do not change with movement.

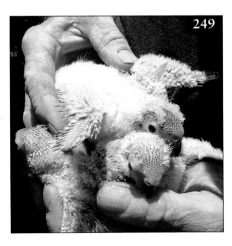

249 Parrot chicks, such as these lorikeets, are altricial and totally dependent on their parents or rearers until weaned.

Conformation

The positioning and conformation of the limbs and the spine should be checked.

Body condition

The toes and elbows are examined. In a well nourished, healthy chick they should be 'plump'. Thin toes and elbows are a good indicator in neonatal chicks of dehydration, malnourishment or disease. Palpatation of the pectoral muscles is helpful; the keel should be well fleshed with soft pectoral muscles.

Behaviour

Young chicks (pre-weaning) should be either sleeping or calling for food. Restlessness could indicate incorrect environmental temperature or stress (e.g. excessive lighting). Older chicks spend a lot of time sleeping, but are more interested in their environment and in socializing with nursery mates.

A feeding response (vigorous extension and bobbing of the head and neck) should be easily elicited by pressing gently at the commissures of the beak. Failure to elicit a response can be an indication of disease, hypothermia or weakness.

Skin

Prior to full feathering the normal chick's skin should be pink or pink–yellow in colour, and soft to the touch. Pallor of the skin can indicate hypothermia, anaemia or illness. Erythematous skin can indicate hyperthermia or illness. Heavily wrinkled skin indicates dehydration (**250**).

Crop

The normal crop should have some food in it at most times. It should not be overdistended, nor should it have significant amounts of air or gas in it. Rhythmic contractions of the crop should be visible in neonatal chicks, and the crop should empty in 4–6 hours in all chicks.

Head

The size of the head should not be excessively large in relation to body size. The beak should have a normal conformation (see Chapter 8, Disorders affecting the beak and cere). There should be no sinus swellings. The nares should be open and symmetrical.

The eyes should be symmetrical and healthy in appearance. They begin to open at 10–28 days and take several days to open completely.

Most Australian and African parrots hatch with their ears open. The ears of eclectus and South American species should be open within 2–3 weeks after hatching.

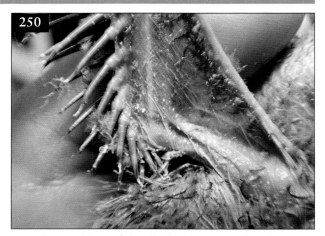

250 The wrinkling of this chick's skin, as well as the poor filling of the basilic vein, are good indicators of dehydration.

Oral cavity

The oral cavity should be examined for diphtheritic plaques or other abnormalities.

Abdomen

In neonatal chicks the abdomen should be large relative to the rest of the body. The liver may be visible through the skin in very young chicks, and rhythmic contractions of the ventriculus should be visible. The duodenal loop may be visible. There should not be bruising or haemorrhage visible. The abdomen can be transilluminated with an intense focal light for closer inspection.

As the chick grows, the abdomen reduces in size relative to the rest of the body. It should be concave when palpated; a convex abdomen could indicate a degree of abdominal distension.

Feather growth

Depending on the species, some chicks are hatched naked or with wispy down feathers. Others are covered in fluffy down feathers. A second wave of down feather growth begins at 1–3 weeks of age and, sometimes, even later in some species.

Pin feathers begin to emerge at 2–3 weeks of age. The body contour feathers emerge over the shoulders first; the pattern of emergence after that varies between species, although usually the body contour feathers emerge at the same time or shortly before the secondary flight feathers on the wings. Primaries may begin to develop before secondary feathers, but usually mature after them. Final feather maturity is usually not complete before the bird has weaned.

Abnormalities include:

- Feathers erupting in a unusual pattern (e.g. in a circular pattern on the crown of the head, rather than running parallel along the line of the body).
- Stress bars in the opened vane.
- Abnormal colouring.
- Haemorrhage in the calamus.
- Dystrophic development.

Droppings

The faecal portion should be relatively well formed and not malodorous. A degree of polyuria is normal, but this should lessen as the chick ages. Excessive or persistent polyuria warrants further investigation.

DIAGNOSTIC TESTING

Microbiology is an important tool in assessing gastrointestinal flora. Gram stains and cultures are frequently used to assess crop or other gastrointestinal problems. Normal bacterial flora includes *Lactobacillus*, *Streptococcus*, *Staphylococcus* and *Bacillus* spp. Low numbers of *E. coli* are often normally cultured as well. Other gram-negative bacilli and *Candida* are rarely cultured from healthy chicks.

Clinical pathology can be used readily on chicks. It is important to note that compared to adults of the same species, chicks normally have:

- Lower PCV and higher white cell count.
- Lower total protein and uric acid.
- Higher CK.

Radiography is an essential tool for assessing the status of the skeletal system.

COMMON PROBLEMS
STUNTING
Aetiology

Stunting is seen in the first 30 days of life. It is usually associated with improper feeding, poor environmental conditions or disease.

Clinical presentation

Signs include subnormal weight gain, reduced muscle mass (toes, wings, back should be checked), abnormal feathering (e.g. head feathers develop in a circular pattern on the crown) and oversized head relative to the size of the body (**251**). Eyelids fail to open normally or when expected, and there is delayed ear opening or narrowing of the ear canal. The affected bird may suffer with chronic, recurrent infections, and be constantly calling and begging for food. As the chick gets older it often develops a globose head with an elongated slender beak. The eyes may appear exophthalmic because of the misshapen skull.

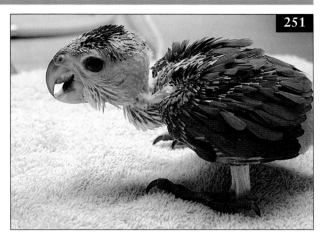

251 A stunted chick. This black-headed caique was suffering from a crop burn. Note the oversized head.

Management

The predisposing cause should be identified and treated. Nutritional inadequacies should be corrected. The prognosis is good if the problem is diagnosed early and treated aggressively.

CROP STASIS ('SOUR CROP')
Aetiology

Causes include:

- Generalized ileus (generalized infection, foreign bodies, chilling, heavy metal toxicosis, dehydration).
- Crop disorders (foreign bodies, overstretched/atonic crop, infectious ingluvitis, fibrous food impaction, crop burns).
- Dietary problems (cold food, excessively watery food, food that settles out in the crop, overfeeding, overly dry food).

Clinical presentation

Signs include the crop failing to empty in more than six hours, regurgitation and loss of feeding response. Signs of dehydration are seen (e.g. erythematous wrinkled skin, tenting of the skin and sunken eyes).

Diagnosis

This is based on crop and faecal cytology (Gram stain) and culture, haematology and biochemistry, and radiography.

Management

The cause should be identified and corrected where possible.

The crop should be emptied with a feeding tube and lavaged with warm saline. (In some extreme cases it may be necessary to perform an ingluviotomy.) It should always be assumed that these chicks are dehydrated. The dehydration should be corrected with parental fluids until crop motility has been restored.

Appropriate antimicrobials should be given as indicated by crop and faecal cytology/culture.

A crop 'bra' can be used if needed. This is a nonadhesive bandage placed under the crop and around the wings to 'lift and support' the atonic crop in order to allow gravity to assist with crop emptying.

Once the crop has been emptied, in many cases it may be advisable to leave it empty for a few hours while dehydration is corrected. Initial feeds should be of small volumes of isotonic saline. If this moves through, solids can be added. Small, watery meals should be fed often. Pre-digesting the hand-rearing formula with a small amount of pancreatic enzymes can liquefy the diet without diluting it.

Motility modifiers (e.g. metoclopramide or cisapride) may assist in restoring motility, although their efficacy is poor if used without other supportive measures.

The prognosis is good, provided prompt and appropriate therapy is provided.

THERMAL INJURIES TO THE CROP
See **252**, and Chapter 13, p. 158.

CROP PERFORATIONS
See Chapter 13, p. 159.

ORTHOPAEDIC PROBLEMS
See Chapter 11.

BEAK MALFORMATIONS
See Chapter 8, p. 125.

INFECTIOUS DISEASE
Definition/overview
Infectious diseases are quite common in young chicks; their low level of immunocompetence combined with often substandard rearing practices leaves them highly predisposed to infection. This same lack of immuno-competence means that the progression of an infectious disease in young birds is often rapid. Prompt and aggressive therapy is needed to save the patient.

Aetiology
Infections may be bacterial (*Pseudomonas, E. Coli,* other gram-negative bacteria); fungal (*Candida, Aspergillus*); viral (polyomavirus, PBFD); *Chlamydophila psittaci*;

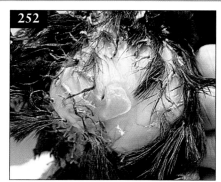

252 Crop burn in a juvenile black cockatoo. Note the initial blanching of the skin prior to necrosis.

parasitic: protozoa (*Cryptosporidia, Trichomonas, Cochlosoma, Coccidia* and *Atoxoplasma* [in young canaries]); and nematodes (ascarids, *Capillaria* and *Acuaria*).

Clinical presentation
Signs include lethargy, loss of feeding response, pallor or erythema of the skin, dehydration, crop stasis, vomiting/regurgitation, weight loss or failure to thrive, subcutaneous haemorrhage, feathering abnormalities and sudden death.

Management
The aetiological agent should be identified and the chick treated accordingly. The patient will require supportive care.

FURTHER READING
Clubb SL (1997) Psittacine pediatric husbandry and medicine. In: *Avian Medicine and Surgery.* RB Altman, SL Clubb, GM Dorrestein, K Quesenberry (eds). WB Saunders, Philadelphia, pp. 73–95.

Flammer K, Clubb SL (1994) Neonatology. In: *Avian Medicine: Principles and Application.* BW Ritchie, GJ Harrison, LR Harrison (eds). Wingers Publishing, Lake Worth, pp. 805–841.

LaBonde J (2006) Avian reproductive and pediatric disorders. In: *Proceedings of the Annual Conference of the Association of Avian Veterinarians Australian Committee,* pp. 229–238.

Schubot RM, Clubb KJ, Clubb SL (1992) *Psittacine Aviculture: Perspectives, Techniques and Research.* Avicultural Breeding and Research Center, Loxahatchee, Fl.

CHAPTER 25
ANALGESIA AND ANAESTHESIA

ANALGESIA
SIGNS AND EFFECTS OF PAIN

It is generally accepted that birds perceive pain along neurological pathways similar to those in mammals. However, as discussed earlier, birds may indicate pain in less obvious ways than domestic mammals. They appear to respond to painful stimuli in one of two ways:

- 'Fight-or-flight' responses:
  - Excessive vocalization.
  - Wing flapping.
  - Decreased head movement.
- Conservation–withdrawal responses:
  - Immobility.
  - Closure of eyes.
  - Inappetence.
  - Fluffing of feathers.

It is thought that the 'fight-or-flight' response is more common when the bird is suffering from sudden or unexpected pain from which it is attempting to escape. In contrast, with chronic or overwhelming pain (which is perhaps more commonly seen in clinical practice) birds appear to be more likely to adopt the 'conservation–withdrawal' responses, perhaps in an attempt to minimize the further pain that struggling would induce and to avoid attracting the attention of potential predators. Care must therefore be taken not to misinterpret lack of movement or vocalization as an indication that the bird is not in pain (253).

In addition to these clinical signs of generalized pain, localized pain may be reflected in feather picking or other self-mutilatory behaviours over or in the vicinity of the painful lesion.

While we know that pain is a response to a noxious stimulus that serves the purpose of alerting an animal to the presence of that stimulus and thereby provoking a response that removes the animal from the stimulus and therefore further injury, we also now know that it is has wider, more far-reaching consequences. Through stimulation of the adrenal gland and subsequent release of corticosterone, pain has an adverse effect on wound healing and the immune system. Survival and recovery rates of birds in pain are much lower than those receiving effective analgesia. As clinicians we therefore have not only a moral obligation to provide effective analgesia, but also sound medical reasons.

PRINCIPLES OF ANALGESIA

There are two underlying principles to consider when developing an analgesic plan for a patient.

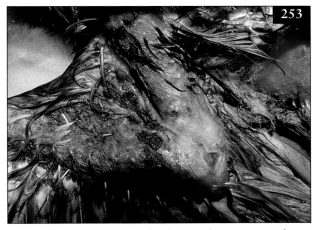

253 Birds are not adept at displaying obvious signs of pain. The clinician should assume that if an injury, such as this bruising, is present, the patient will benefit from analgesia.

Pre-emptive analgesia

Learning to anticipate when a patient will be painful is helpful, as pain is easier to control if the patient is treated before it becomes painful and upset. A painful event stimulates peripheral nociceptors, which transmit the 'pain' signal to the brain via central spinal nociception pathways. Continued stimulation facilitates these pathways and evokes a painful response, a process known as 'wind up'. This facilitation may outlast the initial stimulus by a prolonged period. The underlying theory of pre-emptive analgesia is to use drugs and techniques before, during and after a painful event in order to block this facilitation, preferably before it occurs. When dealing with patients who are already experiencing pain, it is not possible to apply a pre-emptive approach, which may explain why it is more difficult to get the pain under control initially, and then it requires less therapy to maintain analgesia if therapy is continued. The use of pre-emptive analgesia before performing any procedure likely to cause pain is therefore a key element in managing pain.

Multimodal therapy

The perception of pain is both a peripheral and a central event, using several types of receptors and pathways, so there is no single drug class of drug or action that can be used as a sole analgesic agent. The concept of multimodal therapy recognizes this and encourages a multi-level approach to analgesia.

Remove the source of pain

This may involve splinting a fractured limb, removing a foreign body or performing surgery with minimal tissue trauma and handling.

Reduce fear and stress

Fear and stress may enhance the nociception pathways. Providing privacy in a warm, quiet environment in order to reduce apprehension and the judicious use of anxiolytics (e.g. midazolam) may serve to relieve fear and stress and therefore enhance analgesic therapy.

Use several classes of drug to treat pain at different nociceptors

As described above, peripheral nociceptors detect a painful stimulus and transmit, via spinal nociceptive pathways, a message to the brain where central nociceptors perceive it as pain. Inflammation in peripheral tissues may sensitize the peripheral nociceptors, invoking a more intense pain response at lower levels of pain. Using drugs that can reduce inflammation (and therefore decrease peripheral nociceptor sensitivity) while other drugs are used to block spinal pathways and/or central nociceptors can provide more comprehensive analgesia than one class of drug alone.

ANALGESICS COMMONLY USED IN AVIAN PRACTICE

The most commonly used analgesics in avian practice are opioids and NSAIDs. Local anaesthesia may also be used in certain circumstances.

Opioids

Some bird species appear to have more kappa opioid receptors in the forebrain than mu opioid receptors, explaining why some birds do not respond to mu agonists such as morphine, buprenorphine and fentanyl in the same manner as mammals. Therefore, kappa opioids such as butorphanol may be the more efficacious analgesics in birds.

Butorphanol (1–4 mg/kg IM or orally q6h) is currently recommended for opioid analgesia in birds. Higher doses may be hyperalgesic.

Side-effects are uncommon, but may include respiratory depression, nausea and vomiting, bradycardia and constipation.

NSAIDs

NSAIDs act on peripheral tissues and therefore are indicated when tissue damage and inflammation are the source of the pain. They may be most effective when acting synergistically with opioids.

NSAIDs are COX inhibitors, inhibiting the production and actions of prostaglandins, prostacyclin and thromboxane (which cause hyperalgesia and sensitize nociceptors). They are arbitrarily divided into COX-1 inhibitors (inhibiting the production of prostaglandins that are important in physical function, e.g. renal perfusion, gut barrier maintenance) and COX-2 inhibitors, which inhibit the production of inflammatory prostaglandins. In theory, COX-2 inhibition will have an analgesic effect, while COX-1 inhibitors are more likely to have adverse side-effects such as renal damage and gastrointestinal damage. However, this division is not clear cut, and all NSAIDs provide analgesia and are potentially nephrotoxic.

Commonly used NSAIDs include:
- Meloxicam 0.2–0.5 mg/kg IM or orally q12h.
- Carprofen 2–4 mg/kg orally q12h.
- Ketoprofen 2 mg/kg IM q8–24h.

Local anaesthesia

Local anaesthesia is seldom used in birds. However, local anaesthetics interrupt the transmission of pain impulses and, when used preoperatively, they can be used to block the site of tissue manipulation, thus helping to reduce central sensitization.

Cardiovascular side-effects appear to be rare at doses below 1–4 mg/kg. It may be necessary to dilute commercially available preparations in order to prevent overdosing the patient.

Although local anaesthesia reduces pain perception, it does nothing to protect the patient from stress. With many avian patients it may be better to induce general anaesthesia rather than stress the bird with restraint and local anaesthesia.

ANAESTHESIA
WHAT MAKES AVIAN ANAESTHESIA DIFFERENT?

There are four fundamental differences between avian and mammalian anaesthesia: the anatomy of the bird; its metabolism; its tendency to lose heat quickly; and finally, that most birds requiring anaesthesia are chronically ill.

Anatomy
Trachea

Birds have complete tracheal cartilage rings and the trachea is therefore not expandable. For this reason, only noncuffed endotracheal tubes should be used. (If cuffed tubes are used, they must never be inflated.) Additionally, some species (notably waterfowl) have either very long, coiled tracheas or diverticula (bullae). These are anatomical adaptations allowing such birds to hold their breath under water. It also may make it difficult to mask induce these species, making intravenous or intramuscular induction advisable.

Voice production arises from the syrinx, the bifurcation of the trachea. This is located within the body and is a common site for obstructions (*Aspergillus* granulomas or inhaled bird seed).

Air sacs, nonexpandable lungs and lack of a diaphragm

Respiration is achieved by movement of the sternum (up and down) and the ribs (in and out). If these movements are restricted, or if enlarged organs, fat or fluids within the body compress the air sacs, respiratory compromise can quickly develop. Therefore:

- Wherever possible place the bird in ventral or lateral recumbency. Birds in dorsal recumbency may require IPPV to properly oxygenate them.
- If any anaesthesia is likely to be prolonged more than 5–10 minutes, the patient should be

intubated and ventilated, regardless of its positioning.
- Birds with ascites should be handled very carefully, and may need diuretic therapy or coeliocentesis before anaesthesia.

If the coelom is opened during surgery, the bird may be able to breathe *through* the abdomen, via the air sacs. This may require increasing the oxygen flow rate and deepening the anaesthesia to overcome this. Catheterization of the caudal thoracic air sac can allow anaesthesia to be maintained without tracheal intubation, leaving the head free to work on.

Metabolism

The avian metabolic rate is much faster than that of mammals. For this reason, lengthy fasting is potentially dangerous, as hypoglycaemia may develop. Conversely, regurgitation and aspiration of crop and proventricular contents are very real risks. It is generally recommended to fast avian patients for 3–4 hours before anaesthesia. If necessary, crop contents should be removed by lavage prior to anaesthesia.

Heat loss

Birds begin to cool down within 20 minutes of induction. Profound hypothermia, resulting in the patient's death, can easily occur. Various techniques have been developed to maintain body temperature including warmed intravenous fluids, heating pads, warmed anaesthetic gases and radiant heat. Undoubtedly, the best prevention is a well thought out surgical plan and rapid surgical techniques.

Chronically ill birds

The masking phenomenon makes it likely that most avian patients requiring anaesthesia will be chronically ill. The stress of physically restraining a bird to examine it may be far greater than the stress of an anaesthetic.

Procedures should be planned, endeavouring to do as much as possible in as short a period as possible. For example, the patient can be anaesthetized, physically examined, radiographed, blood and swabs taken, fluids given and initial treatment started all in less than ten minutes. This can be done with minimal stress to the patient and maximum return to the clinician.

The ideal requirements for avian anaesthetic agents and techniques are:

- Rapid induction and recovery in order to minimize stress and heat loss.

- Rapid metabolism and excretion, avoiding 'hangover' effects that may delay the bird's return to eating and its normal metabolic rate.
- Minimal cardiac and respiratory depressant effects, combined with good ventilation.
- Operator health and safety must remain an important consideration.

INHALATION ANAESTHETIC AGENTS
Halothane
Halothane manufacture is being scaled down and it is unlikely to be available in the near future. It is soluble in blood, fat and other soft tissues and therefore takes longer to reach effective concentration in the brain. This results in longer induction and recovery times than for isoflurane. It is excreted through the respiratory tract. Marked cardiac arrhythmias (ventricular tachycardia and ventricular fibrillation) frequently occur.

Halothane has a low anaesthetic index, meaning that higher concentrations are required to induce apnoea. Although at first this suggests greater safety, the effect is that the patient continues to breathe and therefore takes in more halothane. When combined with its solubility in the body and its cardiac effects, the result is that apnoea and cardiac arrest during deep halothane anaesthesia are often simultaneous.

Isoflurane
This is poorly soluble in blood, fat and other soft tissues, therefore induction and recovery times are rapid and controlling the depth of anaesthesia is easier to achieve. It is excreted through the respiratory tract. It does cause some cardiac arrhythmias, but not as severe or as life threatening as those seen with halothane.

Isoflurane has a higher anaesthetic index than halothane, meaning that apnoea occurs much earlier in deep anaesthesia, preventing the spontaneous inhalation of more isoflurane. This lessens the probability of fatal cardiac arrhythmias developing, making it a safer anaesthetic agent.

Sevoflurane
This produces a more rapid induction and recovery than isoflurane, but not so much as to be clinically significant. It must run at a higher concentration than isoflurane to maintain surgical anaesthesia. Cardiac arrythmias are not noted. The anaesthetic index is higher than for isoflurane, but again this is not of clinical significance. The higher concentrations required mean that sevoflurane is significantly more expensive than isoflurane, but there are only small clinical advantages.

INTRAVENOUS OR INTRAMUSCULAR AGENTS
Intravenous or intramuscular agents can be used, but it must be recognized that induction and recovery are variable. Recovery is often prolonged, and there can be a significant 'hang-over' effect, with the bird not regaining its normal metabolic rate and appetite for several hours or longer. It is therefore recommended that these agents only be used as an induction agent where mask induction is not feasible (e.g. waterfowl, large ratites) or in the field where gas anaesthesia may be unavailable. Clinicians must be aware of the hazards of using intravenous or intramuscular anaesthesia, and be prepared to deal with adverse effects and prolonged recovery times.

Ketamine
Ketamine alone is not recommended for anaesthesia. Although it does not appear to cause pulmonary depression or cardiovascular depression, ketamine (at anaesthetic doses) gives inadequate analgesia and muscle relaxation and is associated with spontaneous movements, muscular rigidity and violent recoveries. It is excreted through the kidneys and the recovery time is prolonged and variable. The dose is 20–50 mg/kg IM or IV.

Xylazine
When used alone, xylazine does not usually produce adequate surgical immobilization. It may be associated with bradycardia, hypotension, arrhythmias and respiratory depression. It frequently causes salivation, excitement, muscle tremors and convulsions, sometimes aggravated by noise.

Recovery is prolonged, but xylazine can be reversed by yohimbine hydrochloride (0.11–0.27 mg/kg). The dose of xylazine is 1 mg/kg IM.

Xylazine–ketamine
This combination is commonly used for restraint and anaesthesia, but waterfowl (especially ducks and Canada geese), owls and accipiters do not respond well. When used together the combination is synergistic, giving a smooth induction and recovery with improved muscle relaxation and possibly enhanced analgesia. The combination can be associated with cardiac arrhythmias and hypotension. The dose is: ketamine 5–20 mg/kg, xylazine 0.5–2.0 mg/kg, IM or IV.

Diazepam

By itself, diazepam is used for sedation or seizure control. The dose is 0.05–0.15 mg/kg slowly IV, or 0.2–0.5 mg/kg IM.

Diazepam–ketamine

This combination can be used as an intravenous induction agent in large ratites, raptors and waterfowl, but it may not be a reliable maintenance agent. It can be used intramuscularly in psittacines and pigeons (with a slow induction and recovery time). The dose is: diazepam 0.2–2 mg/kg, ketamine 10–40 mg/kg.

Midazolam

This can be used as a sedative and anxiolytic, or as a premedication for anaesthesia. At sedative doses it has minimal effects on blood pressure, heart rate and body temperature. The dose is 0.8–3 mg/kg IM or IV.

Midazolam–ketamine

The dose for this combination is: midazolam 0.2–4 mg/kg, ketamine 10–40 mg/kg, IM.

Medetomidine–ketamine

This is a useful combination for intravenous induction of waterfowl, giving rapid induction and recovery. It is reversible with atipamezole. The dose is: medetomidine 60–85 µg/kg; ketamine 1.5–2.0 mg/kg.

Zolazepam–tiletamine

This is not recommended in birds due to violent recoveries.

Propofol

This can be used as an intravenous induction agent following sedation with medetomidine–ketamine. Apnoea is common following intravenous induction. The dose is 1–5 mg/kg IV. Intubation and IPPV are strongly recommended.

ANAESTHETIC TECHNIQUE
Patient preparation

An accurate weight is obtained of the patient. Psittacines should be fasted for no more than 3–4 hours. Larger birds, especially raptors, may require periods of fasting up to 12 hours. The patient's respiration is assessed by distant examination, looking for mouth breathing, tail bobbing, bilateral wing drooping and exaggerated sternal lift as evidence of dyspnoea. If dyspnoea is present, this must be factored into the anaesthetic plan, or the anaesthesia postponed.

The patient's crop and abdomen should be palpated. If the crop is full, it must be emptied by crop gavage. If there is abdominal distension it must be determined if there is ascites present. If so, preanaesthetic coeliocentesis may be advantageous.

PCV, total plasma protein and blood glucose should be measured as minimal preanaesthetic testing.

If painful procedures are anticipated, pre-emptive analgesia (see above) should be given 20–60 minutes before the procedure commences.

Induction
Parrots and other small birds

Where appropriate or necessary, the patient should be wrapped loosely in a towel to prevent wing flapping and excessive struggling. Mask induction is carried out with 5% isoflurane; induction usually takes approximately 20–30 seconds (**254**).

Waterfowl and other large birds

An intravenous catheter is placed in an accessible vein (e.g. the medial tarsal vein in waterfowl, basilic vein in ratites). Induction is with intravenous drug(s) as described above.

Maintenance

For short procedures (e.g. radiography) maintenance of anaesthesia via a face mask may be all that is required. The mouth and nares should be encased in the mask, which should be sealed around the head to prevent the escape of anaesthetic gas and to assist in ventilation if required. For small patients this can be achieved by stretching a rubber glove over the mask and making a small hole for the patient's head.

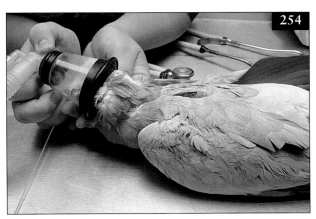

254 Mask induction is suitable for most companion birds.

For procedures longer than five minutes, for compromised patients or for rare or valuable birds, intubation is advisable (**255**). It should be remembered that the avian trachea is composed of complete cartilage rings and the lumen diameter decreases caudal to the glottis (**256**). Therefore, endotracheal tubes should be:

- Noncuffed or, if cuffed, never inflated.
- Relatively shorter than those used in mammals.
- Smaller diameter than the width of the glottis would suggest.

Once intubated, ventroflexion of the neck must be avoided. This can bring the tip of the endotracheal tube into contact with the tracheal mucosa, causing pressure necrosis.

If the patient's condition precludes intubation (e.g. tracheal obstructions), an air sac catheter should be placed as described in Chapter 3, Clinical techniques (**257**).

Once a stable plane of anaesthesia has been reached, the isoflurane concentration can be reduced, usually to 1.5–3%. Oxygen flow rates are typically high, usually 1–3 litres/minute even for small patients.

The patient should, wherever possible, be maintained in lateral or ventral recumbency. When placed in dorsal recumbency the weight of the viscera can compromise the ability of the air sacs to function correctly. Sternal lift, necessary to expand the air sacs, also becomes more difficult for the patient in dorsal recumbency. The patient's head should be elevated to prevent reflux of crop and other intestinal contents and potential aspiration. This is easily achieved by placing a pad under the head to lift it above the level of the crop.

It should be noted that if a surgical procedure is being performed that opens an air sac to room air, spontaneous ventilation through the open air sac will result in a lightening of the anaesthetic depth.

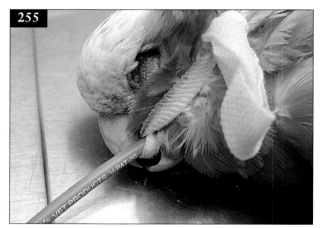

255 Wherever possible, anaesthetized birds should be intubated for anything other than very short procedures.

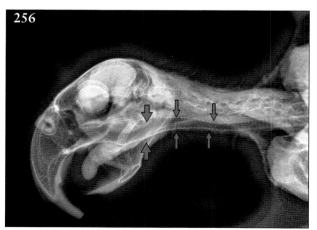

256 This lateral view of the head and neck of a macaw shows the trachea (arrows) narrowing as it progresses caudally. (Photo courtesy L Nemetz)

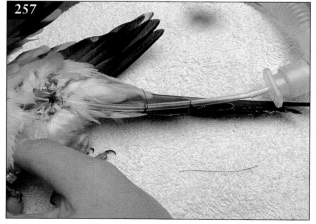

257 When working around the head and neck, anaesthesia can be maintained via an air sac catheter.

Support
Body temperature
Birds have a high surface to body volume ratio and will lose body heat quickly when not active or when their metabolic rate slows. The rate and amount of heat loss is directly proportional to the size of the patient (the smaller the bird, the faster and greater the heat loss). Numerous techniques have been devised to prevent hypothermia in anaesthetized patients and they are listed below. It must be noted, though, that regardless of the thermal support provided, the patient's body temperature will start to decline after approximately 20 minutes of anaesthesia. One of the most important means of minimizing this heat loss is to have a plan and preparations in place before inducing anaesthesia in order to minimize the anaesthetic time. Other techniques that have been advocated include:
- Warmed intravenous fluids throughout the procedure.
- Warmed and humidified anaesthetic gases.
- Radiant heat from overhead heat lamps.
- Heated air units (e.g. the Bair Hugger®).

Heat pads do not appear to be overly effective in providing heat support to avian patients.

Circulatory support
Anaesthesia, especially when associated with surgical blood loss and/or pre-existing dehydration, can lead to decreased vascular perfusion. Warmed fluids given subcutaneously, intravenously or intraosseously will provide both circulatory and thermal support. Balanced electrolyte solutions such as lactated Ringer's solution, given at a rate of 10 ml/kg/hr and even up to 30–60 ml/kg/hr, appear to be safe and effective in most birds (**258**).

Respiratory support
With prolonged anaesthesia (especially in patients that develop hypothermia, hypoglycaemia or hypovolaemia), the patient's respiratory rate may slow and even stop. Cardiac arrest usually follows soon after. Adequate respiratory support, in the form of supplemental ventilation, is therefore essential for most avian anaesthetics. IPPV, performed either manually or by a ventilator, should be instituted early in the anaesthetic process, rather than waiting for problems to develop (**259**). Birds that are breathing by themselves while under anaesthesia will benefit from IPPV at a rate of 4–6 respirations per minute, with sufficient pressure to create normal inspiratory depth. (Excessive pressure should be avoided.) If the

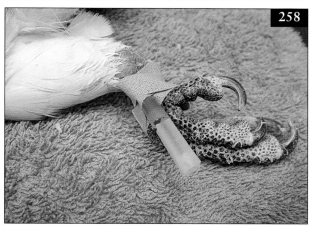

258 Intravenous fluid access into the medial metatarsal vein.

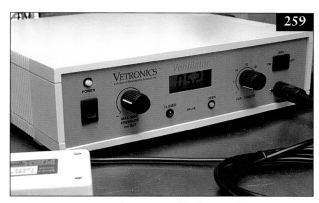

259 Respiratory ventilators suitable for small patients can ease the anaesthetist's work load by ensuring that the patient is well ventilated without resorting to manual IPPV.

bird is apnoeic, IPPV should be given at a rate of 10–12 respirations per minute.

Monitoring
Monitoring of anaesthesia is vital in avian surgery. For this reason all anaesthetic procedures should be monitored by a staff member assigned to this task only. Safe and effective anaesthetic monitoring is a multimodal procedure, relying on visual assessment as well as monitoring equipment.

Manual assessment of the depth of anaesthesia requires monitoring of:
- Respiratory rate and character. The anaesthetized bird should breathe at least once every 2–7 seconds. At a light plane of anaesthesia the respiratory rate and character can be rapid and deep. As the anaesthetic plane deepens, the respiration slows and becomes shallower.

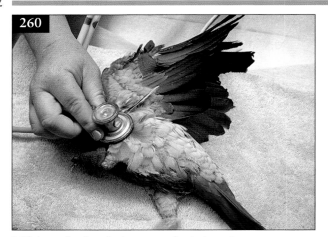

260 Auscultation during anaesthesia is an important monitoring tool.

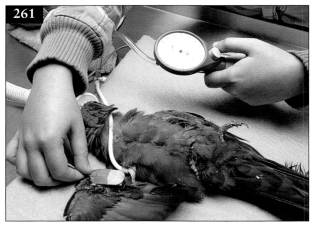

261 Monitoring indirect blood pressure through the use of a Doppler ultrasound. The pressure cuff has been wrapped around the humerus and the crystal over the ventral aspect of the radius and ulna.

- Heart rate and rhythm. Decreases or changes in heart rate and rhythm are often mirrored and preceded by changes in respiration. Auscultation should be performed frequently, if not continuously (260).
- The palpebral reflex (eyelid closure induced by stimulation of the ocular medial canthus or cere) disappears quickly as the anaesthetic plane deepens.
- The pedal (toe withdrawal) reflex and the corneal reflex (third eyelid movement in response to corneal manipulation) slow, but can remain present even at surgical planes of anaesthesia.
- At deep anaesthetic planes, breathing becomes slow and shallow and all reflexes disappear.

Blood pressure monitoring is becoming increasingly recognized as a valuable tool in anaesthetic monitoring. Although direct arterial pressure measurement is ideal, it is usually not practical in private practice. Indirect blood pressure measurement techniques, based on the detection of blood flow beneath an inflated cuff, are therefore recommended (261). Systolic blood pressure determination via ultrasonic Doppler flow detection has been found to correlate well with direct blood pressure. The blood pressure of various avian species under gaseous anaesthesia lies between 90 and 140 mmHg systolic. (See Chapter 3, Clinical techniques.)

Pulse oximetry is generally considered to be unsuitable in birds because of the lack of calibration for avian blood. It may, however, provide some information on trends in blood oxygenation in avian patients.

Electrocardiography has been employed in several avian practices, and has been reported to be a useful tool in monitoring the heart rate and rhythm, especially when auscultation is difficult to perform without interfering with the surgery.

Recovery

Depending on the type and duration of the anaesthetic, recovery to standing and perching usually takes 5–10 minutes. Full recovery usually takes 30–60 minutes.

Following anaesthesia, birds should be:
- Lightly wrapped in a towel to prevent injury from wing flapping or excessive movement during recovery.
- Placed in a darkened, quiet, heated cage and monitored closely until able to perch.
- Extubated only when voluntary head movements are noted.
- Offered food and water as soon as the patient is fully recovered.
- Monitored for bleeding, regurgitation, dyspnoea.

ANAESTHETIC EMERGENCIES

Careful monitoring of respiration, heart rate and blood pressure will usually alert the avian anaesthetist to impending critical emergencies. Cardiac arrest, in many cases, is irreversible and fatal in the anaesthetized bird. However, prompt recognition and treatment of abnormalities can prevent this cardiac arrest in many cases.

Early signs of impending disaster include:
- Changes in respiratory rate and character.
- Changes in cardiac rate and rhythm.
- Hypotension.

Changes in respiratory rate and rhythm

Tachypnoea (increased respiratory rate) can be due to:
- Lightening of the anaesthetic depth.
- Pain perception in the lightly anaesthetized patient.
- Pulmonary haemorrhage.
- Hyperthermia.

Dyspnoea (difficult or laboured breathing) can be due to:
- Airway obstruction (e.g. mucus plugs in the trachea or endotracheal tube).
- Poor circulatory perfusion due to heart disease, anaemia or haemorrhage.
- Restriction of body movement by internal organ enlargement, improper restraint or positioning during the anaesthetic.
- Pulmonary haemorrhage or oedema.
- Pre-existing respiratory disease.

Apnoea (complete cessation of breathing), usually preceded by a slowing of the respiratory rate, can be due to:
- Prolonged or very deep anaesthesia.
- Hypothermia.
- Inadequate ventilation.
- Hypovolaemia.

Management

Upon identifying an unexpected change in the patient's respiratory rate and rhythm, the anaesthetist should firstly check that the anaesthetic machine is functioning correctly and at what concentration the anaesthetic is being delivered. Connections to the patient should be checked to confirm that they are, in fact, connected and patent. The anaesthetist must alert the surgeon to the situation and ask if air sacs have been opened or if there is significant haemorrhage visible.

The patient should be assessed via auscultation (of the heart, lungs and trachea) and monitoring devices such as Doppler blood pressure and ECG.

If tachypnoea is due to a lightening of the anaesthetic plane or perception of pain, the anaesthetic depth should be increased. If air sacs have been opened, the surgeon may have to temporarily 'close' the surgical site until a deeper plane of anaesthesia has been reached.

Tachypnoea or dyspnoea due to pulmonary haemorrhage or oedema does not respond to changes in anaesthetic depth or other treatments. Consideration should be given to terminating the procedure and recovering the patient. If dyspnoea is believed to be due to a mucus plug in the endotracheal tube, the tube should be removed and replaced. If the plug is in the trachea, placing an air sac catheter may be necessary.

Apnoea or a slowing of the respiratory rate should be treated by turning the anaesthetic down or off, leaving the oxygen on and commencing IPPV at 10–12 breaths per minute. Gentle movement of the sternum ventrally and dorsally may assist ventilation if no endotracheal tube or sealed face mask is being used.

If hypovolaemia is suspected, fluid rates should be increased.

Changes in cardiac rate and rhythm

Changes in cardiac rate and rhythm are usually preceded by changes in rate and depth of respiration. Tachycardia usually occurs as a result of decreased anaesthetic depth.

Bradycardia should be treated similarly to apnoea (i.e. the anaesthetic is turned down or off, IPPV is begun or increased and fluid rates are increased). Sternal compression may assist circulation and ventilation. The sternum makes direct cardiac massage difficult, if not impossible. Epinephrine (1:1,000) can be used at a rate of 0.5–1.0 ml/kg IM, IV, intraosseously or intratracheally.

Once cardiac arrest has occurred, resuscitation is unlikely to be successful.

Hypotension

Hypotension occurs after prolonged or deep anaesthesia or severe blood loss. Increasing the fluid rate while lightening the anaesthetic depth and commencing IPPV should be implemented once a significant drop in blood pressure is noted.

FURTHER READING

Acierno MJ, Smith J, Tully TN, Migallon-Guzman D, Mitchell MA (2007) Evaluation of indirect blood pressure measurement techniques (Doppler) and the comparing point of care blood gas analyzer (I-STAT) values. In: *Proceedings of the Annual Conference of the Association of Avian Veterinarians Australian Committee*, pp. 15–16.

Acierno MJ, da Cunha A, Smith J, Tully TN, Migallon-Guzman D, Serra V, Mitchell MA (2008) Agreement between direct and indirect blood pressure measurements obtained from anesthetized Hispaniolan Amazon parrots. *Journal of the American Veterinary Medical Association* **233**(10):1587–1990.

Boedeker NC, Carpenter JW, Mason DE (2005) Comparison of body temperatures of pigeons (*Columba livia*) anesthetized by three different anesthetic delivery systems. *Journal of Avian Medicine and Surgery* **19**(1):1–6.

De Matos REC, Morrisey JK, Steffey M (2006) Postintubation tracheal stenosis in a Blue and Gold macaw (*Ara ararauna*) resolved with tracheal resection and anastomosis. *Journal of Avian Medicine and Surgery* **20**(3):167–174.

Edling TM (2006) Updates in anesthesia and monitoring. In: *Clinical Avian Medicine, Vol 2.* GJ Harrison, TL Lightfoot (eds). Spix Publishing, Palm Beach, pp. 747–760.

Heard DJ (1997) Anesthesia and analgesia. In: *Avian Medicine and Surgery.* RB Altman, SL Clubb, GM Dorrestein, K Quesenberry (eds). WB Saunders, Philadelphia, pp. 807–828.

Klaphake E, Schumacher J, Greenacre C, Jones MP, Zagaya N (2006) Comparative anesthetic and cardiopulmonary effects of pre- versus postoperative butorphanol administration in Hispaniolan Amazon parrots (*Amazona ventralis*) anesthetised with sevoflurane. *Journal of Avian Medicine and Surgery* **20**(1):2–7.

Lichtenberger M (2005) Determination of indirect blood pressure in the companion bird. *Seminars in Avian Exotic Pet Medicine* **14**(2):149–152.

Lumeij JT, Deenik JW (2003) Medetomidine-ketamine and diazepam-ketamine anesthesia in racing pigeons (*Columba livia domestica*) — a comparative study. *Journal of Avian Medicine and Surgery* **17**(4):191–196.

Machin KL (2005) Avian pain: physiology and evaluation. *Compendium on Continuing Education for the Practicing Veterinarian* **27**(2):98–109.

Paul-Murphy J (2006) Pain management. In: *Clinical Avian Medicine, Vol 1.* GJ Harrison, TL Lightfoot (eds). Spix Publishing, Palm Beach, pp. 233–240.

Paul-Murphy J, Hess JC, Fialkowski JP (2004) Pharmacokinetic properties of a single intramuscular dose of buprenorphine in African Grey parrots (*Psittacus erithacus erithacus*). *Journal of Avian Medicine and Surgery* **18**(4):224–228.

CHAPTER 26
SURGERY

INTRODUCTION

An understanding of surgical principles is necessary before operating on a bird. Even though there are many anatomical and physiological differences between birds and mammals, surgical principles and techniques remain similar. As discussed in Chapter 25 (Analgesia and anaesthesia), birds are prone to anaesthetic complications associated with pain perception, hypothermia, hypovolaemia and hypoxia. These anaesthetic complications are closely linked with surgical principles. In order to maximize surgical success, the following principles must be understood and applied:

- Minimize haemorrhage.
- Minimize tissue trauma.
- Minimize anaesthetic time.
- Minimize anaesthetic and metabolic complications.
- Provide postsurgical support and analgesia.

To comply with these principles, the surgeon should:

- Ensure that the patient is in the best possible condition prior to surgery.
- Develop an analgesia and anaesthetic plan that maximizes patient safety and comfort (see Chapter 25, Analgesia and anaesthesia).
- Plan the procedure so as to minimize anaesthetic and surgical time.
- Ensure that surgical preparation and patient support procedures are in place to maximize patient safety.
- Use instruments, techniques and suture materials that minimize tissue damage, blood loss and inflammatory responses.

PRESURGICAL ASSESSMENT AND CONDITIONING
Assessment
Physical examination

This should include a comprehensive physical examination, weighing and respiratory recovery time (a healthy patient should return to normal respirations within 3–5 minutes following capture).

Diagnostics

- Haematology and biochemistries: ideally preoperative PCV, total plasma protein, and blood glucose should be measured for most routine surgical procedures.
- Clotting time (crude estimate): a pin prick of the basilic vein should clot after one minute of direct pressure.

Preconditioning the patient

Clinical pathology parameters that may necessitate postponing surgery include:

- PCV <0.2 l/l or >0.6 l/l.
- Total plasma protein <20 g/l.
- Glucose <11 mmol/l.
- Uric acid >700 μmol/l.
- AST >650 IU/l (in the presence of a normal CK).
- Cholesterol >18 mmol/l.

Medical conditions that may necessitate postponement of surgery include respiratory distress, obesity and concurrent disease problems unrelated to the surgical condition (e.g. cardiovascular disease, infectious conditions).

If any of these abnormalities are detected, appropriate medical therapy should be instituted (e.g. fluid therapy, blood transfusion, tube feeding, diet conversion, weight reduction). Vitamin supplementation may be of benefit in mildly malnourished birds, but should be given several days in advance of the surgery to be of benefit. If a coagulopathy is suspected, vitamin K1 may be of benefit, but it must be administered at least 24 hours prior to the surgery.

If the patient's medical condition is critical and surgery cannot be postponed, the owner must be informed of the increased risks prior to commencing surgery.

MINIMIZING ANAESTHETIC TIME

A surgical plan should be developed. Although exploratory surgery is performed in birds, surgical time can be reduced if a surgical plan has been developed by the surgeon. This should include:

- Revision of the appropriate anatomy if necessary.
- Determination of the extent of the lesion or disease process prior to the procedure. This can be achieved through careful physical examination, radiography and endoscopy.
- Discussion with theatre and nursing staff about the procedures, so that all personnel involved in the procedure know what is happening and what their role is to be.

Prior to anaesthetizing the patient the surgeon should check that all equipment and materials likely to be used in the procedure are accessible and fully functional. The author finds that a verbal rehearsal with all involved personnel at this stage detects and corrects preparation errors that could have resulted in a delay during surgery.

SURGICAL PREPARATION AND PATIENT SUPPORT PROCEDURES
Preparation of the surgical site

Feathers should be plucked; they should not be cut if at all possible. This encourages new feather growth sooner than waiting for cut feathers to moult. Soaking the feathers to be removed with the skin preparation solution prior to plucking will minimize the amount of loose feathers that can potentially contaminate the surgical site. Feather removal can be minimized by using either water-soluble lubricating gel or adhesive tape to hold back surrounding feathers.

Chlorhexidine or povidone–iodine can be used to prepare the surgical site. Alcohol-based disinfectants should not be used, as evaporative heat loss can be significant.

Draping the surgical site

Transparent drapes allow visualization of the patient and have heat retaining characteristics (**262**). If adhesive drapes are not used, towel clamps may be placed around large feathers instead of through the skin.

Patient support

The provision of supportive measures, as discussed in Chapter 25 (Analgesia and anaesthesia), should be factored into the surgical plan. These measures include:

- Thermal support.
- Circulatory support.
- Respiratory support.

MINIMIZING TISSUE TRAUMA AND BLOOD LOSS
Instrumentation

Microsurgical and ophthalmic instruments allow for delicate and atraumatic handling of tissue (**263**). Magnification, using either binocular loupes or an operating microscope, allows for much finer work than can be achieved with the naked eye. Most binocular loupes and operating microscopes come with in-built illumination that complements and enhances the magnification achieved.

Haemostasis can be achieved through the use of radiosurgery (see below) (**264**) and vascular clips

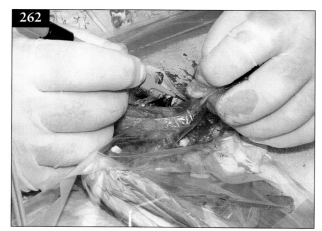

262 Sterile plastic drapes limit contamination of the surgical site.

(e.g. Hemoclips®). Sterilized cotton buds or swabs are useful for swabbing blood and other fluids, as well as gently manipulating tissues. They can also be used for gentle blunt dissection (**265, 266**).

Radiosurgery

High-frequency radiowaves are modified by a waveform adaptor and then focused from the active electrode tip to the indifferent plate (antenna). These radiowaves produce alternating electromagnetic fields that generate heat due to resistance in the tissue. This localized heat volatilizes intracellular fluids, causing cell disruption along the path of the electrode. A frequency of 3.8–4.0 MHz has been found to be optimal for tissue incision, as it focuses the energy into a minimal area.

The waveform can be:
- Fully rectified, fully filtered: pure cutting, suitable for biopsies.
- Partially rectified: coagulation, no cutting.
- Fully rectified, unfiltered: 50% cutting, 50% coagulation.
- Fulguration: destruction of tissue.

Tissue damage (lateral heat) is determined by:
- Electrode size: the greater the size, the more lateral heat and therefore the more tissue damage.
- The time the tissue is exposed to the electrode: the longer the time, the more lateral heat is created.

Radiosurgery therefore offers both haemostasis and minimal tissue damage when used correctly.

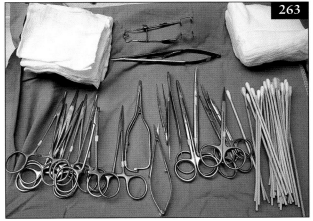

263 Surgical kit for avian surgery. This kit includes ophthalmic instruments and wooden cotton applicators.

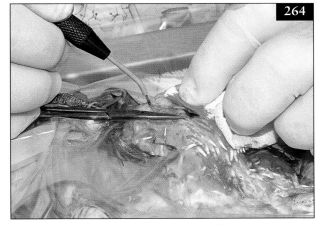

264 The use of radiosurgery minimizes blood loss.

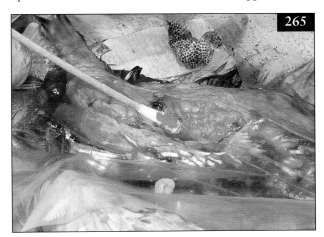

265 Sterilized wooden cotton applicators can be used to apply pressure for haemostasis and to swab a surgical site.

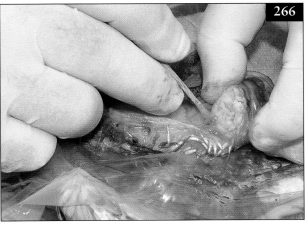

266 Wooden cotton applicators can also be used for blunt dissection.

Carbon dioxide and diode laser surgery

This is slowly replacing radiosurgery. The light emitted from a laser has a wavelength of light that is absorbed by fluid in the cells, thus creating a thermal effect. The degree of penetration can be controlled, allowing for fine, controlled dissection of tissue. Advantages include:

- Haemostasis. The laser cuts and coagulates blood vessels up to about 0.5 mm in diameter. Larger vessels may have to be cauterized or ligated.
- Analgesia. As the laser cuts, it seals nerve endings and axons, reducing the sensation and transmission of pain.
- Decreased postoperative swelling. The laser seals lymphatic vessels, decreasing the extravasation of lymphatic fluid into the surgical site postoperatively.

Endosurgery

Endoscopy has traditionally been used as a diagnostic tool in avian medicine to examine and biopsy internal organs. Recent developments have seen it used as a surgical tool. These developments have included:

- Triangulation of various instruments using multiple ports or entry points.
- The use of radiosurgery and/or laser surgery to ablate lesions and provide haemostasis.
- The combination of these techniques to provide haemostasis during surgical procedures.

Advantages include:

- The combination of both diagnosis and treatment at the same time.
- Reduced surgical stress, pain and time.
- Decreased risk of infection.
- Increased anaesthetic safety.
- Faster postoperative recovery.

Suture choice

Requirements of a suture material include:

- Minimal tissue reaction.
- Absorbable.
- Monofilament sutures are preferable to braided sutures, which sometimes act as a wick to allow transport of serum and bacteria.
- Good knot security.

Choices include:

- Chromic gut produces a marked, granulocytic inflammatory response with a prolonged presence (>120 days).

- Polyglactin 910 (Vicryl) is a synthetic, braided, absorbable suture of glycolic acid and lactic acid. It produces an intense inflammatory reaction but is readily absorbed (60 days).
- Polydioxanone (PDS) is a monofilament, synthetic, absorbable polymer of paradioxanone. It has minimal reactivity, but retains its integrity for long periods.
- Nylon is a monofilament suture. It produces some degree of fibrosis, haematoma, seroma and caseogranuloma formation.
- Newer suture materials (e.g. Vicryl Rapide) are becoming available, but have not been evaluated fully in avian surgery as yet.

COMMON SOFT TISSUE SURGICAL PROCEDURES

INGLUVIOTOMY

Indication

Ingluviotomy is indicated for retrieval of foreign objects, endoscopic access to the proventriculus, placement of feeding tubes and biopsy.

Technique

The bird is positioned in dorsal/lateral recumbency, with the head elevated. The bird should be intubated. The skin is incised over the left lateral wall of the crop, close to the thoracic inlet. The skin edges are gently and bluntly dissected free of the underlying crop. A relatively avascular area is selected for an incision into the crop.

Closure

The crop is closed with two layers of 4–0 or 6–0 PDS in an inverting pattern. The skin is closed separately.

CROP FISTULA REPAIR

Indications

Crop fistulae occur after crop burn due to microwaved or excessively heated and/or inadequately mixed hand-rearing food, or ingestion of caustic substances.

Clinical presentation

Signs include slow crop emptying and erythema or blanching over the crop. In most cases it will be 3–5 days before the delineation between healthy and devitalized tissues becomes apparent, and it may take as long as 7–14 days. At this stage the fistula forms and food leaks out.

Technique

Analgesia, nutritional support and antibiotics/antifungal medications should be provided as appropriate until the demarcation between live and dead tissue is apparent.

Once the fistula has formed, the crop mucosa will have adhered to skin, forming a raised rim of granulation and fibrous tissue around the fistula. The skin is incised around the edges of this rim and the incision is continued for a short distance both cranial and caudal to the fistula. The skin edges are bluntly dissected off the crop. The fistula is excised completely, leaving fresh crop edges (**267–270**). The crop and skin are then closed as for an ingluviotomy (**271**).

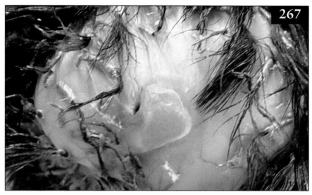

267 Crop burn in a juvenile black cockatoo. Note the blanching of the now avascular skin and the surrounding erythema.

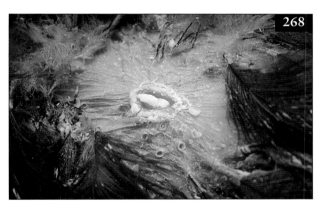

268 Crop burn in a black cockatoo chick, a few days after the photograph in **267**. Note the limit of the burn. Crop necrosis has now become evident.

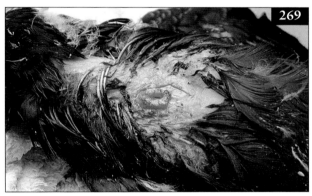

269 Surgical repair of a crop burn in a black cockatoo chick. The skin is dissected away from the crop and the fistula is excised.

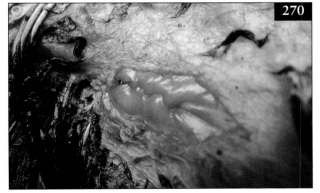

270 After excising the necrotic and granulating edges, the crop is repaired with a double-layer, continuous inverting suture pattern using a monofilament absorbable suture material (polydioxanone).

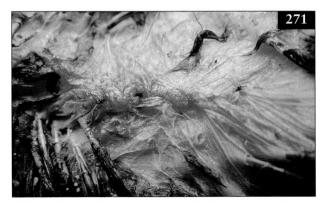

271 Finally, the skin is closed in a single layer with the same suture material.

LEFT LATERAL COELIOTOMY
Indications
This procedure provides access to the gonads, left kidney, oviduct, proventriculus and ventriculus.

Technique
The bird is placed in right lateral recumbency, with the cranial end of the body elevated 30–40° to prevent fluid entering the lungs. The wings are extended dorsally and secured into place. The left leg is abducted and drawn slightly forwards. The inguinal skin web is incised between the abdominal wall and the left leg and the leg is abducted further. This incision is continued from the sixth rib to the level of the left pubic bone (**272**).

The superficial medial femoral artery and vein are cauterized where they transverse (in a dorsoventral direction) the lateral abdominal wall medial to the coxofemoral joint. The muscles (external, internal abdominal oblique and transverse abdominal muscles) are tented up and a stab incision is made with pointed scissors while protecting the viscera. This incision is extended from the pubic bone to the eighth rib. This will require transecting the last two ribs. This is done by passing a bipolar forceps around the ribs, cauterizing the intercostal blood vessels and then cutting the ribs with scissors, in turn.

A small retractor is placed to allow visualization of the internal organs (**273**).

Closure
The muscle and skin are closed in separate layers with absorbable sutures in a continuous or interrupted pattern. No attempt is made to rejoin the transected ribs.

VENTRAL MIDLINE COELIOTOMY
Indications
This procedure is used as an approach to the cloaca for cloacopexy, an approach to the oviduct or testes, or for biopsy of the liver and pancreas.

Technique
The bird is placed in dorsal recumbency and the legs are abducted caudally. The skin is tented and incised in the ventral midline (**274**).

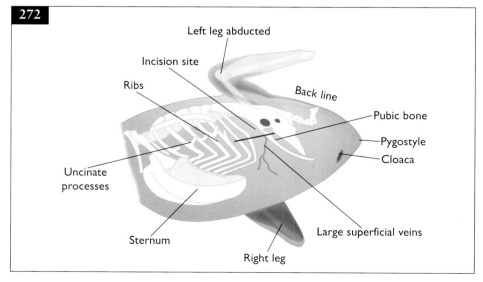

272

Left leg abducted

Incision site

Ribs

Back line

Pubic bone

Pygostyle

Cloaca

Uncinate processes

Large superficial veins

Sternum

Right leg

272 Landmarks for a left flank coeliotomy.

273 View inside the coelum: left flank coeliotomy.

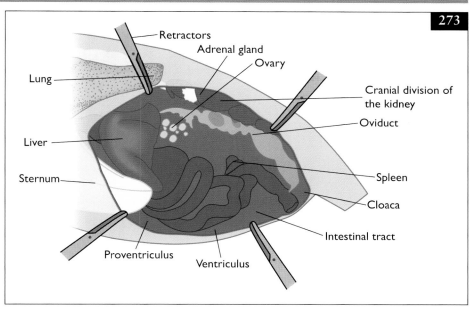

274 Ventral midline coeliotomy: sites for incision.

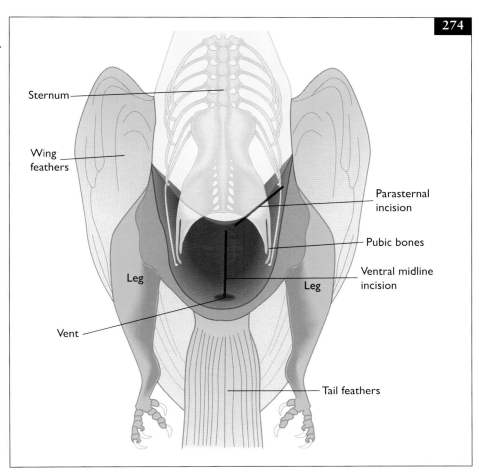

The linear alba is tented and incised in a craniodorsal direction, avoiding iatrogenic damage to the underlying viscera (**275**). If this gives insufficient exposure, the incision can be extended by creating flaps by incising laterally along the sternum cranially or the pubis caudally.

Closure

The muscle and skin are closed in separate layers with absorbable sutures in a continuous or interrupted pattern.

PANCREATIC BIOPSY
Indications

This is used for diagnosis of pancreatic disease.

Technique

With the bird in dorsal recumbency, a midline coeliotomy is performed as described above. The duodenal loop, found on the right side of the abdominal cavity, is gently exteriorized. Care must be taken not to pull too hard on the duodenal loop as this may damage the blood supply to both the duodenum and the splenic lobe of the pancreas.

The pancreas is examined for gross focal lesions. If seen, they are carefully biopsied. If no focal lesions are visible, the distal edge of the ventral lobe of the pancreas, at the apex of the duodenal loop, is carefully reflected to reveal underlying vasculature. Once these

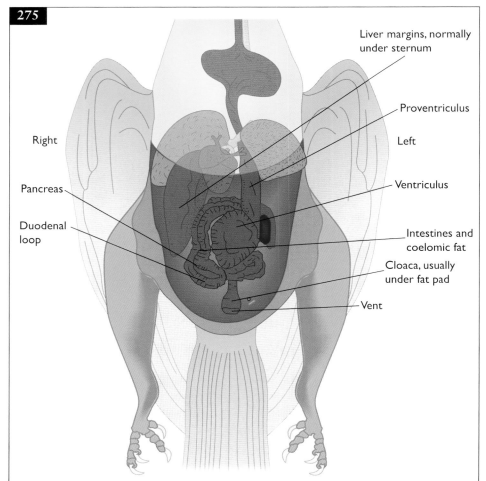

275 View inside the abdomen through the ventral midline incision.

Liver margins, normally under sternum

Proventriculus

Right

Left

Pancreas

Ventriculus

Duodenal loop

Intestines and coelomic fat

Cloaca, usually under fat pad

Vent

blood vessels are located and avoided, the end of the ventral lobe is removed with iris scissors and fixed in formalin. Minimal bleeding usually results.

The duodenum is then replaced into the abdomen, and the skin and muscle are closed as described above.

PROVENTRICULOTOMY

Indications
This is used for retrieval of foreign bodies from the proventriculus or ventriculus.

Approach
A left flank coeliotomy is performed as described above. The proventricular suspensory ligaments are broken down. Two stay sutures are placed in the tendinous part of the ventriculus and it is brought up into the surgical field and attached to the skin. If possible, the rest of the abdomen is packed off with saline-soaked gauze. The triangular lobe of liver overlying the proventricular isthmus is identified and gently reflected with a sterile cotton swab.

A stab incision is made into the isthmus and extended with iris scissors. Suction is used to empty fluid from the proventriculus and ventriculus. If necessary, an endoscope can be placed in the incision to ensure all foreign objects have been removed.

Closure
The proventricular incision is closed with 6–0 or 8–0 synthetic monofilament absorbable suture in two layers: the first should be appositional, the second inverting. The liver is tacked down over the incision. The abdomen is closed routinely.

ABDOMINAL HERNIA

Aetiology
Abdominal hernia is caused by a combination of increased intra-abdominal pressure (fat, ascites, organomegaly) and weakened muscles due to hormonal influences, obesity, lack of exercise and chronic malnutrition. It is commonly associated with females during the breeding season, as enlargement of the ovary and oviduct increases intra-abdominal pressure. Although most hernias occur on the ventral midline, they can also be seen on the lateral body wall and dorsal to the vent.

Precautions
If possible, the bird should be converted to a formulated diet before surgery in order to achieve significant weight loss. Reproductive activity can be reduced by hormonal and behavioural manipulation before surgery. These two treatments may be sufficient to reduce the size of the hernia and avoid surgery.

The veterinarian should be aware that viscera may underlie and be attached to the skin. Replacing viscera back into the abdomen may compromise the air sacs and lead to dyspnoea.

Technique
The bird is positioned according to the location of the hernia. The skin is incised over the hernia, taking care not to cause iatrogenic trauma to underlying viscera (which may have adhered to the skin). The skin over the hernia is gently and bluntly dissected until the borders of the body wall around the hernia are identified. Any adhesions to these borders are dissected away to free them from the hernia contents.

If possible, a salpingohysterectomy is performed and as much intra-abdominal fat as possible is removed before closing.

Closure
The hernia is closed with a monofilament absorbable suture in a simple interrupted pattern. The veterinarian should watch closely at this stage for any changes in the bird's respiratory pattern, indicating excessive pressure on the abdominal and thoracic air sacs.

Very large hernias, or those that cannot be closed without respiratory compromise, may require the use of nonabsorbable mesh inside the body wall, attached to the muscles, last ribs, sternum and pubis.

The skin is closed routinely.

CLOACOPEXY

Indication
This is indicated for chronic cloacal prolapse, associated with hypersexuality in cockatoos, or excessive straining due to:
- Intestinal parasites.
- Retained egg.
- Adenomatous polyp.
- Bacterial enteritis.
- Neoplasia.
- Abdominal mass.
- Cloacal hyperplasia.

Technique
A ventral midline incision is made as described above. The cloaca is replaced. An assistant should place a gloved finger (large birds) or cotton bud (small birds) into the cloaca to define its extent and to lift it to the abdominal wall. Intra-abdominal fat ventral to the cloaca is removed.

Using monofilament nonabsorbable material sutures are placed through the full thickness of the cloacal wall and then around the last rib (at the junction of the sternal and vertebral portions) on each side, or through the cartilaginous border of the sternum. All sutures are pre-placed and tied once all are in position, anchoring the cloaca in a reduced position with the cloacal wall apposed to ribs, albeit more cranial than normal.

Following the placement of these sutures, the ventral cloacal serosa is incised to the level of the submucosa and tacking sutures are placed through the abdominal wall to suture the submucosa to the abdominal muscle. Some of these sutures are incorporated into the abdominal wall closure.

Prognosis

This technique attaches the ventral aspect of the cloaca to the ribs and body wall. However, the dorsal cloaca is not dealt with. Therefore, if the bird continues to strain, this tissue can still prolapse. As time goes on, with continued straining, the sutures may break or cut through the attached tissues and prolapse of all the cloacal tissue can occur.

CLOACOPLASTY/VENTOPLASTY
Indications

This procedure provides temporary or permanent narrowing of the vent opening as treatment for cloacal prolapse (**276**) or atony. A purse-string suture is contraindicated in birds, as the vent closes in a dorsoventral direction, not circular.

Technique

If a permanent narrowing is required, the muco-cutaneous border on the lateral third of the dorsal and ventral vent lips is trimmed on both sides. If a temporary closure is required, this step is not indicated. The lateral third of the vent is closed on both sides with one to two vertical mattress sutures (**277**).

CLOACOTOMY
Indications

Cloacotomy is used for debriding cloacal papillomas or removing cloacoliths.

Technique

The bird is placed in dorsal recumbency. A moistened cotton bud is inserted into the cloaca to outline the structure. An incision is made through the skin, cloacal sphincter and cloacal mucosa from the vent to

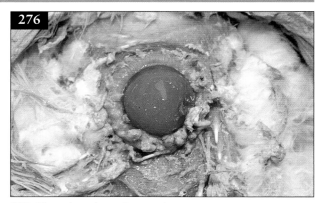

276 Cloacal prolapse in a cockatoo.

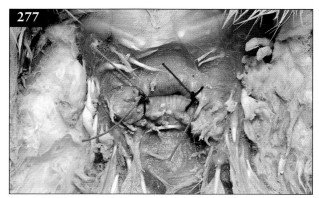

277 Temporary ventoplasty achieved through placing two simple interrupted sutures.

the cranial end of the cotton bud. This opens the ventral wall of the cloaca, exposing the coprodeum, urodeum and proctodeum.

Closure

The mucosa is closed with a continuous suture pattern, the sphincter is closed with a single mattress suture and the skin is closed routinely.

SALPINGOHYSTERECTOMY
Indications

This is indicated for chronic egg laying and any oviductal disease that cannot be managed medically.

Presurgical evaluation and conditioning

Yolk peritonitis and underlying liver, lung and kidney disease all carry a higher risk of surgical complications. An enlarged oviduct (due to hormonal influences) fills the left coelom and makes surgery difficult. Therefore, if time permits, the patient's nutritional status should be improved and the reproductive cycle 'turned off' through behavioural, social and environmental modification and hormonal therapy.

Technique
The left lateral approach gives best exposure, but the ventral midline approach can be used. The ovary is left alone; the blood supply is tightly adherent to major blood vessels, making removal without an operating microscope extremely dangerous.

The infundibulum is identified and gently retracted out through the incision. A large blood vessel running between the infundibulum and ovary must be identified and ligated the ventral suspensory ligament is broken down. The dorsal suspensory ligament blood vessels are cauterized or ligated as needed (the cranial, middle and caudal oviductal arteries). This is done as the ligament is broken down by sharp dissection.

The oviduct is retracted through the incision and the junction with the cloaca is identifed (if necessary, a cotton bud or gloved finger is inserted into the cloaca to delineate the structure). Two haemoclips or sutures are placed across the oviduct near this junction, and the oviduct is removed. Closure is routine.

Follow-up
Continued ovulation with subsequent yolk-related peritonitis has been reported in several birds following routine salpingohysterectomy.

ORCHIDECTOMY
Indications
This procedure may be carried out to treat orchitis or testicular neoplasia, or for behavioural modification.

Technique
The approach is via either a left lateral or bilateral coeliotomy or a ventral midline coeliotomy with cranial flaps. The testis is gently retracted ventrally and a haemoclip is placed across the dorsal blood supply (mesorchium). A radiosurgery unit is used to free the testis from the haemoclip. The incision is closed routinely.

Follow-up
If all testicular tissue is not removed, regrowth is common. Some male characteristics are retained, indicating that testosterone may be produced in other tissues.

ENUCLEATION
Indications
Enucleation is indicated for severe, irreversible panophthalmitis, perforating corneal ulcer or neoplasia.

Precautions
This procedure is more difficult in birds than in mammals because of the relatively larger globe compared with the size of the orbit. The optic nerve is short; excessive traction can result in contralateral blindness. The area is very vascular and the surgeon should anticipate haemorrhage.

Technique
The lids are sutured together in a simple continuous pattern. A circumferential incision is made through the skin (not the conjunctiva) 1–2 mm from the lid margins. Note that the ligamentous attachments at the medial canthus are firm. Haemorrhage can be expected in this area and at the lateral canthus.

Dissection is carried out between the palpebral conjunctiva and the bony orbit, as it is not feasible to identify and transect each individual muscle. The sutured eyelids are manipulated to provide traction on the globe.

In some birds with a large globe, it may be necessary to collapse the globe prior to enucleation. In some species with thin orbital bone, it is feasible to extend the skin incision from the lateral canthus to the auditory meatus and transect the orbital rim at the lateral canthus. This opens the orbit and allows easier retraction of the globe.

Where feasible, a vascular clip is applied blindly to the optic stalk (incorporating the nerve and blood vessels). Care must be taken to apply minimal traction to the globe at this point to avoid damage to the contralateral optic nerve.

After the stalk is clipped, it is transected and the eye removed. If it is not feasible to place a vascular clip, the globe is retracted with the use of sharp dissection. Haemorrhage can be expected at this stage, and can usually be controlled by placing a vascular clip directly on to the now visible optic stalk. If this is not feasible, packing the orbit with absorbable gelatine sponges (Gelfoam®) is usually effective.

Closure
The eyelids are sutured in a simple interrupted pattern.

ORTHOPAEDICS
GENERAL CONSIDERATIONS
Bones
Avian bones are lightweight, but possess great aerodynamic strength. They have thin brittle cortices, which will not provide sufficient holding power for bone screws. Fractures are frequently open and comminuted due to minimal soft tissue coverage.

The blood supply to bones arises from periosteal, medullary, metaphyseal and epiphyseal blood vessels. The periosteal blood supply is very important in callus formation, and its importance may exceed that of the medullary blood supply.

Joints
If joints are immobilized for long periods of time, contracture of ligaments and tendons can result in a permanently reduced range of movement. Fracture callus may impinge on joint range of motion, as may adhesions of ligaments and tendons.

Muscles
Powerful flight muscles can cause rotational deformity of long bones during the early healing phase.

BONE HEALING
The rate of healing is dependent on:
- Displacement of bone fragments. Segmental fractures will heal well so long as periosteal blood supply is intact. If devitalized, the fragment can be incorporated into the fracture site as a cortical bone graft. Healing is slower, as cancellous bone first bridges the gap, then the segment is demineralized and becomes cancellous itself. Healing may take 9–18 weeks.
- Damage to blood supply.
- Presence of infection. Sequestra can add to the stability of a fracture and should not be removed until a bony callus has formed.
- Movement at the fracture site creates a large haematoma and a large cartilaginous bridge.

Healing of bones is a combination of:
- Primary healing. Bone to bone healing through the Haversian system, with minimal callus formation. This is only achieved with rigid fixation with perfect bone apposition.
- Endosteal callus formation. This occurs rapidly where bones are well aligned. It is the most important part of bone healing.
- Periosteal callus formation. This occurs when fractures are not aligned and there is movement at the fracture site.

Stable, well aligned fractures heal faster in birds than in mammals. Clinical stability of a fracture (2–3 weeks) may precede radiographic evidence that bone is healed (3–6 weeks).

Healing times are approximately as follows:
- External coaptation:
  - 1 week: palpable callus, movement still palpable.
  - 2 weeks: movement considerably reduced.
  - 3 weeks: no movement, endosteal callus present.
  - 5–8 weeks: healed, remodelling beginning.
- Internal fixation:
  - 2 weeks: union present.
  - 3 weeks: remodelling beginning.

PRINCIPLES OF ORTHOPAEDIC SURGERY
Orthopaedic surgery should aim for:
- Minimizing of soft tissue damage.
- Accurate alignment.
- Rigid stabilization.
- Maintenance of length and rotational and angular orientation.
- Immobilization, but encouragement of early return to normal function to prevent 'fracture disease' (permanent contracture of muscles, tendons, ligaments and joints).

TYPES OF FRACTURE REPAIR
External coaptation
Benefits of external coaptation (**278–283**) include:
- Decreased chance of infection.
- Less damage to regional vascularity.

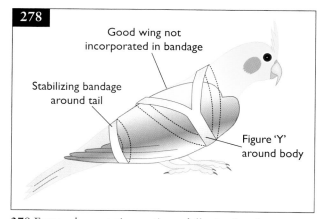

278 External coaptation options: full wing bandage.

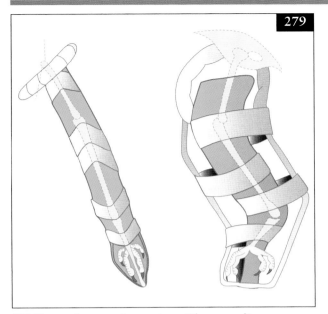

279 External coaptation options: Thomas splint.

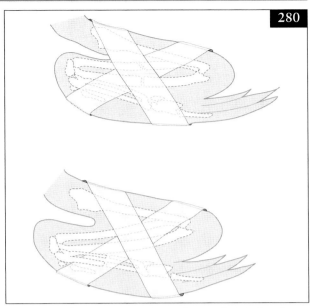

280 External coaptation options: figure-of-eight bandage for metacarpal/radius–ulna fractures.

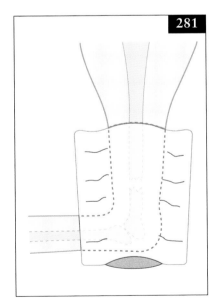

281 External coaptation options: tape splint.

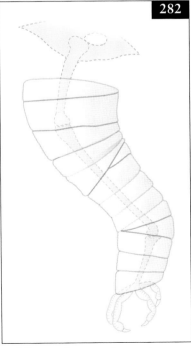

282 External coaptation options: Robert Jones bandage.

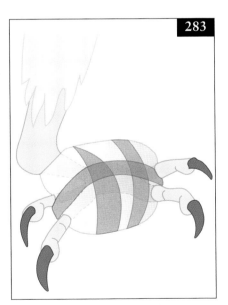

283 External coaptation options: bandaging feet.

- Inexpensive and rapid.
- Minimal surgical and anaesthetic risk in high-risk (e.g. trauma) patients.
- Can be used in patients too small to feasibly operate on.

Disadvantages include:
- 'Fracture disease' is common (restricted joint motion and soft tissue contraction).
- Healed bone may be malaligned.
- Joint ankylosis.
- Shortened bone length.
- Tendon contraction.
- Bone rotation.
- Healing is slower, usually by periosteal callus.

Internal fixation
Intramedullary pins
Stainless steel pins or polymer rods can be used. (Polymer rods are introduced in a retrograde fashion and held in position with bone cement). Intramedullary pins maintain alignment and length of the bone, but may lack rotational stability (**284**). This can be overcome by:
- Combining the pinning with semi- and full-cerclage wire, but great care must be taken not to disrupt the periosteal blood supply.
- Stack pinning with several small pins (most applicable to fractures of the humerus and femur).
- Combining with an external skeletal fixator to create a 'tie-in' fixation (see below).

Pin diameter should equal half to two-thirds of the medullary canal. Excessively large pins can interfere with endosteal blood supply, which may cause avascular necrosis or iatrogenic fractures.
Intramedullary pins can be placed either:
- Retrograde. From the fracture site and advancing the pin out either the proximal or distal end of the bone. Usually used for femoral, humeral and ulnar fractures.
- Normograde. Beginning at a natural end of the bone and advancing the pin toward the fracture site. This is usually used for tibiotarsal, proximal humeral or distal ulnar fractures.

Stainless steel pins should be removed when the bone has healed.

Plates
Advantages of plates include:
- Early return to function.
- Minimal fracture disease.
- Primary bone healing.
- Rigid immobilization.
- Rotational stability.

Disadvantages include:
- The cortices provide poor screw-holding power.
- Plates are often too large and heavy for avian bones.
- Longer surgical time, therefore increased tissue compromise and prolonged anaesthesia.
- Technical difficulties for placement and removal.
- No properly sized implants are available for most birds.
- Expensive.

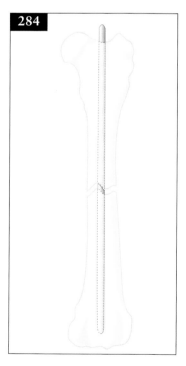

284 Intramedullary pin placed in the femur.

Technique

Bone cement is placed to fill the medullary canal. The intramedullary bone cement is extended at least 1 cm past the end of the plate. Lightweight veterinary cuttable plates are used. There must be a minimum of four screw–bone cortex contacts on each side of the fracture.

External skeletal fixation

External skeletal fixation (ESF) (285) is lightweight, strong, inexpensive and adaptable to many fractures. In closed fractures, it can reduce the risk of osteomyelitis. It provides both rotational and lengthening stability.

The equipment includes:

- Transfixation pins. Positive-profile threaded pins inserted through the predrilled holes have been found to maintain solid bone-to-pin interfaces for prolonged periods (up to three months) in some birds.
- Connecting bar.
- Means of connecting pins to bar. Clamps are available, but dental acrylic and similar hardware materials have been used successfully.

Types commonly used in birds are the type I device, with half pins connected on one side of the limb only (286), and the type II device, with full pins running through the bone and connected on both sides of the limb.

The most distal and proximal pins are inserted first in a medial to lateral direction. Three pins are placed each side of the fracture at a 30–40° angle to the bone, and the connecting bar is then applied.

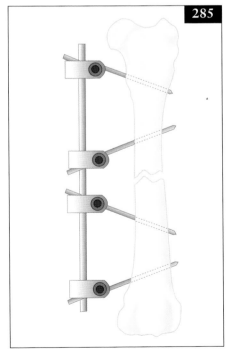

285 Type I external skeletal fixation.

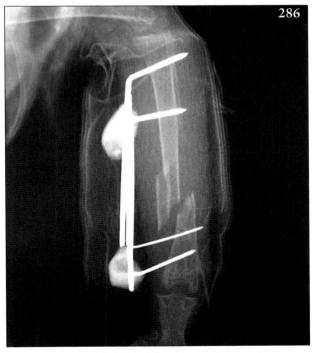

286 Type I external skeletal fixation used to repair a tibiotarsal fracture in a cockatoo.

Tie-in fixator

A tie-in fixator (TIF) is a combination of an intramedullary pin linked to external fixator pins. It can be used to repair diaphyseal and periarticular fractures of all avian long bones except the tarsometatarsus (**287**). The intramedullary pin selected should fill 50–65% of the medullary cavity. It is inserted in a normograde technique past the reduced fracture (**288–290**). Positive-profile ESF pins are inserted perpendicular to the bone at locations where they will not be interfered with by the intramedullary pin (**291**). The protruding end of the intramedullary pin, where it

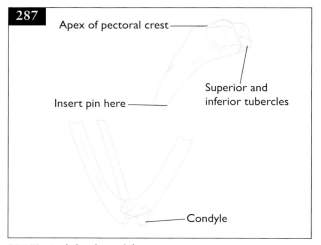

287 Typical diaphyseal fracture.

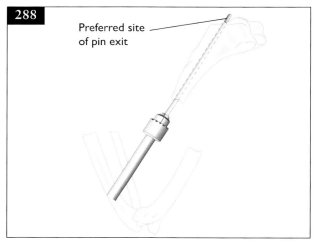

288 Step one. Retrograde placement of an intramedullary pin into the proximal fragment.

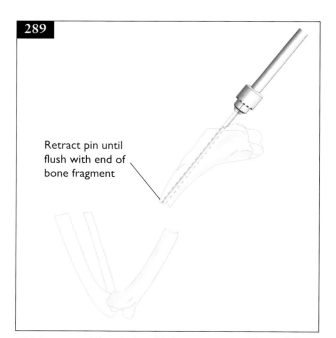

289 Step two. The pin is withdrawn proximally until the pin is flush with the fracture line.

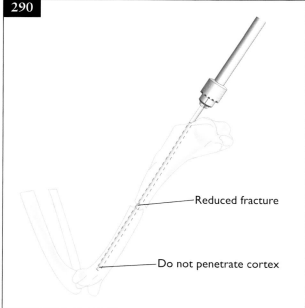

290 Step three. The fracture is reduced and the pin advanced into the distal fragment.

emerges from the skin, is bent at 90° and rotated so that it is in the same plane as the ESF pins (**292**).

All pins are joined by a connecting bar (**293**). The connecting bar can be formed from the intramedullary pin, if long enough, bent again at 90° to run down the length of the limb (**294**).

Primary bone healing often results (i.e. no periosteal callus).

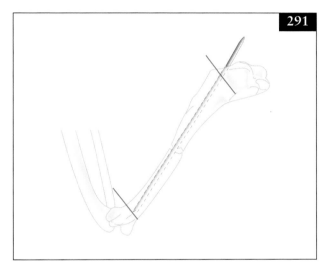

291 Step four. Positive profile threaded ESF pins or K-wires are placed at both ends of the bone, perpendicular to the bone.

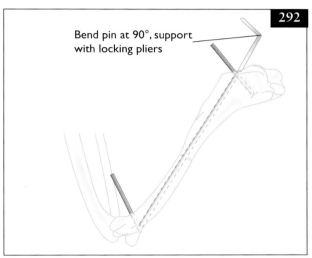

292 Step five. The proximal end of the pin, protruding from the bone, is bent at 90° in the same plane as the ESF pins.

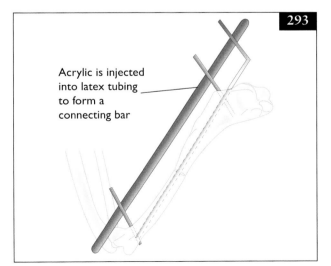

293 Step six. A connecting bar (pin or latex tube filled acrylic) is used to join the ESF pins and the end of an intramedullary pin that has been bent over.

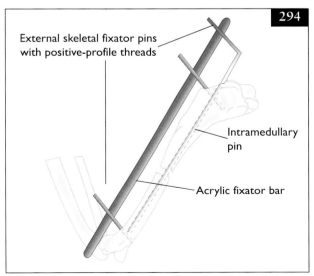

294 The completed tie-in fixator.

SELECTION OF MEANS OF FIXATION

Distortion produced by the powerful flight and leg muscles makes external coaptation a poor choice for humeral and femoral fractures. Antebrachial fractures involving both radius and ulna will do better if surgically repaired. External coaptation often results in a synostosis joining the two bones, making pronation of the antebrachium difficult and thereby restricting flight.

Coracoid, scapula, clavicle

Conservative treatment may be best. Surgical reduction of the coracoid may be indicated if it is distracted.

Proximal humerus

ESF is difficult due to the lack of room in the proximal fragment. A tension band method using semicerclage wire has worked.

Midshaft humerus

TIF is ideal.

Distal humerus

Cross-pinning is recommended, perhaps combined with ESF.

Antebrachium

External coaptation may be used if the ulna or radius is still intact. Otherwise intramedullary pin, ESF or TIF are required.

Metacarpus

External coaptation, ESF type I or TIF are indicated.

Proximal femur

Tension band using semicerclage wire is recommended.

Midshaft femur

TIF is indicated.

Distal femur

Cross-pinning is used combined with ESF.

Tibiotarsal

Fixation may be achieved with type II ESF, TIF or external coaptation.

Tarsometatarsus

External coaptation (**295**) or type II ESF are used.

POSTOPERATIVE MANAGEMENT AND COMPLICATIONS

Antibiotic coverage is provided using:
• Cephalosporins or enrofloxacin for five days postoperatively for uncomplicated fracture repairs.
• Clindamycin or amoxicillin–clavulanic acid can be used for open, comminuted and infected fractures.
• Antibiotic-impregnated methylmethacrylate beads can be used in some fractures if infection is likely.

Analgesia should be provided (see Chapter 25, Analgesia and anaesthesia). Physical therapy (passive range of movement) may have to be done under anaesthesia, starting at at two days (for humeral fractures) or ten days (for other fractures). Five-minute sessions should be given twice weekly for two weeks.

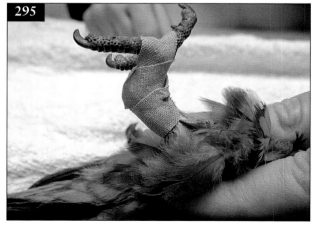

295 External coaptation of a tarsometatarsal fracture.

Patagial contraction is common and can restrict the ability of the bird to extend its wing. This can be overcome by use of rigid fixation (allowing early return to function), passive physical therapy, ultrasound massage and physical massage.

The fracture should be radiographed at seven days and again at three weeks. If re-alignment is necessary, it must be done before ten days. Dynamic destabilization (partial dismantling of fixation) can be started at 21 days if healing is well underway. Sequestra can be seen radiographically at 21 days and can be removed surgically when their extent is clear.

Healing should be complete by six weeks and all fixation removed.

APPROACHES TO THE BONES OF THE WING
Coracoid and clavicle
A ventral approach is used. A skin incision is made along the caudal edge of the furcula starting laterally and continuing medially along the lateral edge of the keel for the first one-fifth or one-sixth of the length of the keel. An incision is made through the superficial pectoral muscle along the caudal edge of the furcula. Cranial and caudal pectoral vessels and nerves are seen between the superficial and deep pectoral muscles. The deep pectoral muscle is incised and reflected along the clavicle and keel. Haemorrhage from the clavicular artery, which supplies part of the pectoral muscles (encountered at caudal midpoint of furcula), must be controlled.

Muscles of the coracoid are now visible: the supracorocoideus and corobrachialis caudalis. These can be separated to get better exposure of the coracoid. Multiple small intramedullary pins are introduced at the fracture site and exteriorized through the point of the shoulder, then the pins are normograded back through the distal fragment taking care not to perforate the pericardium and heart.

The supracorocoideus and corobrachialis caudalis are sutured if separated. The pectorals are reattached to the periosteum in separate layers. The skin is closed.

Proximal humerus
A dorsal approach is used in fractures of the proximal third. The feathers are plucked over the proximal, medial and ventral humerus. In raptors the scapular coverts insert into a fascia, which continues from the cutaneous costohumeralis muscle. This should be maintained if possible, as they may be involved in critical aspects of flight. The skin is incised along the shaft of the humerus.

WARNING:
- The axillary nerve is deep to the propatagialis complex in the proximal third of the humerus.
- A branch of subscapular artery is medial and cranial to nerve.
- The radial nerve crosses the humerus two-thirds of the way down the shaft, near the site of insertion of the deltoideus major muscle.

The propatagialis muscle can be transected in the distal third or one can bluntly dissect through it, avoiding the muscle branch of the axillary nerve. The deltoideus may be retracted proximally, but it needs to be reattached to bone when the procedure is completed.

There are two techniques for repair: stack pinning in birds <300 g or tension band in birds >300 g. In the latter technique, two K-wires are inserted retrograde dorsally and ventrally to the pectoral crest, then the fracture is reduced and the pins are advanced into the distal fragment. Two holes are drilled, one in the humerus 1 cm distal to the fracture, the other through the pectoral crest proximal to the K-wires. Cerclage wire is passed through the holes, made into a figure-of-eight and tightened.

If the deltoideus was elevated, a hole is drilled through the bone to allow a suture to reattach the muscle to the bone. The propatagialis muscle is sutured if it was transected.

Distal humerus
There are two approaches, both of which can be used to reduce and fix internally fractures of the humerus in the midshaft to distal third. The dorsal approach is more commonly used.

Dorsal approach

The bird is placed in sternal recumbency with the affected wing extended. The feathers are plucked from the pectoral crest to the proximal radius/ulna.

The radial nerve should be palpated before making the skin incision. The skin is incised from the proximal third of the humerus to the olecrannon fossa and ventral epicondyle, or even more caudally (296a–d). The deltoideus and triceps insertions on the caudal aspect of the humerus are identified, with the radial nerve emerging between them. The biceps brachii and the tendon of the tensor propatagialis pars

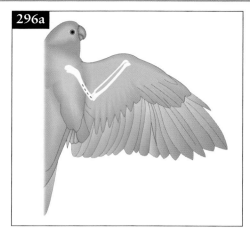

296a Dorsal approach to the distal humerus.

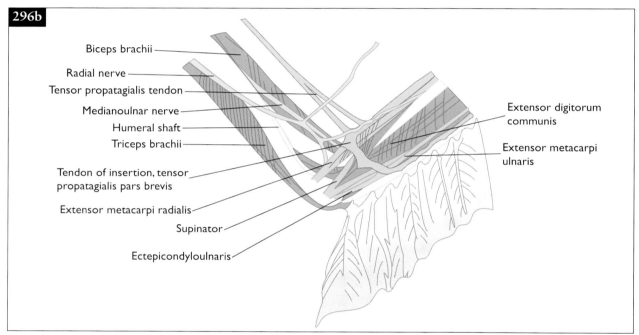

296b Anatomy of the distal humerus (dorsal view).

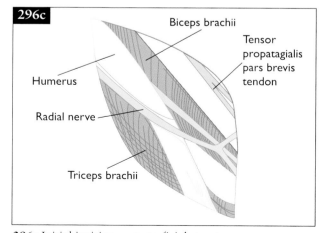

296c Initial incision — superficial structures.

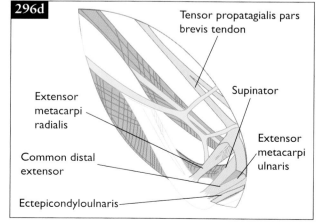

296d Extending the incision distally to reveal structures overlying the dorsal elbow.

brevis are identified on the cranial side of humerus. Distally, three tendons are identified originating from the antebrachium: cranially, the extensor metacarpi radialis; caudally, the extensor metacarpi ulnaris; and between them, the supinator and common digital extensor.

In distal fractures, two K-wires can be used to cross-pin through the dorsal and ventral epicondyles. These can then be tied into an ESF.

Ventral approach

This is used for distracted fractures of the distal two-thirds of the humerus (**297a–c**).

The bird is placed in dorsal recumbency with the affected wing extended. The feathers are plucked from the ventral humerus and dorsally and cranially over the pectoral crest.

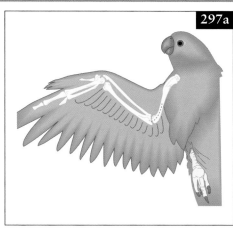

297a Ventral approach to the distal humerus.

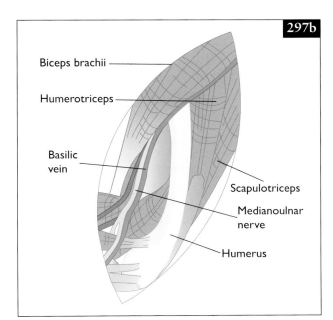

297b Initial incision — superficial structures.

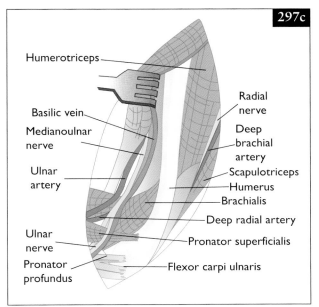

297c Reflection of the biceps brachii gains better exposure of the humeral shaft. If necessary, the humerotriceps can be dissected off the caudal humeraus for more exposure.

The biceps brachii muscle is palpated cranial to shaft of humerus. The ulnar and radial vessels and medianoulnar nerve run deep to or on the caudal edge of this muscle, as does the superficial basilic vein. To avoid these structures, the skin incision is made either over the belly of the biceps muscle or over the humeral shaft caudal to the vessels and nerves. The excision is continued distally to the elbow. The biceps is elevated and retracted with the vessels and nerve. The triceps can be elevated caudally for better exposure.

Closure is by simply suturing skin and superficial fascia as a single layer.

Proximal radius and ulna

A dorsal approach is used for proximal radius and ulna fractures and elbow dislocation (**298a–d**).

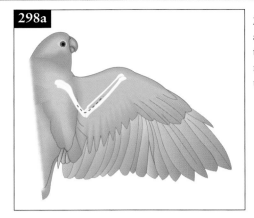

298a Dorsal approach to the proximal radius and ulna.

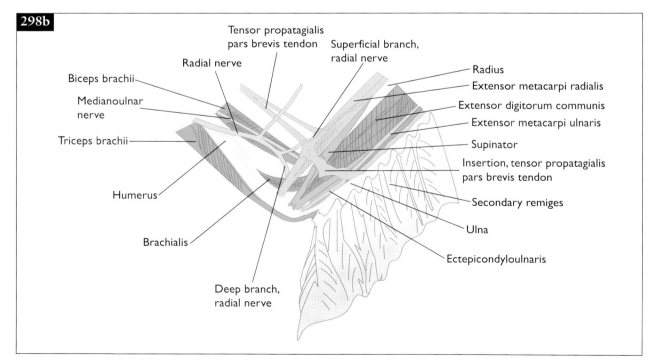

298b Anatomy of the elbow and proximal radius and ulna (dorsal view).

The bird is placed in ventral recumbency and the affected wing is extended. The feathers are plucked from mid humerus to the distal antebrachium.

A curvilinear skin incision is made from the distal humerus, between the radius and ulna, and extending as far as needed for exposure. Care should be taken to avoid branches of the radial nerve and the insertion of the tensor propatagialis pars brevis tendon. The supinator muscle is retracted cranially and the extensor digitorum muscle is retracted caudally. For better exposure of the radial head, the tendon of insertion of the tensor propatagialis pars brevis must be transected. If there is still not enough exposure, the supinator muscle is transected at its distal third, avoiding the deep radial nerve. The ulna can be exposed by incising between the retinaculum of the extensor metacarpi ulnaris and the muscle itself. The branch of the deep radial nerve and the interosseous dorsalis artery and vein that emerge here and run along caudal aspect of ulna should be avoided.

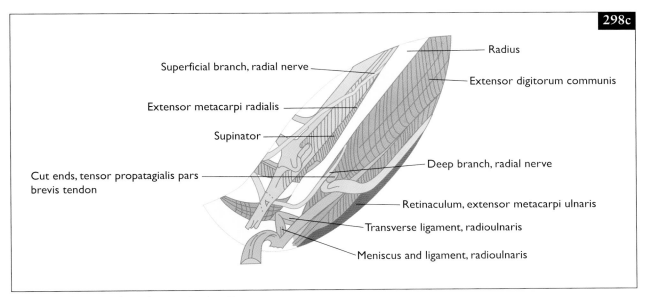

298c Dorsal approach to the proximal radius.

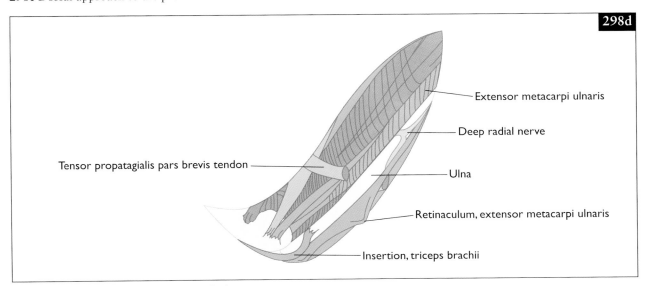

298d Dorsal approach to the proximal ulna.

Distal radius and ulna

A dorsal approach is used for open reduction of fractures of the radius and ulna and luxations of these bones (**299a–c**).

The bird is placed in ventral recumbency and the affected wing is extended. The feathers are plucked from the bone, but the secondaries are left intact.

The skin is incised between the radius and the ulna. If necessary, the extensor metacarpi radialis, on the cranial surface of the radius, and the extensor metacarpi ulnaris, on the dorsal surface of the ulna, can be retracted. If it is necessary to repair the ulna, the calamus of the secondary feathers between bone and skin can be cut, avoiding the follicle.

For ulnar fractures, intramedullary pins are introduced through the fracture site, retrograded out of the olecranon (avoiding the elbow) and normograded into the distal fragment. They can then be tied into a TIF.

Radius

A ventral approach is used for distal radial fractures only (**300a–d**). The dorsal approach is preferred for proximal fractures or ulnar fractures.

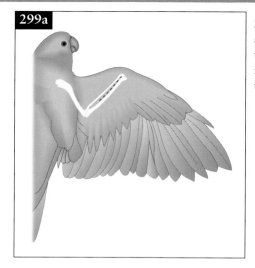

299a Dorsal approach to the distal radius and ulna.

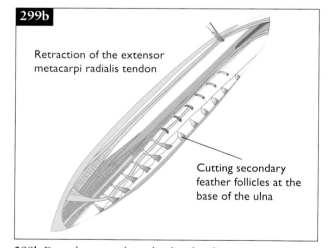

Retraction of the extensor metacarpi radialis tendon

Cutting secondary feather follicles at the base of the ulna

299b Dorsal approach to the distal radius.

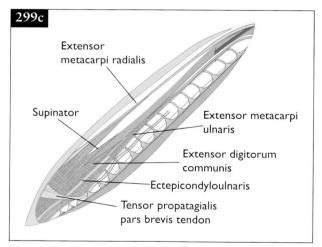

Extensor metacarpi radialis

Supinator

Extensor metacarpi ulnaris

Extensor digitorum communis

Ectepicondyloulnaris

Tensor propatagialis pars brevis tendon

299c Dorsal approach to the distal ulna.

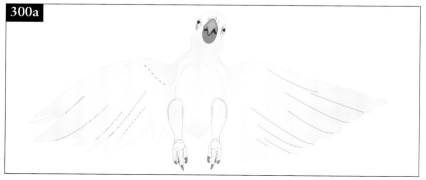

300a Ventral approach to the distal radius and ulna.

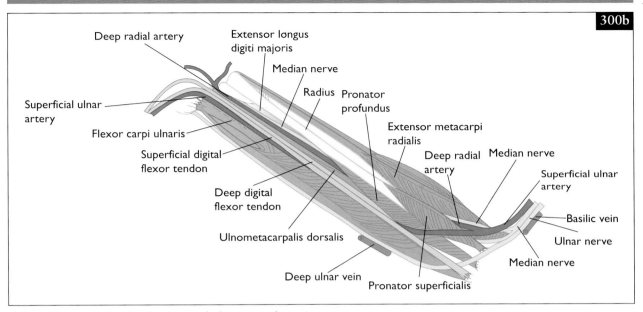

300b Anatomy of the distal radius and ulna (ventral view).

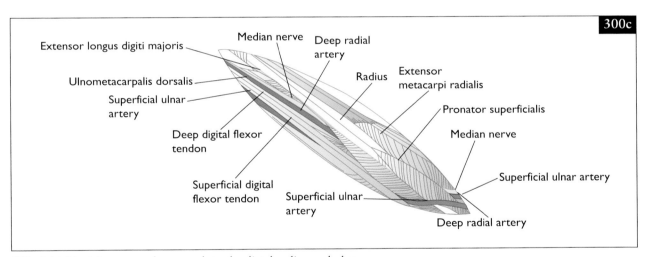

300c Initial incision, ventral approach to the distal radius and ulna.

300d Deeper dissection to expose the distal radius.

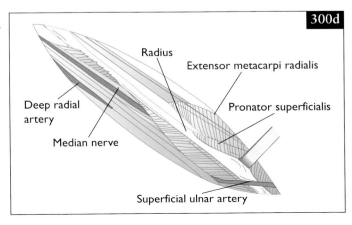

The bird is placed in dorsal recumbency and the affected wing is extended. The feathers are plucked from the ventral antebrachium.

The superficial ulnar artery is palpated distal to the elbow joint. Starting distally to this artery, an incision is made over the caudal aspect of the radius between the extensor metacarpi radialis muscle anteriorly and the extensor digitorum communis over the intraosseous space. Numerous major arteries, veins and nerves, as well as muscle bellies and tendons, are in this area. Care must be taken not to damage them. In order to expose the radius, the belly of the pronator superficialis must be reflected cranially away from the pronator profundus, taking care to avoid the arteries, veins and nerves in this area.

If the fracture is displaced, intramedullary pins are inserted through the fracture site out toward the carpus (avoiding the joint) and then retrograded back through the proximal fragment.

Ulna

A dorsal approach can be used for simple ulna fractures.

The bird is placed in ventral recumbency. Covert and down feathers are plucked from the caudal and dorsal aspect of antebrachium, leaving the secondaries in place.

An intramedullary pin is inserted at right angles to the skin on the caudal aspect of the ulna between the second and third last secondary feathers. As the trochar of the pin cuts into the cortex, the angle of the pin is gradually changed so that it becomes aligned with the ulna as it penetrates into the medullary cavity. The pin can then be manipulated, either closed or open, into the distal fragment.

A slight variation of this technique is to use a larger pin to gain entrance to medullary cavity, and then introduce a blunt-tipped smaller pin. This prevents accidental penetration of the carpal joint.

Metacarpus

A ventral approach is preferred due to the insertion of primary feathers on the dorsal surface (**301a–d**).

The skin is incised between two metacarpals. The abductor digiti majoris muscle lies between two major tendons (deep and superficial digital flexors). These two flexor tendons are retracted cranially and the muscle transected and reflected. Soft tissues tendons, and blood vessels are separated in order to approach the main, or primary, metacarpal bone.

APPROACHES TO THE BONES OF THE LEG
Coxofemoral joint

This approach is used for stabilization of the coxofemoral joint or excision arthroplasty of the femoral head.

The bird is placed in lateral recumbency and feathers are plucked over the dorsolateral femur and pelvis.

A skin incision is made over the dorsolateral crest of the ilium, extending over the femoral trochanter. The iliotibialis lateralis muscle (cranially) and iliofibularis muscle (caudally) are separated from distal to proximally to the iliac crest, cutting the common tendinous insertion of these muscles on the ilium. The musculotendinous insertion of the iliofemoralis externus and the iliotrochantericus caudalis is transected, leaving enough tissue for reattachment. These two muscles lie dorsal to the acetabulum.

The bird is turned 180° to view the transparent membrane covering the joint, being aware of the

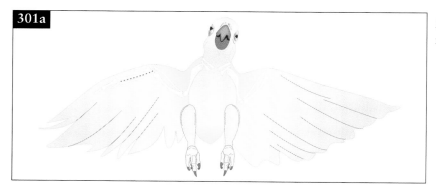

301a

301a Ventral approach to the metacarpus.

branch of the femoral artery crossing this membrane and the femoral vein and nerve deep to it.

Luxations can now be reduced and the joint capsule sutured in two to three locations. Transected muscles and tendons are reattached to close.

Femur

Two approaches are described. Cathartidae (vultures) and gallinaceous birds have a well developed iliotibialis lateralis muscle that covers the underlying structures.

Cathartidae and galliformes

The bird is placed in partial sternal or lateral recumbency. The femoral shaft is palpated and an incision made over it. The iliotibialis lateralis is bluntly separated, being careful not to go too far caudally and damage the sciatic nerve. Retraction of the iliotibialis lateralis reveals the femorotibialis externus (cranial) overlying the femoral shaft, and the iliofibularis lying caudal to it. The femorotibialis externus can be retracted cranially to expose the femur.

301b Anatomy of the metacarpal region, ventral view.

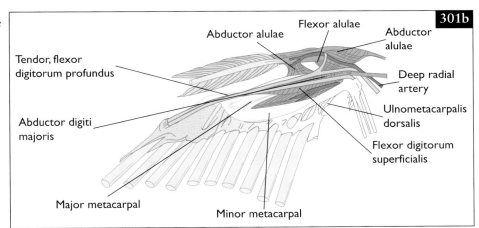

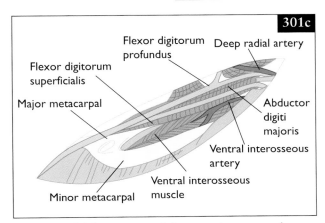

301c Superficial structures of the ventral metacarpal region.

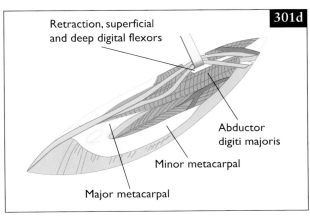

301d Retraction of the deep and superficial digital flexors to expose the major metacarpal bone.

Psittacids, accipiters and stringiformes

The iliotibialis lateralis is not as well developed in these birds.

A skin incision is made from the femoral trochanter to the lateral condyle (**302a–c**). This exposes the iliotibialis lateralis (cranially, overlying the femorotibialis externus) and the iliofibularis (caudally, overlying the sciatic nerve). These two muscles are separated, and the iliotibialis lateralis and femorotibialis externus are retracted together cranially. This exposes the femoral shaft. The ischiatic vein lies caudal to the femur in the middle third.

Tibiotarsus

There are four repair methods:
- Intramedullary pins retrograded out of the hock, then back up towards the stifle.
- Intramedullary pins are introduced from the tibial crest and normograded down through the proximal fragments and then into the distal fragments.
- ESF.
- TIF incorporating the latter two techniques.

A medial approach is used because of the muscle bulk on the lateral side (**303a–c**). Care must be taken, as the medial metatarsal vein crosses the hock and then runs caudally behind the tibiotarsal. Incise over the shaft of the tibiotarsus from just cranial to the hock to the medial femoral condyle.

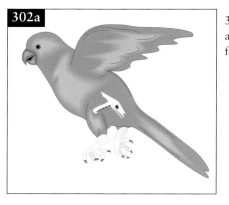

302a Lateral approach to the femur.

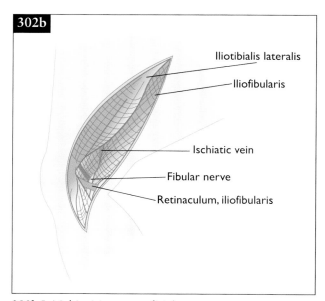

302b Initial incision: superficial structures.

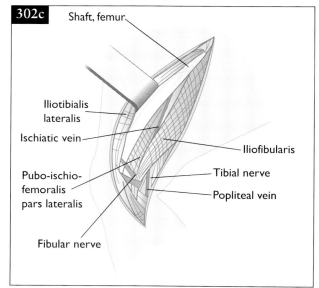

302c Exposure of the shaft of the femur.

303a Medial approach to the tibiotarsus.

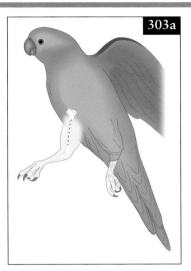

303a

The cranial complex of muscles (fibularis longus and tibialis cranialis) are separated from the medial head of the gastrocnemius. This division is easier to see in raptors than in psittacines. To close the surgery site, this attachment is sutured before closing the skin.

Tarsometatarsus

Fractures of the tarsometatarsus tend to be open fractures and are best repaired with ESF. If intramedullary pins are used, they should be introduced through the fracture and exteriorized retrograde laterally or medially to the joint, then passed normograde back into the distal fragment.

A lateral approach is used. An incision is made along the shaft. The bone is U-shaped, with a groove up the back. Flexor tendons run in this groove; extensor tendons, arteries and nerve supply run on the cranial aspect of the shaft; veins are on the medial and lateral sides.

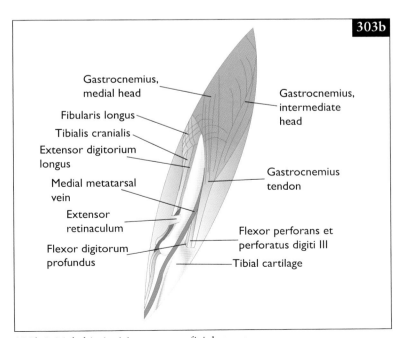

303b

Gastrocnemius, medial head

Gastrocnemius, intermediate head

Fibularis longus

Tibialis cranialis

Extensor digitorium longus

Gastrocnemius tendon

Medial metatarsal vein

Extensor retinaculum

Flexor perforans et perforatus digiti III

Flexor digitorum profundus

Tibial cartilage

303b Initial skin incision — superficial structures.

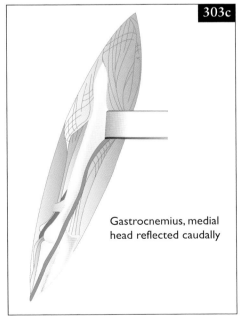

303c

Gastrocnemius, medial head reflected caudally

303c Exposure of the proximal shaft by retraction of the medial head of the gastrocnemics.

FURTHER READING

Altman RB (1997) General surgical considerations. In: *Avian Medicine and Surgery*. RB Altman, SL Clubb, GM Dorrestein, K Quesenberry (eds). WB Saunders, Philadelphia, pp. 691–703.

Altman RB (1997) Soft tissue surgical procedures. In: *Avian Medicine and Surgery*. RB Altman, SL Clubb, GM Dorrestein, K Quesenberry (eds). WB Saunders, Philadelphia, pp. 704–732.

Altman RB (1997) Radiosurgery (Electrosurgery). In: *Avian Medicine and Surgery*. RB Altman, SL Clubb, GM Dorrestein, K Quesenberry (eds). WB Saunders, Philadelphia, pp. 767–772.

Bennett RA (1997) Orthopedic surgery. In: *Avian Medicine and Surgery*. RB Altman, SL Clubb, GM Dorrestein, K Quesenberry (eds). WB Saunders, Philadelphia, pp. 733–766.

Bennett RA, Harrison GJ (1994) Soft tissue surgery. In: *Avian Medicine: Principles and Application*. BW Ritchie, GJ Harrison, LR Harrison (eds). Wingers Publishing, Lake Worth, pp. 1096–1136.

Bowles HL, Odberg E, Harrison GJ, Kottwitz JJ (2006) Surgical resolution of soft tissue disorders. In: *Clinical Avian Medicine, Vol 2*. GJ Harrison, TL Lightfoot (eds). Spix Publishing Inc, Palm Beach, pp. 775–830.

Helmer P, Redig PT (2006) Surgical resolution of orthopedic disorders. In: *Clinical Avian Medicine, Vol 2*. GJ Harrison, TL Lightfoot (eds). Spix Publishing Inc, Palm Beach, pp. 761–774.

Hernandez-Divers SJ (2005) Minimally invasive endoscopic surgery of birds. *Journal of Avian Medicine and Surgery* **19(2)**:107–120.

Martin HD, Ritchie BW (1994) Orthopedic surgical techniques. In: *Avian Medicine: Principles and Application*. BW Ritchie, GJ Harrison, LR Harrison (eds). Wingers Publishing, Lake Worth, pp. 1137–1170.

Orosz SE, Ensley PK, Haynes CJ (1992) *Avian Surgical Anatomy: Thoracic and Pelvic Limbs*. WB Saunders, Philadelphia.

Chapter 27
Formulary

ANTIBIOTICS

Class	Drug	Dose and route	Comments
Penicillins Bactericidal. Well distributed in extracellular spaces, especially in inflamed tissues. Do not readily penetrate the eye and CNS. Excreted by the kidneys, largely unchanged, therefore high concentrations can be found in the urine. Allergic reactions (anaphylaxis) have been reported, possibly from the procaine component in procaine penicillin. Potentially synergistic in combination with aminoglycosides.	Amoxicillin	100 mg/kg q8h 200–800 mg/l of water	Effective against gram-positive bacteria, especially *Staphylococcus*; most (all) gram-negative bacteria are resistant.
	Ampicillin	100 mg/kg IM q6h	
	Amoxicillin/ clavulanic acid	125 mg/kg PO q8–12h 60–120 mg/kg IM q12h	Clavulanic acid inhibits beta-lactamase (bacterial enzyme that inactivates many penicillins).
	Carbenicillin	100–200 mg/kg IM q8h	Improved spectrum against *Pseudomonas* and other gram-negative bacteria. Oral form has poor bioavailability.
	Ticarcillin	200 mg/kg IM q8h	Similar to carbenicillin; much more active against *Pseudomonas*. Also found in combination with clavulanic acid and used at the same dose. Parenteral administration only. (*Penicillins continued over*)

ANTIBIOTICS *Continued*

Class	Drug	Dose and route	Comments
Penicillins *continued*	Piperacillin	100–200 mg/kg IM q8–12h	Good activity against most gram-negative bacteria including *Pseudomonas*, *Klebsiella* and *Enterobacter*. Piperacillin with tazobactam is commonly used in practice, at the same dose. Parenteral administration only.
Cephalosporins Three generations effective against both gram-positive and gram-negative bacteria. Well distributed in extracellular spaces. Do not readily penetrate eye and CNS, except for cefotaxime and ceftazidime. Synergistic with aminoglycosides.	Cephalothin	100 mg/kg IM q6h	First generation. Effective against most gram-positive cocci, many gram-negatives and some anaerobes.
	Cephalexin	50–100 mg/kg IM or PO q6–12h	
	Cefoxitin	75–100 mg/kg IM q8–12h	Second generation. Increased gram-negative activity.
	Ceftazidime	50–100 mg/kg q6–8h IM	Third generation. Penetrates CSF.
	Ceftiofur	10–20 mg/kg IM q12h	Third generation with activity against *Pasteurella*, *E coli*, *Streptococcus*, *Staphylococcus* and *Salmonella* spp.
	Cefotaxime	75–100 mg/kg IM q8–12h	Third generation. Expanded gram-negative spectrum. Penetrates CSF.

ANTIBIOTICS *Continued*

Class	Drug	Dose and route	Comments
Chloramphenicol Bacteriostatic. Highly lipid soluble, therefore good tissue penetration, including CNS and eye; tissue concentrations often exceed serum levels. Reversible dose-related anaemia, CNS depression and loss of appetite have been reported in chickens, turkeys and ducks. Caution with people handling the drug. Not to be used in food-producing animals.	Chloramphenicol palmitate (oral); chloramphenicol succinate (injectable)	50–75 mg/kg IM or PO q6–12h	Broad spectrum against *Chlamydophila*, mycoplasma, gram-positive and gram-negative bacteria and some protozoa; many avian gram-negative isolates are resistant. Oral form (palmitate ester): erratic blood concentrations. Injectable forms (succinate, propylene glycol based): more predictable serum concentrations.
Aminoglycosides Bactericidal. Synergistic with penicillins and cephalosporins. Excellent spectrum against gram-positives and gram-negative bacteria; ineffective against anaerobic bacteria and in proteinaceous environments such as abscesses and exudates. Poor penetration into CNS and eye. Nephrotoxic; in dehydrated birds and birds with compromised renal function the dose should be reduced or a less toxic drug selected.	Amikacin	10–20 mg/kg IM q12h	Greater activity against gram-negative bacteria including some resistant to gentamicin and tobramycin. Achieves higher serum concentrations than gentamicin, but is less toxic so levels are better tolerated. Less toxic side-effects and is the aminoglycoside of choice for use in birds.
	Gentamicin	5–10 mg/kg IM q12h	More toxic than amikacin. Not generally recommended due to narrow margin of safety. (*Aminoglycosides continued over*)

ANTIBIOTICS *Continued*

Class	Drug	Dose and route	Comments
Aminoglycosides *continued*	Tobramycin	5 mg/kg IM q12h	Pharmacology is similar to gentamicin, but has greater activity against *Pseudomonas*. Neurotoxicity and nephrotoxicity may develop.
Quinolones Bactericidal. Most avian gram-negative pathogens, some gram-positive pathogens, most mycoplasma and possibly *Chlamydophila* are sensitive. Not effective against anaerobes. Achieves high levels everywhere, especially in the liver and urinary tract; tissue concentrations may exceed serum concentrations. May cause permanent articular defects in juveniles; use with extreme caution in growing birds. Scattered anecdotal reports of aggressive, irritable behaviour in Amazon parrots treated with quinolones. IM injection causes pain and necrosis at the site of injection. Toxic reactions may be species-specific.	Enrofloxacin	10–30 mg/kg IM or PO q12h	Excellent activity against mycoplasma, some gram-positive and most gram-negative bacteria. However, *Pseudomonas* resistance is common. May have anti-chlamydial activity, but while treatment eliminates clinical signs it may not clear the carrier state. Can cause vomiting in raptors when given orally. If given in water, enrofloxacin may not achieve therapeutic levels except for highly susceptible bacteria. Only a single IM injection should be given, as repeated injections cause significant bruising and muscle necrosis.
	Ciprofloxacin	15–40 mg/kg PO q12h	Antibacterial spectrum similar to enrofloxacin.
	Marbofloxacin	2.5–15 mg/kg PO or IM q24h	Used in raptors, as it does not appear to cause nausea.

ANTIBIOTICS *Continued*

Class	Drug	Dose and route	Comments
Trimethoprim–sulphonamide derivatives Bacteriostatic. Excellent gram-positive and gram-negative spectrum. *Pseudomonas* and some strains of Enterobacteriaceae are resistant. May be effective against some coccidia. Has been used in combination therapy for *Sarcocystis* infection. Wide extracellular distribution. Some birds (especially macaws) suffer gastrointestinal upset and will regurgitate 1–3 hours after an oral dose. Incidence can be reduced if the drug is added to a small amount of food. Sulphonamides are excreted via the same pathway as uric acid. In dehydrated birds and those with compromised renal function sulphas may form crystals and damage renal glomeruli. Therefore, if serum uric acid is elevated, select another drug.	Trimethoprim—sulphadiazine (veterinary formulations)	50–100 mg/kg (of combined product) PO q12h or 8–20 mg/kg IM q12h or 475–950 mg/l of water for 5–7 days	Sterile abscesses and irritation have been reported following the use of the injectable veterinary products.
	Trimethoprim—sulphamethoxazole (medical formulation)	100–200 mg/kg (of combined product) PO q12h	

ANTIBIOTICS *Continued*

Class	Drug	Dose and route	Comments
Tetracyclines Bacteriostatic. Spectrum includes many gram-positive organisms; poor efficacy against most avian gram-negative isolates. Used for *Chlamydophila* and *Mycoplasma*. Wide volume of distribution. Side-effects: • Anorexia, vomiting, diarrhoea. • Immunosuppression. • Hepatotoxicity (rare). • Localized tissue reactions to doxycycline injection formulations. Alteration of gut flora especially yeast overgrowths and secondary bacterial infections. Chelates calcium in gut and bone; dietary calcium interferes with the oral uptake of tetracyclines. Use cautiously in baby birds for extended periods of time.	Oxytetracycline	10–50 mg/kg IM once every 3–5 days	Poorly absorbed when given orally, therefore oral formulations are not recommended. IM well absorbed and widely distributed, but is irritating and will cause necrosis at the injection site.
	Chlortetracycline	40–50 mg/kg PO q12h or 1,500 ppm in food or water	Poor acceptance. Immunosuppressive. Can be used for flock treatment of chlamydiosis, but doxycycline is preferred.
	Doxycycline	25–50 mg/kg PO q24h or 100–500 mg/l of water (African greys may require up to 800 mg/l of water) or 60–100 mg/kg IM once weekly	More lipophilic than other tetracyclines; absorbed better through the gastrointestinal tract and greater bioavailability. May offer significant advantages over other tetracyclines for treating chlamydiosis. Rapid gastrointestinal absorption.

ANTIBIOTICS *Continued*

Class	Drug	Dose and route	Comments
Macrolides and lincosamides Bacteriostatic. Indicated for *Pasteurella*, *Bordetella*, some mycoplasma, *Campylobacter spp.*, *Clostridia spp.* and obligate anaerobic bacteria. Often used for susceptible upper respiratory tract infections and osteomyelitis. Active against gram-positive organisms and anaerobes, but virtually all aerobic gram-negative bacteria are resistant.	Erythromycin	60 mg/kg PO q12h	Active against chlamydiosis in people, but not effective at the dose levels used in birds. Injectable form may cause severe tissue irritation.
	Clindamycin	25–150 mg/kg PO q12h	Used occasionally to treat osteomyelitis caused by susceptible gram-positive pathogens. Only oral forms are used in avian medicine because of injection site necrosis with injectable formulations.
	Lincomycin	75–100 mg/kg IM or PO q12h or 500–750 mg/l of water	Usually combined with spectinomycin. Has been used to treat respiratory and gastrointestinal infections caused by gram-positive bacteria and mycoplasma.
	Azithromycin	50–80 mg/kg PO q24h	New generation macrolide; appears to be active against intracellular infections including *Chlamydophila*, *Toxoplasma*, *Plasmodium* and *Cryptosporidium*.
	Tylosin	10–40 mg/kg IM q12h or q8h or 200–500 mg/l of water	Used predominantly for suspected mycoplasma infections and *Pasteurella*. IM injections can be very irritating.

ANTIFUNGAL DRUGS

Class	Drug	Dose and route	Comments
Metronidazole Bactericidal. Effective against many gram-positive and most gram-negative obligate anaerobes. Ineffective against aerobic bacteria. Highly effective against many protozoa. Well absorbed from the gastrointestinal tract, highly lipophilic and penetrates bones, CNS and abscesses.	Metronidazole	10–50 mg/kg PO q12–24h	Frequently used for anaerobic infections (including clostridial infections) and motile protozoa (*Trichomonas, Giardia and Cochlosoma*).
Azoles Inhibit ergosterol synthesis. Fungistatic, so months of therapy are often required. Takes several days to reach steady-state concentrations.	Ketoconazole	20–30 mg/kg PO q12h for 10–30 days. Should be administered with food	For *Candida* infections. Probably not as effective with *Aspergillus* infections as other azoles. Widely distributed to tissues, but is highly protein-bound and does not penetrate CNS or eye fluids. Water insoluble unless dissolved in acid first. Toxic side-effects seen in mammals are rarely seen in birds, but may be associated with hepatotoxicity.
	Enilconazole	Nebulization solution; enilconazole 100 mg: 9 ml DMSO: 90 ml NaCl Topically: dilute 1:10 and apply q12h	Administered topically or nebulized.

ANTIFUNGAL DRUGS *Continued*

Class	Drug	Dose and route	Comments
Azoles *continued*	Fluconazole	1.5–10 mg/kg PO q12h or 10–20 mg/kg PO q24–48h	Effective against *Candida* (especially mycelial form), *Aspergillus* and *Cryptococcus*. Penetrates eye, CNS and CSF. Best safety margin of the azoles.
	Itraconazole	5–10 mg/kg PO q24h given with food for at least 1 month after signs have resolved	Used for gastrointestinal and cutaneous candidiasis and dermatophyte infections. Maybe more effective than other azoles and amphotericin B in *Aspergillus* infections. Poorly distributed to CSF, ocular fluids and plasma (tissue concentrations are higher than in plasma). Although less toxic than amphotericin B, it appears that African greys may be sensitive to this drug, causing anorexia and depression. Itraconazole is not recommended for use in this species, but to use at 2.5–5 mg/kg PO q24h if necessary.
	Miconazole	5 mg/kg intratracheally q12h for 5 days or apply topical gel q12h	Can be used topically, intratracheally or via nebulization. Many toxic side-effects (cardiac arrhythmias, cardiac arrest) if given IV too quickly. (*Azoles continued over*)

ANTIFUNGAL DRUGS *Continued*

Class	Drug	Dose and route	Comments
Azoles *continued*	Clotrimazole	2 mg/kg intratracheally q24h or 10 mg/ml NaCl as a nasal flush q12h	Poorly absorbed, therefore topical use or nebulized only. Effective against *Aspergillus*. It may cause local irritation.
	Voriconazole	12–18 mg/kg POq12h	Voriconazole has dose-dependent pharmacokinetics and may induce its own metabolism. Used for the treatment of African grey parrots infected with *Aspergillus* or other fungal organisms that have a minimal inhibitory concentration for voriconazole < or = 0.4. Higher doses may be needed to maintain plasma voriconazole concentrations during long-term treatment. Safety and efficacy of various voriconazole treatment regimens in this species require investigation.
Terbinafine Inhibits ergosterol synthesis.	Terbinafine	10–15 mg/kg PO q12–24h or nebulization (1 mg/ml; 500 mg terbinafine + 1 ml acetylcysteine + 500 ml distilled water)	*Aspergillus* and dermatophytes Good oral absorption; distributed well to fat and skin.

ANTIFUNGAL DRUGS *Continued*

Class	Drug	Dose and route	Comments
Polyenes Act on fungal membrane sterols.	Amphotericin B	1.5 mg/kg IV q8h for 3–5 days or 1 mg/kg intratracheally q12h or nebulize at 0.3–1 mg/ml for 15 minutes q6–12h or 100 mg/kg PO q12h for 10–30 days for the treatment of megabacteria (*Macrorhabdus ornithogaster*)	Fungicidal. Active against both yeast and hyphal fungi. Used orally for the treatment of megabacteria (*Macrorhabdus ornithogaster*). Not absorbed orally; for aspergillosis it must be administered IV, topically or by nebulization Widely distributed when given IV, but only minor systemic absorption with aerosol or topical administration. Nephrotoxicity is common in mammals, but uncommonly reported in birds. Topical solutions must be diluted before flushing into closed spaces (e.g. sinuses) to prevent irritation. Combine with itraconazole for best response.
	Nystatin	200,00–300,000 units/kg PO q8–12h	Not systemically absorbed. Must come into contact with yeast to be effective, therefore tube feeding may bypass oral lesions. Do not mix with hand-rearing formula to ensure concentration and contact time are maximized.
Fluorinated pyrimidines Inhibit macromolecule synthesis.	5-Fluorocystine (Flucytosine)	60 mg/kg PO q12h for birds >500g; 150 mg/kg PO q12h for birds <500g	Rarely used. Can be used with amphotericin B to treat aspergillosis. Resistance develops rapidly when used alone.

MYCOBACTERIAL TREATMENT PROTOCOLS

Protocols involve combinations of antituberculous drugs, as resistance to a single drug can develop rapidly. Because these organisms can only be killed during replication, which occurs once every 16–20 hours, treatment often lasts nine months or longer. Organisms can also persist for months in caseous lesions and macrophages where replication seldom occurs. Therapy is aimed at achieving the highest possible blood levels of drug rather than maintaining constant blood levels. Therefore, the highest tolerable doses of drugs are given once daily. Treatment protocols include the following combinations of drugs, most given orally once daily:

- Amikacin 20 mg/kg q24h IM, enrofloxacin 30 mg/kg.
- Enrofloxacin 30 mg/kg, ethambutol 30 mg/kg, rifabutin 15 mg/kg.
- Clarithromycin 55 mg/kg, rifabutin 6 mg/kg, ethambutol 30 mg/kg, enrofloxacin 30 mg/kg.
- Clarithromycin 55 mg/kg, rifabutin 15 mg/kg, ethambutol 30 mg/kg, enrofloxacin 30 mg/kg.
- Clarithromycin 55 mg/kg, rifabutin 15 mg/kg, ethambutol 30 mg/kg.

ANTIVIRAL DRUGS

Class	Drug	Dose and route	Comments
Acyclovir Used for treating outbreaks of herpesvirus infection.	Acyclovir	80–330 mg/kg PO q8h for a minimum of 7 days	Works better on in-contact birds rather than affected birds. Injectable form is very irritant.
Interferon Group of small protein and glycoprotein cytokines naturally produced by the immune system following natural infection or vaccination. Interferons protect the bird by suppressing cell proliferation, inhibiting viral replication and augmenting the activity of macrophages and T lymphocytes. They are species specific and a mammalian interferon would not be expected to have a significant action in birds. However, cross-species reactivity has been reported in birds.	Avian interferon	1,000,000 units IM q24h for 90 days or 1,000,000 units IM every 2–7 days for 3 treatments	Initially, the use of interferon was limited due to the difficulty in manufacturing the protein in large enough quantities, but the recent development of recombinant DNA technologies has made interferon economic and easy to produce. Not commercially available at time of writing.

ANTIPROTOZOAL DRUGS

Class	Drug	Dose and route	Comments
Nitroimidazoles Used against motile protozoa (*Trichomonas, Giardia, Cochlosoma, Spironucleus, Histomonas*). *Candida* overgrowth after prolonged therapy can occur, especially in cockatiels.	Carnidazole	20–30 mg/kg PO once	Safe with good efficacy, but must be given on an empty stomach, as vomiting may otherwise occur.
	Ronidazole	6–10 mg/kg PO or 60–600 mg/l of water for 7 days	Treatment of choice for *Trichomonas*; dose can be increased to 600 mg/l of water if resistance develops.
	Dimetridazole	200–400 mg/l water for 5 days	Toxic if overdosed: depression, anorexia, ataxia, seizures (incorrect water preparation or excessive water intake [e.g. hot weather, feeding chicks]). Do not use in pekin robins and finches. Use with care in lorikeets and mynahs (use lower dose).
	Metronidazole	50 mg/kg PO q12–24h or 40–80 mg/l of water for 3 days	Frequently used for motile protozoa (*Trichomonas, Giardia and Cochlosoma*).
Sulphonamides Used to treat coccidia.	Sulphachlorpyridazine	100–400 mg/l of water for 3–5 days	Contraindicated with dehydration, liver disease, renal disease. Treatment periods >2 weeks may require supplementation with folic acid. All treatments should be repeated after five days to allow for the prepatent period of coccidia. (*Sulphonamides continued over*)
	Sulphadimethoxine	20–50 mg/kg PO q12h for 3–5 days or 250–500 mg/l of water for 5–7 days	
	Sulphadimidine	50–150 mg/kg PO q12h or 3330–6660 mg/l of water for 5 days	

ANTIPROTOZOAL DRUGS *Continued*

Class	Drug	Dose and route	Comments
Sulphonamides *continued*	Sulphamethazine	75–185 mg/kg PO q24h for 3 days or 125 mg/l of water for 3 days	
	Sulphaquinoxaline	100 mg/kg PO q24h for 3 days or 250–500 mg/l of water for 5–7 days	
Benzeneacetonitrile derivatives Used to treat coccidia. All treatments should be repeated after five days to allow for the prepatent period of coccidia.	Clazuril	2.5 mg tablet per pigeon or 7 mg/kg PO q24h for 2–3 days	Single dose may suppress oocyst excretion for two weeks.
	Diclazuril	10 mg/kg PO q24h on days 0, 1, 2, 4, 6, 8 and 10 or 5 mg/l of water	Can be used for treating *Toxoplasma*.
	Toltrazuril	25–75 mg/l of for 5 days or 7–15 mg/kg q24h for 3 days or 20–35 mg/kg PO once	Has also been used to treat *Atoxoplasma* in canaries.
Amprolium and **amprolium–ethopabate** Used to treat coccidia. Inhibits the active transport of thiamine into the cell. Coccidia are 50 times as sensitive to this inhibition as the host.	Amprolium; amprolium–ethopabate	15–30 mg/kg q24h for 1–5 days or 50–100 mg/l of water for 5–7 days	Resistance is common. Treatment periods >2 weeks may require supplementation with folic acid. All treatments should be repeated after five days to allow for the prepatent period of coccidia.

ANTIPROTOZOAL DRUGS *Continued*

Class	Drug	Dose and route	Comments
Pyrimethamine Used for *Toxoplasma, Atoxoplasma, Sarcocystis, Leucozytozoon.*	Pyrimethamine	0.5 mg/kg PO q12h 30 days	
Quinacrine HCl Used for *Atoxoplasma, Plasmodium.*	Quinacrine HCl	5–10 mg/kg PO q24h 10 days	Overdosage may cause hepatotoxicity.
Chloroquine Used for *Plasmodium* and other blood parasites.	Chloroquine	10–25 mg/kg PO as a first dose, then 5–15 mg/kg at 6,18 and 24 hours	Use in conjunction with primaquine.
Primaquine Used for *Plasmodium*, in combination with chloroquine, and *Sarcocystis.*	Primaquine	0.3–1 mg/kg PO q24h for 3–10 days	Use in conjunction with chloroquine.
Mepacrine HCl Used for *Plasmodium* in canaries.	Mepacrine HCl	0.24 mg/kg PO q12h	

INTERNAL PARASITICIDES

Class	Drug	Dose and route	Comments
Fumarate reductase inhibitors Benzimidazole derivatives. Used mainly for treating nematodes. Interfere with energy metabolism; prevent the parasite from using sugars.	Albendazole	10–50 mg/kg PO once	Can be used for treating microsporidia, as well as some nematodes. Can be toxic in raptors at doses over 25 mg/kg. (*Fumarate reductase inhibitors continued over*)

INTERNAL PARASITICIDES *Continued*

Class	Drug	Dose and route	Comments
Fumarate reductase inhibitors *continued* Usually requires several days of treatment, although single high doses can be effective. Low toxicity, but can affect haematopoietic cells and intestinal epithelium. Do not use during breeding, as embryotoxic effects have been observed. Toxicity varies with species and drug.	Thiabendazole	40–100 mg/kg q24h for 7 days or 100–500 mg/kg once	Less effective than fenbendazole.
	Cambendazole	60–100 mg/kg q24h for 3–7 days	
	Fenbendazole	25–50 mg/kg once or 8–10 mg/kg daily for 3–4 days or 50 mg/kg/day for 3 days (may treat *Giardia*)	May also be effective against some cestodes, trematodes and *Giardia*. Can interfere with feather growth during moulting. Can be toxic to bone marrow, causing leucopenia.
	Mebendazole	10–25 mg/kg q12h for 5 days or 10–20 mg/l of water for 3–5 days	Effective against some cestodes and trematodes.
	Oxfendazole	10–40 mg/kg once	
	Febantel	30 mg/kg once	
Imidithiazoles Used against nematodes. Stimulates cholinergic receptors, causing paralysis of the parasite. Regurgitation, anorexia, diarrhoea and neurological signs (ataxia, head tilt and torticollis) are occasionally seen.	Levamisole	20–40 mg/kg PO once or 100–200 mg/l of water for 3 days, repeat in 2 weeks	Not recommended in finches, lories or debilitated birds.

INTERNAL PARASITICIDES *Continued*

Class	Drug	Dose and route	Comments
Gamma amino butyric acid (GABA) interfering drugs Macrocyclic lactones. Used against ascarids and other nematodes, blood-sucking external parasites and *Cnemidocoptes* microfilaria. Toxicity is low, but overdosing and idiosyncratic reactions include severe depression, inactivity, excessive sleeping and neurological signs. Budgerigars, African finches and European finches may be more sensitive.	Ivermectin	200–400 µg/kg IM or PO once	Toxicity may be higher if the drug is injected (particularly via the IM route).
	Milbemycin	2 mg/kg PO once	
	Moxidectin	200–400 µg/kg IM or PO once	
Adenosine triphosphate synthesis blockers Block synthesis of ATP and produce paralysis by interfering with energy metabolism.	Niclosamide	50–100 mg/kg PO once, repeat in 10–14 days	Used for treating cestodes and trematodes. Praziquantel is more effective.
	Rafoxanide	10 mg/kg PO	Used for treating trematodes and cestodes.
Miscellaneous	Praziquantel	10–20 mg/kg PO or IM once	Used for treating cestodes and trematodes. Caution with IM in finches; sudden death has been reported. Very unpalatable. *(Miscellaneous continued over)*

INTERNAL PARASITICIDES *Continued*

Class	Drug	Dose and route	Comments
Miscellaneous *continued*	Piperazine	100–250 mg/kg PO once or 1,000–2,000 mg/l of water for 3 days	Used for ascarids only. Resistance is common.
	Pyrantel tartrate, pyrantel pamoate, pyrantel embonate	7–25 mg/kg PO once	Used for nematodes. Poorly absorbed from the gastrointestinal tract. Good safety margin.
Paromomycin	Paromomycin	100 mg/kg PO q12h for 7 days	Used for treating *Cryptosporidium*.

EXTERNAL PARASITICIDES

Class	Drug	Dose and route	Comments
Pyrethrins and synthetic pyrethroids	Pyrethrin, permethrin	Spray or wash	Often combined with insect growth regulators.
Piperonyl butoxide	Piperonyl butoxide is usually combined with a pyrethrin or permethrin	Spray or wash	
Organophosphates	Malathion, maldison	Spray or wash	Toxic; use is not recommended because of hazards to birds and owners.

EXTERNAL PARASITICIDES *Continued*

Class	Drug	Dose and route	Comments
Fipronil	Fipronil	3 mg/kg spray or spot-on application	Not registered for use in birds. Spray works better than spot-on application. Beware of inhalation or dermal absorption of the alcohol base. Beware of the drying effect the alcohol base may have on feathers.
Carbaryl 5%	Carbaryl	Dust lightly or add 1–2 teaspoonfulls to nesting material	Carbamate flea powder.
Gamma amino butyric acid (GABA) interfering drugs Macrocyclic lactones. Used against blood-sucking external parasites and *Cnemidocoptes*. Toxicity is low, but overdosing and idiosyncratic reactions include severe depression, inactivity, excessive sleeping and neurological signs. Budgerigars, African finches and European finches may be more sensitive.	Ivermectin	200–400 µg/kg topically, IM or PO once	Toxicity may be higher if the drug is injected (particularly via the IM route).
	Moxidectin	200–400 µg/kg topically, IM or PO once	

HORMONAL THERAPIES

Class	Drug	Dose and route	Comments
Reproductive hormones			
	Deslorelin	Long-acting implant	See leuprolide acetate (below)
	Human chorionic gonadotropin (HCG)	500–1,000 units IM on days 1, 3 and 7 and then every 2 weeks as required	Continued use is limited by formation of anti-HCG antibodies.
	Leuprolide acetate	100–700 µg/kg every 2 weeks for three treatments, then as required	GNRH agonist. Must be combined with environmental, behavioural and dietary changes for effect.
	Medroxyprogesterone acetate	5–25 mg/kg IM every 4–6 weeks	Often used for feather picking behaviour. Side-effects include polyuria/polydipsia, polyphagia, diabetes mellitus, hepatopathy, weight gain, sudden death. At very low doses it may be useful in suppressing ovulation.
	Megestrol acetate	2.5 mg/kg PO q24h for 7 days, then weekly as required	Seldom used because of severe side-effects, similar to medroxyprogesterone.
	Oxytocin	0.5–1.0 IU/kg repeated every 30–60 minutes	Used to stimulate oviductal contractions, but is not a naturally occurring hormone in birds. Use is contraindicated if uterovaginal sphincter is not dilated. Should be used in conjunction with calcium gluconate injections.

HORMONAL THERAPIES *Continued*

Class	Drug	Dose and route	Comments
Reproductive hormones *continued*	Prostaglandin E2 (Dinoprost)	0.02–0.1 mg/kg applied topically into the cloaca	Used to induce egg laying in egg-bound birds; simultaneously relaxes uterovaginal sphincter while contracting oviduct.
Thyroxine	Levothyroxine	5–200 µg/kg PO q12h	May induce moult. Monitor for cardiotoxicity.
Insulin	Short-acting insulin, NPH insulin, ultralente insulin	The immediate use of short-acting insulin (0.1–0.2 U/kg) can initially stabilize the patient, but long-term control at home usually required. Longer-acting insulin (NPH or ultralente): dose rates vary considerably, and should be based on the observed effects; they range from 0.067–3.3 U/kg q24h or q12h	For insulin-dependent diabetes.
Glucocorticoids Previously recommended for the treatment of shock and as an anti-inflammatory drug. Side-effects are severe: polyuria/polydipsia, catabolism, immunosuppression. Topical application seems to be as severe as, or worse than, parenteral administration.	Dexamethasone	2–4 mg/kg SC, IM or IV	With the possible exception of prednisolone sodium succinate, the use of glucocorticoids in birds is dangerous and cannot be recommended.
	Hydrocortisone	10 mg/kg IM q24h	
	Methylprednisolone acetate	0.5–1 mg/kg IM	
	Prednisolone	0.5–1 mg/kg IM once	
	Prednisolone sodium succinate	2–4 mg/kg IV once	
	Triamcinolone	0.1–0.5 mg/kg IM once	

DRUGS USED TO TREAT LIVER DISEASE

Class	Drug	Dose and route	Comments
Anti-inflammatory Anti-fibrotic and anti-inflammatory.	Colchicine	0.04–0.2 mg/kg PO q24h	May cause nausea and vomiting in some birds.
Chelating agent Chelates iron.	Deferoxamine	100 mg/kg PO, IM or SC q24h	Preferred iron chelator for iron storage disease. Avoid in birds with renal disease.
Diuretic Reduce ascites.	Furosemide	0.15–2 mg/kg IM, SC or PO q12–24h	Overdose can lead to dehydration and electrolyte abnormalities. Lorikeets are very sensitive to this drug; use with caution.
Lactulose Does not treat liver disease. Reduces absorption of ammonia from intestine by altering the pH of the intestinal lumen and promoting an osmotic catharsis. This reduces the ammonia levels presented to the liver. Best results are seen in carnivorous birds (e.g. raptors) as vegetable protein lacks many encephalopathic precursors.	Lactulose	150–650 mg/kg PO q8–12h	Can cause diarrhoea.

DRUGS USED TO TREAT LIVER DISEASE *Continued*

Class	Drug	Dose and route	Comments
Anti-oxidant Unproven remedy that offers good promise in avian medicine. Anti-oxidant. Enhances protein synthesis and hepatocellular regeneration. Protective effect against hepatotoxins. Suppresses fibrogenesis. Promotes fibrolysis.	Silibinin (Silymarin, milk thistle)	50–75 mg/kg PO q12h	Use a low alcohol or alcohol-free base.
Hepatoprotective drugs	Ursodeoxycholic acid	10–15 mg/kg PO q24h	Bile acid. Cytoprotective. Reduces involvement of hepatocytes and biliary epithelium in inflammatory process. Changes mix of bile acids to eliminate toxic bile acids from liver.

DRUGS USED TO TREAT KIDNEY DISEASE

Class	Drug	Dose and route	Comments
Decrease production of uric acid	Allopurinol	10–15 mg/kg PO q12–24h	May worsen renal disease. Maintain good hydration.
Reduce inflammation associated with articular gout	Colchicine	0.04–0.2 mg/kg PO q24h	May cause nausea and vomiting in some birds.

DRUGS USED TO TREAT KIDNEY DISEASE *Continued*

Class	Drug	Dose and route	Comments
Increase secretion of uric acid	Probenecid	–	Not currently recommended for use in birds. May exacerbate the condition.
Anti-inflammatory	Aspirin	1 mg/kg PO q24h	Used together for the treatment of membranous glomerulonephritis.
	Omega 3 and 6 fatty acid supplementation, mixed in a ratio of Omega 6:Omega 3 of 6:1	0.1 ml/kg PO q12h	

DRUGS USED TO TREAT CARDIOVASCULAR DISEASE

Class	Drug	Dose and route	Comments
Angiotensin converting enzyme (ACE) inhibitors Block the formation of angiotensin II, thereby blocking the renin–angiotensin–aldosterone system. They also have a diuretic effect.	Enalapril	0.5–1.25 mg/kg PO q12h	Side-effects could include hypotension, reflex tachycardia, dehydration, gastrointestinal disorders, renal dysfunction and hyperkalaemia.
	Benazapril	0.5 mg/kg PO q12h	
Cardiac glycoside Indicated for myocardial dysfunction, chronic mitral insufficiency and chronic volume overloads. Contraindicated for hypertrophic cardiomyopathy, ventricular tachycardia and sinus or AV node disease.	Digoxin	0.02–0.05 mg/kg PO q24h	Adverse effects relate to myocardial toxicity, therefore patients should be monitored for clinical improvement and via ECG for prolonged PR time. Serum concentrations should be measured after one week of therapy or one week after the dose is changed. The dose can be increased if the serum concentration is <0.8 ng/l 8–10 hours after dosing.

DRUGS USED TO TREAT CARDIOVASCULAR DISEASE *Continued*

Class	Drug	Dose and route	Comments
Positive ionotrope Similar in effect to digoxin, but with less risk of adverse effects.	Pimobendan	0.15 mg/kg PO q12h	
Diuretic Reduce ascites.	Furosemide	0.15–2 mg/kg IM, SC or PO q12–24h	Overdose can lead to dehydration and electrolyte abnormalities. Lorikeets are very sensitive to this drug; use with caution.

GASTROINTESTINAL DRUGS

Class	Drug	Dose and route	Comments
Intestinal motility modifiers Used for gastrointestinal motility disorders including slow emptying crops, crop stasis and regurgitation or vomiting.	Metoclopramide	0.5–2 mg/kg PO or IM q6–12h	Increases force and frequency of gastric contractions, relaxes pyloric sphincter, and promotes peristalsis in the duodenum and jejunum
	Cisapride	0.5–1.5 mg/kg PO q8–12h	Stimulates gastrointestinal motility
Intestinal protectants Used when proventriculitis or gastric ulceration is present.	Cimetidine	5 mg/kg PO	Reduces gastric secretion of HCl and pepsin. May impair the metabolism of concurrently administered drugs. Potential side-effects: depression, diarrhoea, tachycardia, respiratory failure. (*Intestinal protectants continued over*)

GASTROINTESTINAL DRUGS *Continued*

Class	Drug	Dose and route	Comments
Intestinal protectants *continued*	Sucralfate	25 mg/kg PO q8h	A complex disaccharide that reacts with stomach acid to form a complex that binds to proteins associated with an ulcer and produces a protective layer that protects the ulcerated mucosa from gastric acids and microbial pathogens.
Laxatives and cathartics Used to remove foreign bodies from the gastrointestinal tract.	Mineral oil (paraffin oil)	5 ml/kg PO	Acts unchanged as an emollient laxative. Care must be taken to prevent aspiration; give by crop gavage. Can be mixed with peanut butter in a ratio of 1 part mineral oil to 2 parts peanut butter.
	Methylcellulose	5 ml/kg PO q12h	Absorbs water and swells. Care must be taken not to mix too thickly or give too much, as it can absorb enough water to block the gastrointestinal tract.
	Magnesium sulphate (Epsom salts)	0.25–1.0 g/kg PO q24h for 1–2 days	Retains or attracts water via osmotic forces. Must be used with caution.

GASTROINTESTINAL DRUGS *Continued*

Class	Drug	Dose and route	Comments
Laxatives and cathartics *continued*	Lactulose	150–650 mg/kg PO q8–12h	Has a laxative effect through osmotic catharsis. In birds with caecae, lactulose passes to the caecae where saccharolytic microflora ferment lactulose to produce acetic, lactic and other organic acids, which lowers the pH of the caecal content.
	Vegetable oils (e.g. castor oil, raw linseed oil, olive oil)	15 ml/kg PO	Act as irritant purgatives; form sodium and potassium salts of released fatty acids after hydrolysis by pancreatic lipase, making them irritant soaps.

ANAESTHETICS AND SEDATIVES

Class	Drug	Dose and route	Comments
Sedatives Used for sedation or to control seizures and convulsions	Diazepam	0.05–0.15 mg/kg IV or 0.2–0.5 mg/kg IM	Can be used as a premedication prior to anaesthesia if given 10–20 minutes before induction. Onset of action 10–20 minutes when given IM. At sedative doses there are minimal effects on blood pressure, heart rate and temperature. *(Sedatives continued over)*
	Midazolam	0.5–1.5 mg/kg IV or 0.8–3 mg/kg IM	

ANAESTHETICS AND SEDATIVES *Continued*

Class	Drug	Dose and route	Comments
Sedatives *continued*	Phenobarbital	1–7 mg/kg PO q12h	Mild sedative effect used for long-term seizure control. May cause deep sedation and ataxia. Dose is best adjusted by response to treatment.
	Potassium bromide	25–80 mg/kg PO q24h	Used for long-term seizure control, alone or in conjunction with phenobarbital. May take up to 90 days to establish steady state.
Anaesthetics See Chapter 25 Injectable anaesthesia is a not recommended in companion birds; regimes and doses are included here to assist veterinarians without access to inhalation anaesthesia.	Ketamine	20–50 mg/kg IM or IV	Ketamine alone is not recommended for anaesthesia. Inadequate analgesia and muscle relaxation. Associated with spontaneous movements and muscular rigidity. Not associated with pulmonary depression or cardiovascular depression. Violent recoveries. Lack of coordination. Excitement. Head shaking. Wing flapping.

ANAESTHETICS AND SEDATIVES *Continued*

Class	Drug	Dose and route	Comments
Anaesthetics *continued*	Xylazine	1 mg/kg IM or IV	Does not usually produce adequate surgical immobilization. May lower the arrhythmogenic threshold to endogenous catecholamines. Respiratory depression. Hypotension. Bradycardia. Excitement and convulsions. Prolonged recovery. Muscle tremors, salivation and movement in response to noise. Reversible with yohimbine 0.11–0.27 mg/kg IM.
	Xylazine–ketamine	K 4.4 mg/kg + X 2.2 mg/kg) IV or K 20–30 mg/kg + X 2.5–4.0 mg/kg IM	Commonly used for restraint and anaesthesia. However, waterfowl (especially ducks and Canada geese), owls and acciptres do NOT respond well to this combination. Combination is synergistic, giving a smooth induction and recovery with improved muscle relaxation and enhanced analgesia.
	Ketamine–diazepam	K 10–40 mg/kg + D 0.2–2 mg/kg IV or IM	Can be used as an intravenous induction agent in large ratites, raptors and waterfowl, but may not be a reliable maintenance agent. Can be used intramuscularly in psittacines and pigeons, with a slow induction and recovery time. *(Anaesthetics continued over)*

ANAESTHETICS AND SEDATIVES *Continued*

Class	Drug	Dose and route	Comments
Anaesthetics *continued*	Ketamine–medetomidine	K 1.5–2.0 mg/kg + M 60–85 µg/kg IV	Useful for inducing waterfowl. Can be reversed with atipamezole.
	Ketamine–midazolam	K 10–40 mg/kg + M 0.2–2 mg/kg IM	
	Propofol	1–5 mg/kg IV	Can be used as an intravenous induction agent following sedation with medetomidine–ketamine. Apnoea is common following IV induction. Intubation and IPPV are recommended.
	Alfaxalone	5–10 mg/kg IV or 10–20 mg/kg IM	Brief apnoea on induction if not given slowly. Short duration. Note that these doses are anecdotal; no controlled studies on the use of alfaxalone in birds have been conducted.

ANALGESICS

Class	Drug	Dose and route	Comments
Opioids Some bird species appear to have more kappa opioid receptors in the forebrain than mu opioid receptors, explaining why some birds do not respond to mu agonists such as morphine, buprenorphine and fentanyl in the same manner as mammals. Therefore, kappa opioids such as butorphanol may be the more efficacious analgesics in birds.	Butorphanol	1–4 mg/kg IM or PO q6–12h	Higher doses may be hyperalgesic. Side-effects are uncommon, but may include respiratory depression, nausea and vomiting, bradycardia and constipation.

ANALGESICS *Continued*

Class	Drug	Dose and route	Comments
Nonsteroidal anti-inflammatory drugs (NSAIDs) NSAIDs act on peripheral tissues and therefore are indicated when tissue damage and inflammation are the source of the pain. They may be most effective when acting synergistically with opioids. All have the potential to cause renal damage and gastrointestinal ulceration.	Carprofen	2–4 mg/kg PO q12h	
	Flunixin	2–4 mg/kg IM or PO q12h	Renal side-effects and gastrointestinal ulceration are common; use with caution in all species.
	Ketoprofen	2 mg/kg IM q8–24h	
	Meloxicam	0.2–0.5 mg/kg IM or PO q12h	Available as a palatable oral suspension or in an injectable form. Oral suspension can be diluted (1:5) with sterile water or methylcellulose to give a stable oral solution for small birds.

ANTIDOTES AND OTHER DRUGS USED IN POISON CASES

Class	Drug	Dose and route	Comments
Antidotes	Atropine	0.01–0.1 mg/kg IM, repeat every 3–4 hr as required	Organophosphate and carbamate toxicosis. Does not cause pupillary dilation.
	Calcium EDTA (edentate calcium disodium)	10–50 mg/kg IM q12h for 3–5 days	Treatment of choice for lead and zinc toxicosis. Often recommended as an oral treatment, but efficacy is uncertain and cannot be recommended. Ongoing therapy may be required for chronic lead toxicosis, (e.g. twice weekly for 6–8 weeks after initial stabilization). (*Antidotes continued over*)

ANTIDOTES AND OTHER DRUGS USED IN POISON CASES *Continued*

Class	Drug	Dose and route	Comments
Antidotes *continued*	Deferoxamine	20–100 mg/kg IM or PO q24h for 3–5 months	Preferred chelator for iron storage disease. May take three months to achieve effect. May cause reddish discoloration of urine.
	Dimercaprol (BAL)	25–35 mg/kg q12h PO for 3–5 weeks	Heavy metals other than lead or zinc. Rarely used.
	Dimercaptosuccinic acid (DMSA)	25–35 mg/kg PO q12–24h for 3 weeks	Oral chelation of lead. Can be used with CaEDTA.
	D-Penicillamine	30–50 mg/kg PO q12h 1–3 weeks	Preferred chelator for copper toxicosis, but can be used for other heavy metal toxicosis. Can cause nausea and vomiting.
	Pralidoxamine	10–100 mg/kg IM, repeat after 6 hours	Organophosphate toxicosis; contraindicated for carbamate toxicosis. Must be used within 24–36 hours of exposure.
	Vitamin K	0.2–2.2 mg/kg IM q6–8h until stable, then q24h orally for 2–4 weeks, depending on toxin	Warfarin toxicosis.
Adsorbents	Activated charcoal	2,000–8,000 mg/kg PO	May be mixed with hemicellulose to form a bulk laxative to remove toxins from the gastrointestinal tract.

PSYCHOTROPIC DRUGS

Class	Drug	Dose and route	Comments
Benzodiazepines Inhibit dopamine and potentiate GABA. Muscle relaxants. Anxiolytic. Can interfere with learning.	Diazepam	0.5 mg/kg PO q8–12h or 0.25–0.5 mg/kg IM or IV	
	Lorazepam	0.1 mg/kg PO q12h	
Butyrophenones Inhibit dopamine. Used for self-mutilation and feather picking.	Haloperidol	0.1–0.4 mg/kg PO q12–24h or 1–2 mg/kg IM every 2–3 weeks	May cause anorexia or depression.
Antihistamines Inhibit histamine receptors, producing sedation.	Diphenhydramine	2–4 mg/kg PO q12h	May work best if feather picking is allergic in origin.
	Hydroxyzine	2 mg/kg PO q8h	
Progestins Potentiate GABA. Have a calming effect and anti-inflammatory effect. Multiple side-effects.	Medroxyprogesterone acetate	5–25 mg/kg IM every 4–6 weeks	Often used for feather picking behaviour. Side-effects include polyuria/polydipsia, polyphagia, diabetes mellitus, hepatopathy, weight gain, sudden death.
	Megestrol acetate	2.5 mg/kg PO q24h for 7 days, then weekly as required	Seldom used because of severe side-effects, similar to medroxyprogesterone.
Tricyclic antidepressants Potentiate serotonin, giving a sedative and anticholinergic activity. Alleviate anxiety and depression. Use with care because of side-effects including constipation and arrhythmias.	Amitriptyline	1–5 mg/kg PO q12–24h	Use for at least 30 days to assess effect.
	Clomipramine	0.5–2.0 mg/kg PO q12–24h	Side-effects may include regurgitation, drowsiness, death (possibly with pre-existing arrhythmias). Adjust dose after 2–3 weeks.
	Doxepin	0.5–1.0 mg/kg PO q12h	Adjust dose after 14 days.

PSYCHOTROPIC DRUGS *Continued*

Class	Drug	Dose and route	Comments
Serotonin specific re-uptake inhibitors Have serotonergic effects. Some effect in birds.	Fluoxetine	0.4–3.0 mg/kg PO q12–24h	May cause sedation.
Narcotic antagonists and agonist/antagonists Act at the opiate centres in the brain, blocking endorphin response to self-injurious behaviour. May be useful in some birds.	Naltrexone	1.5 mg/kg PO q8–12h for 1–18 months	Contraindicated if liver disease is present. May need to increase dose to effect.

NUTRITIONAL SUPPORT

Class	Drug	Dose and route	Comments
Calcium Used to treat hypocalcaemic diseases including hypocalcaemic tetany, egg binding and metabolic/nutritional bone disease.	Calcium borogluconate	50–100 mg/kg IM or slowly IV	
	Calcium carbonate	3–7 mg/kg feed	Calcium requirements vary considerably between species and according to reproductive status (e.g. budgerigars have very low calcium requirements compared with chickens; egg-laying hens require more calcium than inactive hens or cocks).
	Calcium glubionate	20–25 mg/kg PO q24h or 750 mg/l of water	
	Calcium gluconate	5–10 mg/kg slowly IV or 10–100 mg/kg IM	For hypocalcaemic tetany or egg binding. Dilute with saline before injecting.

NUTRITIONAL SUPPORT *Continued*

Class	Drug	Dose and route	Comments
Iodine	Lugol's iodine	0.2 ml/l of water	Used to treat thyroid hyperplasia (goitre) in budgerigars.
Iron	Iron dextran	10 mg/kg IM repeated weekly	Used for treating anaemia, although not used as frequently as it once was. Use with caution in species prone to iron storage disease (e.g. mynahs, toucans, lorikeets).
Vitamins	Vitamin A	There is considerable variation in recommended doses for vitamin A. Species susceptible to vitamin A toxicosis (e.g. cockatiels and budgerigars) should be dosed at 2,000–5,000 IU/kg IM weekly; those less susceptible may benefit from doses of 20,000–30,000 IU/kg IM weekly	Dietary sources include fruit (caretenoids — provitamin A), spinach, fish, rodents. Seed and insects are low in vitamin A. Beware of over-supplementing vitamin A.
	Vitamin B1 (thiamine)	1–2 mg/kg IM or PO q24h	Dietary sources are grains and leafy green plant material.
	Vitamin B7 (biotin)	0.05 mg/kg PO q24h for 1–2 months	
	Vitamin B12	0.25–0.5 mg/kg IM weekly	May cause orange/pink urine and urates. (*Vitamins continued over*)

NUTRITIONAL SUPPORT *Continued*

Class	Drug	Dose and route	Comments
Vitamins *continued*	Vitamin D3	3,000–6,000 IU/kg IM weekly	Requires 11–45 minutes of unfiltered sunlight (or UVB at 290–320 nm) per day to activate vitamin D3 synthesis in the skin. Beware of over-supplementation.
	Vitamin E	0.06 mg/kg IM weekly	Dietary sources include green plants. Sunflower oil, hazelnuts and almonds have insufficient levels of Vitamin E and the effect of the Vitamin E is negated by polyunsaturated fatty acids. Low in whole prey (rodents and fish).
	Vitamin K1	0.025–2.5 mg/kg IM q12h or 0.2–2.2 mg/kg IM q6–8h until stable, then q24h orally for 2–4 weeks, depending on toxin	Dietary sources include apple peel, spinach leaf and termites. Large fig parrots (*Psittaculirostris* spp.) require vitamin K supplementation in their diet.

CHAPTER 28
REFERENCE INTERVALS FOR COMMONLY KEPT COMPANION BIRDS

Species	Amazon	Budgerigar	Caique	Canary	Cockatiel	Cockatoo
PCV (l/l)	0.41–0.53	0.44–0.58	0.47–0.55	0.45–0.55	0.43–0.57	0.40–0.55
WBCs (x10⁹/l)	5–17	3–10	8–15	3–10	5–11	5–13
H (%)	31–71	40–68	39–72	21–60	46–72	45–72
L (%)	20–67	22–60	20–61	20–65	26–60	20–50
E (%)	0	0	0	0–1	0–2	0–2
M (%)	0–2	0–2	0–2	0–1	0–1	0–2
B (%)	0–2	0–2	0–1	0–1	0–1	0–1
AST (IU/l)	150–350	150–375	120–365	130–350	120–400	140–360
CK (IU/l)	120–425	120–370	120–390	55–350	160–420	150–420
Bile acids (μmol/l)	30–150	30–120	10–110	20–90	40–110	30–110
Uric acid (μmol/l)	130–620	285–765	150–630	245–750	200–650	225–655
Glucose (mmol/l)	14–21	12–25	9.4–21	8.9–20	12.6–24.4	11.4–23.2
Total protein (g/l)	26–45	20–45	25–35	30–45	20–50	25–49
Calcium (mmol/l)	2–3.4	2–2.8	2.1–2.8	1.5–3.4	2–2.7	2–2.9

H = heterophils; L = lymphocytes; E = eosinophils; M = monocytes; B = basophils. (SI units)
Adapted from: Fudge A (2000) *Laboratory Medicine: Avian and Exotic Pets*. WB Saunders, Philadelphia

(*Continues on page 322*)

Species	Conure, *Aratinga* spp.	Conure, *Pyrrhura* spp.	Eclectus, red-sided	Grey parrot	Lories	Lovebirds
PCV (l/l)	0.42–0.55	0.42–0.55	0.45–0.55	0.45–0.53	0.47–0.55	0.44–0.55
WBCs (x10⁹/l)	6–11	5–10	9–15	6–13	8–13	7–16
H (%)	44–72	46–71	46–70	45–73	39–60	40–56
L (%)	20–49	22–53	23–57	19–50	22–70	20–53
E (%)	0	0–1	0–1	0–1	0–1	0–2
M (%)	0–1	0–2	0–1	0–2	0–2	0–1
B (%)	0–2	0	0–1	0–1	0–1	0–1
AST (IU/l)	140–350	140–270	140–340	110–340	140–370	130–360
CK (IU/l)	150–370	140–280	130–410	140–410	180–400	160–400
Bile acids (µmol/l)	10–90	10–90	30–110	10–100	20–100	10–90
Uric acid (µmol/l)	130–690	190–740	120–650	120–650	120–700	195–635
Glucose (mmol/l)	9.3–21	11.9–22	12–22	14.2–20	10.5–21.5	12.2–22
Total protein (g/l)	24–45	35–50	30–45	25–45	19–40	18–35
Calcium (mmol/l)	2–2.8	2–3.1	2–3	2–3.5	2–2.9	2.1–2.9

H = heterophils; L = lymphocytes; E = eosinophils; M = monocytes; B = basophils. (SI units)

Adapted from: Fudge A (2000) *Laboratory Medicine: Avian and Exotic Pets*. WB Saunders, Philadelphia

Species	Macaw	Mynah	Pionus	Quaker (monk parakeet)	Ring-neck parrot (Indian)	Senegal
PCV (l/l)	0.42–0.56	0.38–0.50	0.45–0.54	0.45–0.58	0.45–0.54	0.45–0.60
WBCs (×10⁹/l)	10–20	8–12	5–13	8–17	8–14	6–14
H (%)	50–75	45–64	55–74	47–70	40–70	44–73
L (%)	23–53	21–55	19–70	20–63	30–55	22–70
E (%)	0	0–4	0–1	0–1	0–1	0–2
M (%)	0–1	0–1	0–1	0–4	0–1	0–1
B (%)	0–1	0–1	0–1	0–3	0–1	0–1
AST (IU/l)	65–170	200–350	130–360	130–380	150–390	120–330
CK (IU/l)	90–360	250–420	120–410	190–400		150–400
Bile acids (µmol/l)	7–100	30–100	15–90	20–90		20–100
Uric acid (µmol/l)	110–700	135–710	120–685	130–710	195–700	135–710
Glucose (mmol/l)	11.7–20	12.5–20.5	12–20.5	11.5–22	12.2–20	14.2–20
Total protein (g/l)	24–44	30–45	20–43	25–35		30–42
Calcium (mmol/l)	2.1–3	2–2.7	2–2.6	2.1–2.7	2.1–2.6	2.1–2.7

H = heterophils; L = lymphocytes; E = eosinophils; M = monocytes; B = basophils. (SI units)

Adapted from: Fudge A (2000) *Laboratory Medicine: Avian and Exotic Pets*. WB Saunders, Philadelphia

CHAPTER 29
BIOLOGICAL VALUES FOR SOME COMMON COMPANION BIRD SPECIES

Species	Weaning age (days)	Sexual maturity	Adult body weight (g)	Life expectancy (years)
Alexandrine parrot	85–100	2–3 years	200–300	25–35
Amazon, blue-crowned	90–120	4–6 years	620–1000	50–70
Amazon, blue-fronted	90–120	4–6 years	360–490	50–70
Amazon, double yellow-headed	90–120	4–6 years	460–700	50–70
Amazon, yellow-naped	90–120	4–6 years	470–800	50–70
Budgerigar	30–40	6–9 months	35–45	7–12
Caique	95–105	2–3 years	120–150	30–40
Canary	21	10 months	15–25	6–12
Cockatiel	40–50	8–12 months	80–100	10–15
Cockatoo, bare-eyed (little corella)	110–120	3–4 years	450–600	30–40
Cockatoo, greater sulphur-crested	120–150	3–4 years	850–950	50–70
Cockatoo, lesser sulphur-crested	80–90	2–3 years	310–380	40–60
Cockatoo, Major Mitchell	80–90	2 years	350–450	40–60
Cockatoo, medium sulphur-crested	100–120	3 years	275–350	40–60
Cockatoo, rose-breasted (galah)	85–95	2–3 years	250–320	20–40
Cockatoo, citron-crested	85–95	2–3 years	300–400	50–60

Species	Weaning age (days)	Sexual maturity	Adult body weight (g)	Life expectancy (years)
Cockatoo, Moluccan	100–120	3–5 years	700–1000	50–60
Cockatoo, umbrella	95–105	5–6 years	550–650	50–60
Conure, *Aratinga* spp.	55–75	2–4 years	110–130	15–25
Conure, *Pyrrhura* spp.	55–75	9–18 months	55–85	15–25
Eclectus, red-sided	80–90	3 years	380–410	25–30
Grey parrot, Congo	100–120	4–6 years	390–500	50–60
Grey parrot, Timneh	95–105	3–5 years	280–360	25–35
Jardine parrot (red-fronted)	95–105	3–4 years	200–250	20–25
Lorikeet, rainbow	60–70	1–2 years	130–150	15–20
Lory, chattering	85–100	2–3 years	160–180	30–35
Lory, red	85–100	2–3 years	100–130	25–30
Lovebirds	45–55	6–12 months	40–50	7–15
Macaw, blue and gold	90–110	5–7 years	1000–1200	50–80
Macaw, green-winged	110–140	3–5 years	1050–1320	60–90
Macaw, Hahn's	70–85	2–3 years	130–150	25–30
Macaw, hyacinth	180–270	5–7 years	1200–1700	60–90
Macaw, military	110–120	2–3 years	860–1100	50–60
Macaw, scarlet	90–110	5–7 years	950–1150	50–80
Meyer's parrot	70–90	2 years	80–110	25–35
Mynah bird	60	2–3 years	180–260	12
Pionus, blue-headed	70	2–3 years	250	20–25
Pionus, white-capped	70–100	2 years	130–160	25–30
Quaker (monk parakeet)	50–60	1 year	120–140	20–30
Ring-neck parrot (Indian)	70–90	2 years	110–120	25–30
Senegal parrot	70	2–3 years	125	15–25

APPENDIX I: SOME COMMONLY KEPT SPECIES OF COMPANION AND AVIARY BIRDS

Amazon parrots
Blue-fronted Amazon	*Amazona aestiva*
Blue-crowned Amazon	*Amazona farinosa guatemalae*
Double yellow-headed Amazon	*Amazona oratrix*
Yellow-naped Amazon	*Amazona auropalliata*

Macaws
Hyacinth macaw	*Anodorhynchus hyacinthinus*
Blue and gold macaw	*Ara ararauna*
Green-winged macaw	*Ara chloroptera*
Hahn's macaw	*Ara nobilis nobilis*
Military macaw	*Ara militaris*
Scarlet macaw	*Ara macao*
Spix's macaw	*Cyanspitta spixii*
Chestnut-fronted macaw (Severe)	*Ara severa*

Pionus parrots
Blue-headed pionus	*Pionus menstrus*
White-capped pionus	*Pionus seniloides*
Bronze-winged pionus	*Pionus chalcopterus*

Cockatoos
Umbrella cockatoo	*Cacatua alba*
Rose-breasted (galah) cockatoo	*Eolophus roseicapillis*
Moluccan (salmon-crested) cockatoo	*Cacatua moluccenensis*
Bare-eyed (little corella) cockatoo	*Cacatua pastinator*
Greater sulphur-crested cockatoo	*Cacatua galerita galerita*
Medium sulphur-crested cockatoo	*Cacatua galerita eleonora*
Lesser sulphur-crested cockatoo	*Cacatua sulphurea sulphurea*
Major Mitchel cockatoo	*Cacatua leadbeateri*
Citron-crested cockatoo	*Cacatua sulphurea citrinocristata*
Slender-billed (long-billed corella) cockatoo	*Cacatua tenuirostris*
White-tailed black cockatoo	*Calyptorhynchus baudinii*
Slender-billed black cockatoo	*Calyptorhynchus latirostris*
Yellow-tailed black cockatoo	*Calyptorhynchus funereus*
Red-tailed black cockatoo	*Calyptorhynchus banksii*
Glossy black cockatoo	*Calyptorhynchus lathami*
Cockatiel	*Nymphicus hollandicus*

Conures
Sun conure	*Aratinga solstitialis*
Jenday conure	*Aratinga jandaya*
Nanday conure	*Nandayus nenday*
Patagonian conure	*Cyanoliserus patagonus*
Green-cheek conure	*Pyrrhura molinae*
Maroon-bellied conure	*Pyrrhura frontalis*

Eclectus parrots
Red-sided eclectus parrot	*Eclectus roratus polychlorus*
Solomon Island eclectus parrot	*Eclectus roratus solomonensis*
Vosmaeri eclectus parrot	*Eclectus roratus vosmaeri*

Grey parrots
African (Congo) grey parrot	*Psittacus erithacus erithecus*
Timneh grey parrot	*Psittacus erithecus timneh*

Other parrots
Quaker (monk) parakeet	*Myopsitta monachus*
Caique	*Pionites* spp.
Alexandrine parakeet (parrot)	*Psittacula eupatoria*
Malabar (blue-winged) parrot (parakeet)	*Psittacula columboides*
Indian ring-neck parrot	*Psittacula krameri krameri*
Kakarikis	*Cyanoramphus* spp.
Eastern rosella	*Platycercus eximius*
Regent parakeet (Rock Pebbler) (Smoker)	*Polytelis anthopeplus*
Australian King parrot (parakeet)	*Alisterus capularis*
Princess parrot (Alexandra's parakeet)	*Polytelis alexandrae*
Jardine (red-fronted) parrot	*Poicephalus gulielmi*
Senegal parrot	*Poicephalus senegalus*
Rainbow (green-naped) lorikeet	*Trichoglossus haematodus haematodus*
Swainson's (blue mountain) lorikeet	*Trichoglossus haematodus moluccanus*
Chattering lory	*Lorius garrulous garrulous*
Red (Moluccan) lory	*Eos bornea*
Black-capped lory	*Lorius lory*
Lovebirds	*Agapornis* spp.
Budgerigar	*Melopsittacus undulatus*

Other commonly kept birds
Canary	*Serinus canaria*
Pigeon	*Columba livia*
Zebra finch	*Poephila guttata castanotis*
Bengalese (Society) finch	*Lonchura domestica*
Red-eared waxbill	*Estrilda troglodytes*
Golden-breasted waxbill	*Amandava subflava*
Orange-checked waxbill	*Estrilda melpoda*
Hill mynah	*Gracula religiosa*

INDEX